Breaking the
Food Seduction

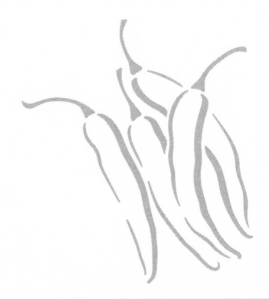

Neal Barnard, M.D.

Breaking the Food Seduction

The Hidden Reasons Behind
Food Cravings—And 7 Steps to
End Them Naturally

WITH MENUS AND RECIPES BY JOANNE STEPANIAK

St. Martin's Press   New York

www.stmartins.com
Design by Kate Nichols

LIBRARY OF CONGRESS CATALOGING-IN-PUBLICATION DATA

Barnard, Neal., 1953–
    Breaking the food seduction : the hidden reasons behind food cravings—
and 7 steps to end them naturally / Neal Barnard.—1st ed.
        p. cm.
    Includes bibliographical references (page 305).
    ISBN 0-312-31493-0
    1. Compulsive eating. 2. Food habits. 3. Reducing diets. I. Title.
RC552.C65B375 2003
616.85'26—dc21
                                                            2003043159

First Edition: June 2003

10   9   8   7   6   5   4   3   2   1

Contents

A Note to the Reader

My goal is to provide you with information about foods and health. However, neither this book nor any other can take the place of individualized medical care or advice. If you are overweight, have any health problem, or are on medication, you should see your doctor before making any changes in your diet or exercise routines, and you should follow your doctor's recommendations, which will be based on your individual needs.

There are many situations in which a diet change can alter your need for medications. For example, individuals with diabetes, high blood pressure, or high cholesterol levels often need less medication when they improve their diets. You should be sure to work with your physician to adjust your regimen as needed.

The science of nutrition grows gradually as time goes on, so I encourage you to consult with other sources of information, including the references listed in this volume.

With any dietary change, it is important to ensure complete nutrition. Be sure to include a source of vitamin B_{12} in your routine, which could include any common multivitamin, fortified soymilk or cereals, or a vitamin B_{12} supplement of five micrograms or more per day.

I wish you the very best of health.

Acknowledgments

I owe a large debt of gratitude to many people whose efforts contributed to this book. First, very special thanks to Mary Ann Naples, an enormously skillful literary agent, and Marian Lizzi, a wonderful editor, who helped shape this book to communicate clearly and effectively.

This book would not have been possible without the efforts of the many research volunteers who have participated in our studies, giving so generously of their time, not to mention many early mornings at the laboratory and late nights in research meetings. I also have had the privilege of working with insightful and skilled coinvestigators: Patricia Bertron, R.D., Jolie Glass, M.S., Judy Harris, Donna Hurlock, M.D., Jennifer Keller, R.D., Amy J. Lanou, Ph.D., Andrew Nicholson, M.D., Paul Poppen, Ph.D., Anthony R. Scialli, M.D., Mark Sklar, M.D., and Gabrielle Turner-McGrievy, M.S., R.D.

Joanne Stepaniak, M.S. Ed., provided delightful recipes and tips that make healthy eating a joy, and Jenifer Howell Clements, R.D., expertly completed the nutritional analyses. Doug Hall provided wonderful graphics. Thank you to Jennie Brand Miller, Ph.D., of the University of Sydney, for kindly providing updated glycemic index data.

Special thanks to my assistant, Juliet Capon, who handled an enormous number of organizational details with unequaled skill.

Simon Chaitowitz, John Murphy, and Joan Higgins have done a brilliant job of conveying the messages of this book to producers, editors, and reporters so that these important concepts will not simply gather dust in libraries.

Mindy Kursban, Esq., and Jay Ukryn, Esq., pried loose from the federal government intriguing and previously unknown information about how industry and government keep less-than-healthy foods on our plates.

Breaking the
Food Seduction

Introduction

Amy starts her day off being "good." She eats a breakfast of instant oatmeal with fruit and heads to work, vowing that today she will stick to her diet. But by eleven A.M., the familiar call from the vending machine starts, and Amy feels powerless. She can't fight the craving for chocolate, and ultimately gives in to temptation—every time.

Paul's doctor has warned him repeatedly that he is risking serious health problems if he does not lower his cholesterol. Time and time again, he has said he would try to cut down on cheese, meat, and other fat-laden foods that contribute to his cholesterol level. Yet he just can't seem to walk past the pizza joint around the corner from his office during lunchtime. The smells and sights lure him in again and again.

Susan has diabetes. Her good health depends upon her eating a diet free of processed junk food like potato chips, candy, and fast-food hamburgers. Even so, these are some of her favorites. She eats foods she knows she shouldn't and feels helpless to improve her life.

How are foods treating *you*? Do any of the stories above sound familiar? Do chocolate or sweets get the better of you more often than you'd like? Has the diet you've grown accustomed to made you gain weight? Has it made your cardiologist nervous, or maybe contributed to high blood pressure, diabetes, joint pains, or migraines?

You might be a willing victim of doughnuts, double bacon-cheeseburgers, french fries, candy bars, or greasy fast-food chicken, whatever their effect on your waistline or health. But, more likely, you watch yourself being dragged down an unhealthy path against your better judgment. It's not that you don't know what kind of diet you'd like to follow, the problem is that it's so easy to be led astray.

You've felt the seduction. "I know I shouldn't," you tell yourself. But tastes and aromas call out like Sirens, leaving you little hope of resisting. We love food—and adore it sometimes—even when it doesn't love us back. Love is supposed to be nourishing and even invigorating, but sometimes our affairs with food pass from love to enslavement.

This book is going to show you a side of this love affair that will surprise you. Perhaps most surprising is that you will end up back in control. If you're not so sure that this is even possible, there are two essential facts you should know:

First, certain food habits are *physical*. It is not gluttony, weak will, or an oral personality that leads you to the refrigerator, at least not for the most part. It is not your fault that foods act as they do. It is a special property of the foods themselves that causes them to be so addicting. Chocolate, for example, has opiate effects, stimulating the release of chemicals within the brain's pleasure center that keep you hooked.

Second, the ability to break bad food habits is mainly physical, too. That is, by adjusting your overall diet and exercise patterns so that your blood sugar stays on an even keel and your appetite-controlling hormones are working *for* you, rather than against you, you can become more resistant to cravings and less likely to snack or binge. You can even reset your tastes in a fundamental way, leaving bad habits behind and starting with a clean slate.

So often we try to muscle our way out of bad habits by willpower alone: "I will *not* have another cookie," "I can say 'no' to chocolate," "I am *not* going to give in to french fries." Of course, that resolve melts within minutes and we are right back where we started.

Think how much easier it would be if you simply were not drawn to unhealthy foods. What if your blood sugar and hormones happened to be in such perfect alignment that you were no longer so attracted to the foods you've been trying to leave behind? That is where we're headed. There will still be a role for making good decisions about what you will eat from day to day. But when you are better balanced physically, changing the way you eat suddenly becomes so much easier.

Breaking the Seduction

This book is based on research studies that have examined how various foods affect our health and how we change from one eating pattern to another. My colleagues and I have conducted these studies over the past several years at our research center in Washington, D.C. People anxious to cut their cholesterol levels, lose weight, control diabetes, or deal with other health concerns come to our offices, where our doctors, dietitians, and nutritionists provide carefully designed diets and then track how these foods affect not only weight, cholesterol, and blood sugar, but also hormone levels and many other biochemical factors. In the process, our team also studies the specific factors that help people break old food habits and start new ones. Over the years, we have found the best ways to help people start down new, healthy paths. Although many doctors are still less than optimistic about people's ability to break bad habits, we have come to exactly the opposite viewpoint. We have found ways to help people revamp their diets with confidence as a matter of routine.

Mary Ann is a real person who is participating in our research. She enthusiastically jumped into the kind of diet adjustments you will read about shortly, and broke out of a rut that had trapped her for years. She was able to set aside foods that had contributed to a chronic weight problem and more or less forget about them. In the process, she lost forty-five pounds almost effortlessly.

Months later, while on vacation, she happened to sample some of those old treacherous foods again. To her surprise, the spell was broken—she was no longer their slave. "When I thought about these observations, it dawned on me that there had been a dramatic change. The best way that I can explain it is to say that the food was just that— food. It seemed as if it no longer had any power over me. This was quite a revelation, and I'm not sure how it happened, but there you are." All she had done was to follow the simple diet adjustments you will read about in this book. It was extraordinarily easy, and it worked like a charm.

And rather than continue to tempt fate, she again left the unhealthy

> ➤I Although many doctors are still less than optimistic about people's ability to break bad habits, we have come to exactly the opposite viewpoint. We have found ways to help people revamp their diets with confidence as a matter of routine.

foods aside and feels better than ever. Many others have had the same experience. And you can, too.

Let me give you an example of how a few easy diet adjustments can make you more resilient in the face of seduction. In 1999, researchers at Boston's Children's Hospital experimented with teenage boys' breakfasts. They fed them typical instant oatmeal and then tracked their snacking later in the day. As boys do, they dug into snacks a fair amount as the day went on. Then, the researchers repeated the experiment with just one change: instead of instant oatmeal, they used the regular variety. Now, oatmeal is, of course, a very healthful food. It is rich in *complex carbohydrates* that, during the process of digestion, release natural sugars into your bloodstream for energy. But oatmeal is made "instant" by chopping the oats very finely. This not only makes it cook very quickly, it also digests a bit too quickly. The result is a rapid rise and fall of blood sugar and a fast return of your appetite. But regular or "old-fashioned" oatmeal leaves the oats more or less intact. They release their sugars into your bloodstream bit by bit, keeping your blood sugar steady and holding hunger at bay.

This was just a simple change of a single food, but it made a big difference. The research team found that, just by selecting regular oatmeal instead of instant, the boys snacked *35 percent less* later in the day. The snack-blocking effect was noticeable all morning long, and, if lunch was chosen with equal care, well into the afternoon.[1]

There is much more to beating food habits and cravings—as you will soon see—but this simple example gives a glimpse of how easy it can be. Instead of struggling to summon the willpower to force yourself to change, an easier way is to make yourself more *physically resilient* to food cravings. Certain foods can do that automatically by reducing hunger for hours, keeping your blood sugar steady, and preventing hormone swings that can spark cravings.

Mary Ann told us what she especially loves about her diet change:

❧ With a simple change at breakfast, research participants snacked 35 percent less later in the day.

"Shopping in the 'Misses' rather than the 'Women's' departments, fitting into subway seats with room to spare, and watching the astonished faces of people who don't recognize me at first glance—these things would have happened, no matter how I lost those forty-five pounds. But it's the improvement in my physical and emotional well-being that brings real satisfaction. After I switched to a healthy diet, my fasting blood sugar dropped from 132 to 85 in just three months. Within six months, my blood pressure had gone from 142/96 to 126/78. I feel great. I'm full of energy. I'm never hungry. I never feel deprived. I haven't become cranky and irritable, as I used to when I was dieting. And I love to look at my plate and know that everything on it is truly good for me!"

She had broken the food seduction. Her experience, and that of the other people you will meet in this book, is wonderful to see, and yours can be very much the same.

When Enough is Enough

Foods are not our enemies. They nourish us and give us pleasure. But sometimes enough is enough. A few years ago, as I was preparing to go on a long trip overseas, one of my staffers came into my office and closed the door. She asked that I not bring back any chocolate, as I had often done on previous trips. Unbeknownst to me, those seemingly harmless bars of *chocolat noir* aggravated the temptations she already faced every day at the food shop downstairs. They perched on her desk like gargoyles, threatening to pack on the pounds at the first bite. It's one thing to have an occasional treat. It's quite another to see your thighs expanding before your very eyes, and she wanted none of it.

Researchers at the University of Michigan brought out the truth about chocolate. In a research study, they gave twenty-six volunteers a drug called *naloxone*. They then offered them a tray filled with Snicker's Bars, M&M's, chocolate chip cookies, and Oreos. Normally, these snacks would have quickly disappeared. But the drug knocked

> ⇥ My job is to help you understand food desires and cravings and to help you fight them on the level where they happen: your biochemistry.

out the desire for chocolate. A candy bar was not much more exciting than a crust of dry bread.[2]

Naloxone is an opiate blocker. That is, it stops heroin, morphine, and other narcotics from affecting the brain. And it blocks the effects of chocolate, too. This research study showed that chocolate's appeal does not come from its creamy texture or deep brown color. Chocolate stimulates the same part of the brain that morphine acts on. For all intents and purposes, chocolate is a drug—not necessarily a bad one and not a terribly strong one, but strong enough nonetheless to keep us coming back for more.

At about the same time, researchers made a similar discovery about cheese and other dairy products. They contain chemical compounds no one ever suspected were there—mild opiates that are released during digestion.[3] Other researchers have added more evidence that there really is something about sugar, chocolate, cheese, meat, and certain other foods that sets them apart. They don't simply tickle the taste buds. It appears that they actually stimulate the brain in such a way that it is easy to get hooked and tough to break free, even if you find yourself gaining weight or lapsing into health problems.

When people try giving up chocolate or cheese to tackle a weight or cholesterol problem, it is a whole different matter from banning, say, apples or pears. Yes, your brain does recognize fruits as nourishing, and even monitors the nutrients they provide. But it does not get giddy with excitement at the prospect of their being on the menu. As far as your neurological circuitry goes, you can take them or leave them.

Seductive foods are like drugs. No, they will not make you sing, dance on a table, or rob a convenience store, but scientific studies suggest that they do affect your brain just enough to keep you hooked. It is a curious thing that some foods have this property, while others do not. In Chapter 1 we will see why this is.

If you are now panicking, imagining that the moral of this frightening story is that you can never enjoy chocolate or other favorites again, relax. My job is to help you understand food desires and cravings, and to help you fight them on the level where they happen: your biochemistry. If you feel that you like chocolate, cheese, potato chips, or cookies a little *too much,* you'll soon see why that is, and exactly what to do about it.

Feeling Healthy Again

For many people, the problem starts with gaining a few pounds. As the bathroom scale becomes more and more discouraging and our clothes no longer fit, our self-esteem takes a bit of a knock. If we start a diet, we soon find that it is not so easy, and our self-esteem takes more pummeling. If we abandon our attempts at dieting we feel even worse. And if our weight gain causes other symptoms—joint pains or diabetes, for example—we just don't feel like ourselves at all. Food habits gone askew also lead us toward high cholesterol levels, high blood pressure, digestive problems, or other conditions, replacing our youthful vigor with a feeling of vulnerability.

When you break the seduction and unwind the downward spiral that food habits can cause, physical problems start to melt away. You feel younger and healthier, with a new sense of control. You have more energy, and it shows. Your family members and friends notice the change and may even be inspired to join you on your highway to health.

Another of our research volunteers, Carole, said, "After having been overweight my whole life, changing the way I eat has finally allowed me to maintain a healthy weight and a healthy lifestyle. Now I eat so much better and am never hungry. I would encourage anyone to give it a try."

For Once in Your Life

If you have ever said, "I know how to eat right; I just don't quite do it," well, now is the time to bring new power into your life. We'll start with a look at some fascinating insights about how sugar, chocolate, cheese, and other foods work their sorcery in your brain. Then in part II we will show them who's boss. If you have been in a love-hate relationship with seductive foods for years and perhaps battling a weight problem at the same time, let me encourage you to read this entire book very carefully, but pay particular attention to part II. It will bring you into a new physical balance, so that, when fattening foods serenade you, you can turn down the volume. We will walk through seven simple steps that will build physical resilience against cravings and unhealthy food habits:

First, we will plan your breakfast to block cravings and snacking later in the day.

Second, we will choose foods that hold your blood sugar steady, so hunger stays in bounds.

Third, we will make sure your natural appetite-taming hormone, *leptin,* is working to its maximal extent.

Fourth, we will break out of craving cycles—whether they occur daily, monthly, or yearly, and whether they are caused by hormonal changes, the darkness of winter, or a hectic work schedule.

Fifth, we will use exercise and rest to restore your natural diurnal rhythm.

Sixth, we will look at whether your social life is contributing to poor eating habits and, if so, what to do about it.

Seventh, we will take a look at extra motivators you can use when you need to boost your resolve.

If you have been struggling with foods with less success than you would have liked, you will want to take full advantage of these seven steps. If, on the other hand, you are not especially hooked on foods or are the kind of person who breaks habits very easily and are anxious to get started with healthier eating habits, you can skim part II and really focus on part III, which includes everything you need to jump in. I strongly recommend using part III's Kickstart Plan. It is designed to quiet cravings and to get you started on a new and healthy path as quickly as possible. It is highly structured and lasts exactly three weeks, and it will change your relationship with food in a very fundamental way.

I wrote this book for several reasons. First, I was surprised to find that foods we eat every day have quite striking chemical effects that virtually no one recognizes. Who would imagine that cheese contains traces of compounds that work like narcotics? Who realized that dieting rapidly depletes a vital appetite-controlling hormone? Who knew that some foods stimulate appetite while nearly identical foods can tame it? Or that revamping the diet from top to bottom is, for many people, easier than making a few minor diet changes?

But, beyond these fascinating facts, I wanted to tackle a clinical problem. People are easily seduced by foods that leave them out of shape and often in poor health, and they tend to be the same foods over and over. No one ever told me they just couldn't get away from radishes or green beans. I never met anyone hooked on spinach, cantaloupe, pears, or romaine lettuce, either. The seductions are sugar, chocolate, cheese, and meat, mainly. Often, people do not recognize the price they pay for these love affairs, but I see them every day on weight charts and in cholesterol test results.

To doctors, food addictions are obvious. They don't generally use that term. But any doctor who recommends a menu change to a heart-attack patient knows full well that the patient will defend the very diet—rich in meat, cheese, and fried foods—that caused his or her problems in the first place. Most doctors are not up to the struggle. It's easier to write a prescription for a cholesterol-lowering drug or blood pressure medicine than confront the force of habit.

But using drugs, when the real problem is diet, is a serious error. Drugs may compensate for some of the ill effects of the food habits that are so common. But they generally control only one problem at a time. More importantly, they are limited in what they can accomplish, they have side effects, and, as a health-care strategy for our population as a whole, they are phenomenally expensive. A change in diet, however, tackles a huge range of health concerns simultaneously—often much more effectively and more safely than drugs can.

Cholesterol-lowering drugs, for example, usually do work, at least to a degree. And sometimes they are essential. But they do nothing for the patient's weight, which has probably climbed over the years as well, or for blood pressure or blood sugar problems, either. The patient may also be troubled by constipation or other digestive problems, and, over the long run, is at a higher risk for certain forms of cancer. As the pharmacy cashier plunks the patient's money into the cash register, no one mentions the fact that all these problems are caused, in large measure, by the same foods that have pushed cholesterol upward. The patient has to go back to the doctor for one prescription after another to treat each diet-related problem. The costs to the patient mount month after month, as do potentially dangerous side effects.

But a diet change, if it is done right and goes far enough, not only reduces cholesterol, it can actually reopen clogged arteries. It can trim your waistline, bring down your blood pressure, and, if you have diabetes, improve it or even make it go away, all at the same time. Diet changes can rapidly knock out digestive problems, and, over the long run, have a dramatically beneficial effect on cancer risk. For some people, diet changes can even ease arthritis, prevent migraines, and reduce menstrual cramps, as we'll see shortly. And the "side effects" are all good ones—more energy, improved endurance, and years added to your life.

Doctors' tendency to focus on prescription drugs, while ignoring patients' diets, has fueled the astounding growth of the pharmaceutical industry in recent decades. Drug companies now employ one full-time sales representative for every fourteen American doctors in order to make sure things stay that way.

Collectively, the medical industry has recognized many of the dangers of food addictions, but it has specifically and deliberately decided to do nothing about them. That is to say, doctors have *presumed* that patients are reluctant to change their eating habits—and drug companies have *depended* on it. A few years ago, my colleagues and I calculated the health care costs attributable to bad diets in the U.S. and found that, in the most conservative possible estimate, these direct medical costs are easily over $60 billion annually.

So, in drafting this book, I wanted to address head-on the pessimism doctors so often feel about patients and their diets. While it is true that everyone is a bit resistant to a diet change, the fact is, resistance can be fairly easily overcome. With a bit of encouragement, even our most timid patients can revolutionize their diets and succeed beautifully.

Time to Begin

Throughout this book I will draw on the experience of our research studies, which have helped people enjoy a new level of health. I'll invite you to join our team by making the same kinds of diet changes our volunteers make. No, this doesn't mean you have to come in for blood tests or any of the other rigors they go through. But we have learned what works to help people get healthier, and you can easily do the same.

So let's get started. If you've found it to be a bit challenging to break old habits and start down a new and healthier path, you'll soon see why this was so and what the answer is. I'll first ask you to set aside the idea that food habits are simply someone's "fault" and that the answer is willpower. We have a much more accurate—and practical—understanding of what it is about chocolate, cheese, and other foods that keeps you hooked. In the next several chapters, we'll survey the foods that tend to hook us the most. I'll address each one in turn to demystify its addictive nature—and I think you will be very surprised at what you read here.

Then I'll explain in detail how breaking free of problem foods can really give a boost to your health, so that when the time comes to make changes you'll have all the motivation you need. After all, if there is no health benefit to be gained in breaking a food habit, why bother? Not everything that is seductive is bad for you. Take hot peppers, for example. There is little doubt that they affect the brain and that they can even be habituating. Over time, people who enjoy them tend to want gradually larger amounts. Even so, there is very little evidence that these foods actually cause any problems whatsoever. On the other hand, some of the most addicting foods really do come with enough calories, fat, or cholesterol to cause health problems, and we'll take an objective look at the value of breaking their spell. Some of the health risks of foods may surprise you—I imagine you'll even find some facts a bit hard-hitting—but I present them, albeit briefly, so that you understand the stakes we are playing for and the enormous benefits you can aim for over the long run.

I'll also include a glimpse of what food industries—and sometimes even government agencies—are doing to keep unhealthy foods in your line of vision. I am not trying to push you to march on the Capitol in protest. Rather, I would like you to understand what you—and all the rest of us—are dealing with as we tackle food issues. Once you understand where certain food promotions and advertisements come from, you'll be better able to resist the lure of their message.

The seven-step plan is easy and is designed to put you in charge, once and for all. If you are like other people who have used these same steps, you'll feel physically different on the very first day you put this plan to work. You'll put the brakes on cravings and will be naturally inclined to make healthier food choices. You'll see the results on the scale and will very likely feel better than you ever thought possible.

This book is designed not only to give you the most powerful tools for losing weight, keeping those pounds away, getting healthy, and staying that way. It is also a guide to the healthiest possible foods. I hope you'll find it to be a road map to health that you can share with your loved ones. It includes a huge collection of carefully developed and delicious menus, recipes, and tips on dealing with fast food, restaurant dining, snacking, and travel—the practical issues we face every day.

Needless to say, there is a great deal of controversy over just what are the most healthful foods. But the preponderance of evidence has led to a reasonably clear picture of what we ought to be eating. So I will present an *optimal* diet—guidelines that bring you to as close to a perfect menu as is humanly possible. Whether you wish to come with me all the way there or just part way, you are likely to reap enormous benefits.

I hope you enjoy what you learn. I also invite you to let me know of your experiences and to join with us in our efforts to encourage better eating habits and better health. My colleagues and I conduct our research studies and educational programs at the Physicians Committee for Responsible Medicine, a nonprofit organization founded in 1985 to promote preventive medicine, good nutrition, and higher standards in research. In our Washington, D.C. offices, PCRM conducts studies of the effect of diet on a variety of health conditions and also focuses on the process of diet change itself—what makes habits easy or difficult to break. Our findings are published in peer-reviewed medical journals. PCRM also publishes *Good Medicine,* a quarterly magazine. PCRM physicians, nutritionists, and dietitians regularly appear on television, radio, and in print and are strong advocates for healthful diets. I would encourage you to join us, work with us, and take advantage of our educational materials. We can be reached at 5100 Wisconsin Avenue, Suite 400, Washington, DC 20016, or visit us on-line at www.pcrm.org.

Part I
The Seductions

When you imagine your absolute favorite foods, which ones come to mind? Sugary treats? Chocolate? Savory cheese? A thick, juicy steak?

In this section, we'll look at some surprising traits of the foods we love as we explore why we sometimes love them a little too much. We'll then size up whether these love affairs are actually doing us any harm. And we'll finish with a look at how food industries work tirelessly behind the scenes to maintain their place in your heart—or at least in your stomach.

Our goal for the moment is to understand our food habits. Then, in parts II and III, we'll see how to break them.

The Seduction Begins:
How Foods Addict You

Y ou're not going to make me give up chocolate, are you?" the young woman asked. She had come to my office to join a research study that demanded some fairly major diet changes. But there was a limit. Chocolate was not negotiable.

"No, we're not," I replied, to her visible relief. "But, very soon you might look at chocolate a bit differently."

She was thirty-five, with a successful career. She was about to begin a series of diet readjustments that would help her lose weight, boost her energy, and make her healthier overall. Unbeknownst to her at the outset, however, these same diet changes were about to knock out food cravings that had been troubling her for longer than she could remember. And that would change her life.

The truth was, even though she loved candy bars, fudge, and chocolate chip cookies, they were not entirely her friends. Each candy wrapper's nutrition label read almost like a confession—ten, twelve, or fifteen grams of fat in a single serving, and every last gram seemed to descend straight to her thighs. She liked chocolate, but she had been desperate to find some way to control it so that she could have it when she wanted, but not be its slave.

Does her situation sound familiar? We all get into food ruts of one kind or another, whether they involve simple daily habits or intense, recurring cravings. At the Physicians Committee for Responsible Medicine, we see their effects all too clearly in our research studies. Of all the things that influence our volunteers' weight, health, or how they feel from day to day, *the number-one factor is the foods they've become hooked on.*

New discoveries have helped us understand why it is that some foods become almost magnetic. It is now abundantly clear that your desire for certain foods—chocolate, potato chips, or cookies, for example—is not simply a choice, like what color socks you'll wear or what movie you might go see. The demand is *physical.*

To return to the case of our research volunteer, whose name, by the way, is Cynthia, she felt an intense craving for something sweet every evening, usually around eight or nine o'clock. It was not that she might *appreciate* a sweet in the way one might like a flower or a pretty picture. This was an overwhelming physical need. And it was specific. Plain table sugar didn't do it. Neither did fruit, raisins, or syrup, sweet as they may be. What she needed was a combination of sweetness and fat, with a bit of chocolate taste as an essential ingredient: a cookie, a chocolate bar, or maybe some ice cream. She might resist it for an hour or two. But sooner or later she would find herself plugging quarters into a candy machine or hurrying off to the convenience store with the same mixture of humiliation and compulsion that people feel as they fall off the wagon into the waiting arms of cigarettes, alcohol, or other addictions.

Over the years she had gained quite a bit of weight. She had dieted, exercised, taken various weight-loss supplements, and even managed to get her meal plan in pretty good shape for short periods at a time. But nothing lasted. Unhealthy foods called her back. Like an old love song, chocolate appealed to her to return to its loving embrace.

Her husband had no interest in sweets. But he fancied himself a pretty good cook, and loved to lay out a big breakfast of omelets made with cheese and bacon, which his father had taught him to make as a child growing up in Chicago. At lunch and dinner he generally avoided red meat, but ate a considerable amount of turkey and salmon, and he had acquired a particular taste for cheese. It did not have to be anything fancy. Cheddar had worked its way into many of his recipes, and he munched on gouda or edam with crackers in the evening while watching TV. He didn't turn up his nose at Velveeta, either, which he thought made a darn good quesadilla.

He had a weight problem of his own, and a serious cholesterol problem, too. His doctor had put him on cholesterol-lowering drugs, which helped—but not as much as either of them had hoped. The doctor also referred him to a dietitian who went over his current diet in elaborate detail and then pronounced his sentence: no more than six ounces of meat per day. One egg yolk per week. *Cottage cheese.* At that point he went blank, while she went on about having at least five servings of fruits and vegetables every day, drinking plenty of water, and blah, blah, blah, blah. If this was living, he would rather die.

In a very real sense, both were addicts, although neither would have used such a strong word. The fact is, they had both become hooked on specific foods that were tremendously compelling and even habituating. And the reason, it appears, is that these foods produce an overly strong reaction in the brain's pleasure center, causing the brain to keep them on its radar screen, so to speak.

Chocolate, Cheese, and Your Brain

The brain's pleasure center is not there just for fun. It is essential for survival. It guides you to eat, rather than waste away, and to reproduce, rather than let your genetic lineage die out. Imagine what would happen if your brain were unable to recognize pleasure, so that, for example, you got no good feeling at all from eating a meal when you were hungry. You would not look after your basic needs. Your brain's pleasure center makes you *want* to eat, exercise, interact with others, and even reproduce.

Whenever an experience provides more pleasure than expected, your brain releases a bit of *dopamine,* the brain's main pleasure-producing chemical. If its name implies that it can make you a bit dopey, that is not far from the truth. Dopamine is central to virtually anything that feels good. An unexpected food treat, a romantic flirtation—or anything your brain takes to be a good thing—causes dopamine to lock onto brain cells and build a permanent memory trace of where pleasure comes from. It keeps flavors, scents, and even sexual experiences alive in your mind, and makes you want to experience them again and again.

So the brain's pleasure center is just doing its job when it guides you to what it thinks you need for survival—an unexpectedly filling food or a receptive mate, for example. In the distant past, food choices were limited, and our pleasure center did not have a particularly challenging job. It helped us remember the difference between luscious, sweet fruits and immature ones, and between plump, fatty nuts and others that had become shriveled and dried. But sugary, fatty, delectable foods are everywhere nowadays, ready to confuse our senses and lead us astray.

What if someone invented a chemical that could trigger the brain's pleasure circuitry—a chemical that did not make you stronger, help you reproduce, or assist you in any other way—but still gave your brain a feeling so warm and pleasant that you would want to repeat it over and over? Well, someone did. Heroin, cocaine, alcohol, nicotine, and, in fact, *all* recreational drugs work on the brain's pleasure center, triggering a greatly exaggerated dopamine response.

Someone also invented chocolate bars, wedges of cheese, cookies, and doughnuts. All of these foods are capable of stimulating precisely the same part of the brain that responds to heroin. And that is why they can be addicting. The fact is, we've been a bit too clever for our own good, refining food products to the point where they provide all the pleasure and very little of the nutrition we need.

Now, being addicted to a food doesn't mean you are going to end up in rehab. What it really means—for foods, drugs, or anything else— is that you have developed an intense motivation to keep taking it. This strongly compulsive quality, which is the basis of an addiction, is different from physical dependency or from having withdrawal symptoms when you quit. For example, a person who is addicted to gambling feels an intense motivation to take dangerous risks, but there are no withdrawal symptoms when the casinos are closed. Yes, many addictive substances have both a compulsive quality as well as withdrawal symptoms when you stop using them—the irritability that smokers feel, the tremors alcoholics experience, or the abdominal cramps heroin addicts have when they go cold turkey. But these symptoms relate to brain centers other than those that control addiction. They may not occur at all. Here's the point: You can be addicted to sugar, chocolate, or cheese slices, even if you don't wake up tremulous and sweating if you've missed your dose.

Addicted to chocolate? Sounds like an overstatement, doesn't it? But the attraction to chocolate is not simply due to its taste and creamy texture. Chocolate hits the brain and causes a habituation that is as real and physical as addiction to narcotics—albeit not so destructive. As we saw in the Introduction, when volunteers take the opiate blocker naloxone, their desire for chocolate falls away almost instantly. Ditto for ice cream and other snack foods.[1] Chocolate stimulates opiate receptors in the brain, and blocking those receptors undoes chocolate's principal attraction.*

Now, in theory, any food that tastes good can trigger the brain's pleasure center at least a little bit, and that applies to strawberries and asparagus—for people who like them—just as it does to cookies or chocolate. It is a question of degree. Some foods, like chocolate, work on the brain's pleasure center much more strongly than others, and alcohol and drugs are off the scale. The effects also differ from one person to another. Some people don't care for alcohol, while others cannot function without it. The same is true of many different foods. Cheese is irresistible to some people, but holds little interest for others.

Many of our research volunteers are beyond passionate about chocolate. One said that a day did not go by without thoughts of the creamy, warm substance melting over her tongue. She knew full well that a Hershey Bar or two packed enough fat to show up on the scale in short order. But for her chocolate was oxygen. During our research study, she set it aside, using diet adjustments you'll see in this book. But, for weeks she continued to carry a chocolate bar with her in her purse, just to know it was there.

It should be said that your body does not always rely on its reward system to guide your choices. When you are thirsty, you crave water. But water does not have to be stunningly delicious to be satisfying. Similarly, oxygen in the air we breathe is not especially exciting, unless you haven't had any for a minute or two. Your body has many ways to regulate how you satisfy your needs. The reward system is just one mechanism for doing that, and, as it happens, one that can easily be fooled.

---

*In case you were wondering, opiate blockers like naloxone are not generally used in weight-loss programs, since they can damage the liver over the long run.

Thrill-Seekers: When Your Brain Makes Less Dopamine Than Other People's

As we have seen, opiate-blocking medications can stop chocolate addiction dead in its tracks. These drugs have also been used to help people control other excesses of the brain's reward system. Researchers at the University of Minnesota gave an opiate blocker to a group of compulsive gamblers. Seventy-five percent of them were much improved, compared to only twenty-four percent taking a placebo.[2] The drug's only side effect was nausea—and even that was probably less than the sick feeling they may have had seeing their money drained away.

Researchers believe that compulsive gamblers have lower-than-normal levels of the brain's dopamine receptors, meaning that they get less pleasure from everyday activities than other people do and seek out extra stimulation just to feel normal.

They are not the only ones. Special brain scans, called *positron emission tomography,* have shown that many overweight people have fewer brain receptors for dopamine, called DRD2 (dopamine receptor D_2), compared to other people. For them, the brain-rewarding chemical has fewer places to attach to brain cells and work its magic. Presumably, they are less able to experience rewarding pleasurable feelings, and will tend to overeat to try to get the stimulation they lack. Another possibility, not yet ruled out, is that these people were not born that way, but that through repeated overeating they have somehow caused the brain to reduce the number of these dopamine attachment sites.[3]

Increasing scientific evidence suggests, however, that many people are, in fact, born that way. With a genetic trait handed down from their parents, their brains have 30 to 40 percent fewer of the brain receptors that are responsible for pleasurable feelings, compared to other people.[4,5] They are on a constant quest to reach the normal, satisfied state other people take for granted. The low-D_2 gene has been amply demonstrated among alcoholics, especially those with serious dependency beginning early in life. It has also been found in people who abuse recreational drugs. And among smokers, those who never manage to quit are more likely to have the low-D_2 gene, compared to those who succeed at quitting, who, in turn, have a higher prevalence of the low-D$_2$ gene compared to people who were never attracted to tobacco in the first place.[6]

Among obese individuals, especially carbohydrate cravers, D$_2$ deficiencies are as common as they are in alcoholics, drug abusers, and smokers—suggesting that, for some, food really acts as a drug.[7] Researchers have found that other genes also influence the brain's response to drugs, alcohol, and other substances, including food.

These observations helped explain why alcoholism, drug abuse, and food compulsions often run in families. What is missing in these individuals is not a part of the brain that copes with alcohol or any specific drug. What is deficient is the brain receptor for normal feelings of pleasure. As a result, they are vulnerable to *anything* that provides it: One family member might be hooked on wine, another on drugs, and another on compulsive overeating, and they may have more than one addiction at the same time.

You may be asking whether you or your loved ones carry this genetic trait. Unfortunately, it is not something doctors routinely check. However, you can get a pretty good idea if the low-D$_2$ gene, or other addiction-fostering genes, may lurk on your chromosomes from a simple glance at your family tree. Think about your parents, grandparents, and siblings. What are/were their drinking and eating habits like? What they drink is not so important as how much and how often, and how young they were when trouble started. A person who drinks only occasionally, or who smoked but managed to quit, is less likely to be responding to a genetic trait than someone who persists in these habits even when things get out of hand.

Whatever your family history, one thing is clear: genes are not destiny. We can overcome the addictive properties of food through bolstering our physical resilience, instead of relying on simple willpower—and this works whether you have addiction genes or not. You can strengthen yourself against an unwanted infatuation with unhealthy foods, as we will see in part II. The fact is, healthy foods can turn on that feel-good dopamine system, too—maybe not in quite the same way chocolate does, but they will do the job. Ditto for exercise. You can get the "runner's high" without leaving the room, as we will see in chapter 10.

Food and Sex

Rather have chocolate than sex? Well, it may not surprise you that the same part of your brain that appreciates chocolate is also responsible for libido, that is, sexual attraction.[8] Your genes are just anxious to reward you for anything that perpetuates their existence. The reason is obvious: if you never felt like eating, you would perish. And if courtship and sex were a complete bore, our species would have died out long ago. So our brains give us a little dopamine, along with pheromones, to keep food on our minds and to make blind dates, ill-fitting clothes, and schmaltzy love songs seem worthwhile.

Here's the problem: Sometimes we use food to stimulate the deepest parts of the brain when what we really need is friendship and love. And if the part of the brain that keeps us interacting with others—talking, flirting, dating, or just being together—can be satisfied with a bowl of chocolate ice cream instead, we can find ourselves becoming more and more alone.

I once had a patient who was remarkably withdrawn. He had virtually no social contacts, and, in fact, had had no friends at all for many years. I asked him about this, and he said, "Well, I have friends. I have my drug friends." He did not mean that he had friends with whom he took drugs. He meant *drugs were his friends*. His "social life" consisted of getting high in total isolation.

Although his was an extreme case, the fact is many people feel a bit the same way. When they are lonely, bored, or stressed, food becomes more than a source of nutrition. Food becomes a friend. A woman whose husband wonders why she binged while he was on another extended business trip tells him, simply, "Chocolate was here. Where were you?" If foods can work on the very parts of our brain that are designed for warmth, friendship, and love, no wonder loneliness leads to overeating, drinking, or drug use. And once addictions start they develop a life of their own, whether people are around to support us or not.

If food can replace love, the reverse is true, too. New lovers don't eat. Lost in a dream land, they lose their appetites for everything except each other. It is as if love is a gastrointestinal disorder, called being "lovesick."

If chocolate and friendship compete for the same part of the brain, we can push chocolate out of the competition by strengthening friendships. In today's society, that can be a challenge, but we'll tackle it in chapter 11.

The Price We Pay for Our Food Addictions

Some people are trapped by vulnerabilities that neither they nor anyone else ever recognized. If you were to test lung cancer patients, for example, you would find that many were born with the low-D_2 gene, a trait that drives them toward tobacco, or, for that matter, alcohol, drugs, food, or anything else that stimulates the brain. They never knew why they had such a hard time quitting smoking.[9] It was the combination of a highly addictive substance—nicotine—and a genetic vulnerability to addiction that led to a terrible but predictable conclusion. Had cigarettes never been invented, they would have turned elsewhere for stimulation—to healthful outlets, like exercise or competition of various kinds, or perhaps to dangerous ones, like alcohol or drugs.

Some food addictions are more or less harmless. Others exact a greater toll than you might imagine. In the harmless category, an occasional chocolate bar is no cause for worry. Hot peppers are habituating, but it is difficult to blame them for any serious bad effects. Caffeinated beverages cause no more than a bit of irritability or sleep disruption, and perhaps headaches when you stop using them.

On the other hand, some habits are not so benign over the long run. In Western countries, people become habituated to diets rich in cheese, meat, sugar, and fat as easily as they might to tobacco, alcohol, or drugs. If that statement sounds exaggerated or alarmist, let me explain, starting with a look at other populations.

In some areas of Latin America laborers routinely chew coca leaves. Each leaf delivers a bit of the pain-killing and mood-boosting effect that has made cocaine such a popular drug. Similarly, in much of the Indian subcontinent, men chew a mixture of betel nut and tobacco. Sidewalks everywhere are splatted with red betel juice stains. The hygiene issues are nothing compared to the potential for oral cancer—something that has worried researchers for decades. But people who use coca or betel consider them entirely normal, and even healthful. They resist advice to leave these habits behind, and campaigns to curtail the use of these substances fall flat.

In Asia, traditional diets are fairly healthy. Rice has been the staple for millions of people, and noodles, vegetables, and bean dishes have made up most of the diet. Meat, if eaten at all, is mainly a flavoring or garnish used in the same way Americans might use a pickle or a slice of tomato. Dairy products have been uncommon; to this day, Asian restaurants do not serve glasses of milk or slices of cheese.

However, things are changing in Asia. McDonald's, Wendy's, Burger King, and KFC have invaded, and meat and dairy products have displaced traditional diets. Where children once favored rice and vegetables, they now eat burgers and fries. Japanese schools have begun emulating the American habit of serving milk, on the naïve assumption that it will help their children build bones. What they are building is a generation of overweight kids and even more overweight adults. Westernization of the diet has made Asian children look more and more like their out-of-shape North American counterparts, and has sparked epidemics of the same diseases that have plagued the western world: obesity, heart disease, diabetes, hypertension, and cancer.

Meanwhile, in North America and Europe, diets have been too high in fat, protein, and cholesterol for generations. During my upbringing in Fargo, North Dakota, a meal was not a meal unless it included meat. Cheese and other dairy products were equally routine. Health researchers lamented our choice of dietary staples, noting that American children typically have the beginnings of artery blockages before they finish high school. Things worsened in the 1970s and 1980s when fast-food restaurants perfected the ability to sell burgers and french fries to an eager public. Americans already fared badly, compared to the rest of the world. Men and women in Boston or Topeka died younger than their counterparts in Tokyo or Osaka, and, as diets have deteriorated further, disease rates have only worsened. Cheese consumption, for example, doubled from 1975 to 1999, and rates of obesity, high cholesterol levels, diabetes, hypertension, and other problems have continued to escalate.

Some people struggling with these health problems might have an unfortunate genetic predisposition. But, in most cases, you would be quite accurate in considering them victims of addiction. They have unknowingly become hooked on foods that made these diseases manifest. Had they been able to keep unhealthy foods at arm's length, very likely their health problems would never have occurred.

Just as coca chewers and betel users don't connect these habits to health problems, many people in Western countries fail to recognize that foods are a major cause of their illnesses, too. They resist efforts to reduce the use of unhealthy, addicting foods and, for the most part, ignore advice favoring healthier choices.

Rather than quitting the offending food, we end up on medications, in the hospital, or worse. Four thousand Americans have heart attacks every day, largely due to bad diets, smoking, and other lifestyle factors that we could potentially control, were we able to conquer our addictions. I cannot tell you how many people tell me their cholesterol problems are genetic. And that may be true for perhaps one in ten. But for the rest, it was not bad genes their parents gave them, but bad recipes, and tastes for foods that drive cholesterol levels up.

Meanwhile, medical services to prevent and treat heart problems have become big business. A recent television commercial depicted a man climbing into a pickup truck driven by his wife who has collected him at the doctor's office. His cholesterol level is up, he tells her. The answer is *Lipitor,* Parke-Davis's wildly popular cholesterol-lowering drug that sells for more than three dollars for a single pill.

But drug prescriptions are a poor substitute for breaking a few habits. Dr. Dean Ornish's program for reversing heart disease, based at the Preventive Medicine Research Institute near San Francisco, showed that lifestyle changes can be much more effective than drugs for patients with heart disease. In his ground-breaking research study, a change in diet and lifestyle promptly opened up coronary arteries to such an extent that the difference was clearly evident on angiograms, special X rays of the heart, in 82 percent of patients in the first year, with no drugs, surgery, or high-tech, artery-busting procedures. And as the years went by they kept getting healthier and healthier. They had broken their addictions to unhealthy foods, and their bodies healed on their own.

The same is true with diabetes. The condition is rare among Asians who continue traditional plant-based diets, and similarly rare among vegetarians. But, once Asians move to Seattle, Los Angeles, Chicago, or Atlanta, and trade traditional rice and vegetables for Western fare, diabetes rates climb 400 percent.

The Diabetes Prevention Program of the National Institutes of

Health tested what drugs or diet changes could do to prevent the disease in a group of 3,234 volunteers who were "pre-diabetic," with blood sugar levels inching toward the danger zone. The popular diabetes drug *Glucophage* (metformin) was able to cut diabetes incidence by 31 percent. That was impressive. But a combination of diet and exercise was nearly twice as effective, bringing a 58-percent drop in diabetes rates.[10]

Sometimes we need medications, and they can indeed be lifesaving. But they are often too weak to stop the full effects of unhealthy food habits, they have side effects, and they are expensive. So many people are on medications for cholesterol problems, diabetes, or hypertension, that drug companies are cashing in to unprecedented degrees, while insurance companies and tax-funded prescription programs are strained more year by year.

Too often, things turn desperate. At any point in time, more than fifty thousand Americans are waiting for another American to die so that they can have a transplanted kidney. Some cases are unavoidable. But in three-quarters of the cases, their kidneys failed due to diabetes and hypertension, and breaking free from addictions to unhealthy foods that aggravate these conditions could have prevented many of them.

What Goes Up Must Come Down

There is another problem that can come with just about any addiction. Stimulating the brain's opiate receptors can bring a bit of a high. But, as an addiction—to food or anything else—becomes established, the brain adjusts so as to *expect* the stimulation to continue. Between doses, feelings of emptiness, anxiety, or depression begin to take hold, and the brain comes to rely on addictive substances to make these feelings vanish. Just as using a crutch when you don't really need one can weaken your leg muscles, addictions weaken your natural mood-maintaining chemistry. Then, if you break the addiction, you'll be left with uncomfortable feelings, and another addiction is likely to leap forward to "solve" it.

If you are leaping ahead to assume that this means that anything that is tasty and pleasurable should be avoided, for fear of some sort of brain damage, let's get a quick reality check. The message of this book is not a puritanical one. The fact is, your brain's pleasure center is there to help you. It responds to love, friendships, sexuality, physical activity, and foods that are good for you. The only problem is that things that push brain chemistry a bit too far in one direction generally lead to a rebound in the opposite direction later on. And moods that go up artificially inevitably come back down, ending up lower than where they started.

Think about people you may know who have had serious addiction problems, say, with alcohol, drugs, or major eating disorders. Their lives often become more and more constricted and empty. Anxieties take over, and they may lapse into depression. And these feelings push them right back into their addiction, which is what their brains need in order to feel "normal." What if ordinary foods—say a couple of hundred calories worth of sugar consumed every day—could do the same thing, ratcheting up the brain's opiate receptors just a notch and distorting our moods ever so slightly? Well, if the brain adjusts accordingly and comes to *expect* a daily boost from sugar or other junk foods, feelings of emptiness, anxiety, and depression may well follow, at least for some of us.

Could it be that many cases of chronic anxiety, depression, or feelings of boredom or emptiness result, not from the existential problems of human life but from too many doughnuts, chocolate bars, and sodas? Sounds a bit silly, doesn't it? But, before you decide that junk food has no effect on any part of our bodies higher than, say, a double chin, let's take a look at the surprising ways these seducers actually work their biochemical mischief, in chapters 2 through 5. But first, an optimistic word about what happens when you set aside a troubling food habit.

Breaking Free

The goal of this book is to help you break free. Yes, foods can be addicting, but there are easy things you can do to regain physical resilience against cravings and unhealthy food habits, and they are far more powerful than simple willpower. If you follow the steps laid out in this book, your body will do the rest.

Miki is a young woman who came to our center, not for herself, but for her husband, who had been diagnosed with a form of cancer. She wanted the very best of nutrition for him, and she joined him in the diet change. Some months later, she wrote to us about how wonderful they both felt. Not only was her husband doing very well, but so was she. "The most amazing things have resulted from this endeavor. I have enjoyed not only the new foods and wonderful tastes, but also a marked improvement in my health. I have lost sixty-seven pounds in one year. For the first time in my life I was not on a diet. I was able to increase my exercise regimen due to the weight loss. My cholesterol is well in control (having dropped significantly in the last year). One of the most amazing results for me has been the near disappearance of all diabetic symptoms. My blood sugar measurements have decreased, on average, 185 points without any medication. I feel fantastic, and for the first time in a long time have gotten a clean bill of health at my annual physical. We started these classes for my husband; however, I have gained as many benefits along the way as he has. You have our profound gratitude."

When we have paid too dear a price for the seductions we have fallen into, gaining new control is like getting a complete refund.

2

Sweet Nothings:
The Sugar Seduction

ere is how to magnetize a baby: Start with a calm infant of nine to twelve weeks of age. Sit face to face, about fifteen inches apart. Dip a pacifier into sugar water (made by stirring a teaspoon of sugar into a cup of water) and put the pacifier in the baby's mouth. If it falls out, dip it again and put it back. Keep it there for three and one-half minutes while maintaining consistent eye contact. That's all it takes. You can then leave the room. When you return, you will find that the baby will look at you, smile, gurgle, and maybe even throw you a coy expression. He or she will follow you with his or her eyes and clearly prefer you over other people. What you have done is to register your face in the baby's memory and connect that image with a sensation in the baby's pleasure circuitry, triggered by sugar. The effect is temporary, lasting for several minutes rather than hours or days, but it is quite noticeable.

Researchers at the University of Massachusetts at Amherst pioneered this peculiar sort of experiment.[1] Apart from its practical value for grandparents, aunts, and uncles, these studies have allowed scientists to explore sugar's druglike effects, as we'll see in this chapter. But we're getting ahead of ourselves. Let's start at the beginning.

Hooked on Sugar

An enormous number of people feel hooked on "carbohydrates." They are drawn to cookies, cake, bread, potato chips, and french fries. But the truth is, what they are hooked on is not carbohydrate at all— at least, not in the way that scientists use that term. After all, there is carbohydrate—that is, starch—in green vegetables, fruits, and beans, too, yet virtually no one is "hooked" on them.

What so-called "carbohydrate addicts" are really hooked on is sugar.[2] In essentially every case, the carbohydrates people crave are those that are either loaded with sugar—like doughnuts and cookies— or that rapidly disintegrate into millions of sugar molecules that rush into the bloodstream during the process of digestion. White bread, potatoes, and, of course, anything with sugar itself in it, are the foods that cause a blood sugar spike, and they are the ones people crave. Unfortunately, on the heels of that blood sugar spike comes a rapid blood sugar drop that can spark a quick return of appetite. And that means a trip back to the fridge for more cookies or cake, or a rush to the nearest doughnut shop. These foods usually have fat—shortening in cookies, or butter on bread—mixed in, too, and the combination causes a pronounced opiate effect, as we'll see shortly.

Most other carbohydrate-rich foods—the healthy choices, including vegetables, beans, and most whole grains—are different. Yes, they will eventually release sugars in the course of digestion, but they do so slowly, in precisely the form your body uses for energy. There is nothing wrong with these starchy foods. In fact, without them you would not have the normal fuel you need for an active life, let alone any sort of athletic endeavor.

The finger of blame, if there is one, ought to point at sugar. That's what gets us hooked and what adds lots of unnecessary calories. Candy counters, soda machines, and convenience store displays all offer sticky treats. And certain kinds of bread, potatoes, and cookies can be sugar bombs, too, propelling late-night binges. Now, there are also healthy choices when it comes to bread and potatoes, and, in this chapter, we'll sort out which are which.

Norma, one of our research participants, felt really hooked. "Once I start, I can't stop," she said. Bread, cookies, and crackers seemed to have no limit, and distractions, like television, only aggravated the

≫ In essentially every case, the "carbohydrates" people crave are those that are either loaded with sugar—like doughnuts and cookies—or that rapidly disintegrate into millions of sugar molecules that rush into the bloodstream.

problem. Sitting in front of a favorite program, she would easily lose track of how much she had eaten. "Before I know it, I've eaten a whole pack of cookies, and I'm still looking for more." Despite other improvements in her diet, her weight-loss efforts were stalled.

How Sugar Affects Your Mind and Mood

What is it about these foods? Well, there are actually several different ways they work their magic on your brain:

First, sugar triggers the release of natural opiates within the brain, just as chocolate does, as we saw earlier. Your brain cells have tiny molecular structures on their surface called *opiate receptors*. When you exercise vigorously, your natural endorphins attach to these receptors, where they act as painkillers and cause the famous "runner's high." Endorphins are cousins of morphine and heroin in their chemical structure, but milder in their action, and they activate the dopamine system within the brain's pleasure center. There is actually a whole family of endorphins and related chemicals. And whether their release is triggered by exercise or by the taste of sugar, the result is a pleasant "feel-good" effect, and whatever physical or psychological troubles might have been bothering you are toned down a bit.

Researchers at the Johns Hopkins University in Baltimore tested sugar's effects in an unusual way. Their test subjects were babies who were just one to three days old. Needless to say, none of these tiny infants had ever tasted a doughnut, seen a television commercial for sugary cereals, or made a trip to a convenience store. But they had a very noticeable reaction to sugar. The researchers first placed the infants in their bassinets for five minutes, and, naturally, some began to whimper a bit during this time. Then they gave each baby either a tiny amount of sugar in water or else just plain water, dribbling the fluid into the baby's mouths with a plastic syringe. The effect was almost immediate. Sugar-water stopped them from crying. Water alone did nothing.[3]

A pacifier can do that, too, but there is a critical difference: If the pacifier is removed, crying can ensue immediately; but sugar's effect lingers for several minutes, even after the taste is gone. The reason is that sugar causes opiates to be released in the infant's brain, and these naturally calming compounds stay on after the sugar is gone.

Infants whose mothers were narcotic addicts during pregnancy react very differently. Sugar is useless. They cry whether they get sugar or not. The fact is, these babies were exposed to narcotic opiates in the womb, and their natural opiate circuitry no longer responds normally; they are resistant to its effects.[4]

The opiate effect is probably triggered by the mere *taste* of sugar, rather than by a rise in the amount of sugar in the bloodstream. A baby's taste buds are set for the slight sweetness of mother's milk, and as sugar—which is far sweeter than mother's milk—touches the tongue, it sets off a chain reaction: The taste buds send impulses through nerves leading to the base of the brain, and from there to the cortex—the outermost layer of the brain. At that point, the baby becomes aware of the sweet taste. And, along the way, nerves stimulate the pleasure center, causing the release of natural opiate compounds that color the experience as an enjoyable one. These opiates also block pain, at least slightly.

Hospitals have taken advantage of sugar's opiate action. When babies' blood samples are drawn by a typical heel-stick, a little sugar given in advance has a noticeable calming effect. The same is true during circumcision.

The pronounced attraction that sugar has for children—suckers, gum, sugary drinks, sweetened cereals, and on and on—suddenly starts to make sense. It doesn't just taste good. It turns on the opiate machinery deep within their brains, which is why it has an essentially magnetic effect on infants. And although, for many of us, sugar's ability to trigger pleasure starts to wane as we reach adulthood, for others, sugar remains a drug of choice.

Although sugar alone trips the opiate machinery, food manufacturers have found that whipping in a bit of fat accentuates its effects. In fact, many of the foods people call "carbohydrates" actually have at least as much fat as carbohydrate, and this fat-carb mixture may cause an even more pronounced opiate effect, similar to that caused by

❧ Although sugar alone trips the opiate machinery, food manufacturers have found that whipping in a bit of fat accentuates its effects.

chocolate. When researcher Adam Drewnowski gave the opiate blocker naloxone to volunteers, as we saw in the Introduction, it not only blocked chocolate cravings, it also cut the craving for potato chips, a classic fat-carb mix.

That First Bite

Sugar causes the release of opiates within the brain. But that opiate response does more than make you feel good. It also has a marked appetite-driving effect. You've experienced it: You had a little bit of an appetite before you took your first bite of sugar. Might taste good, you thought. But once it touches your lips, sugar's opiate effects break through the dam holding back your appetite, and an army of dietitians could not save you from the binge that sweeps you away. Inside your brain, the opiates triggered by the sweet taste are busily resetting all your internal priorities to make you care about one thing and one thing only: eating more of what has just passed your lips.

Some people have a special yen for carbohydrate-rich foods in the wintertime. As the days become shorter, especially at northern latitudes, some people lapse into depression. Many discover that sweet or starchy foods bring them out of it. Far from being a problem, these carbohydrate-rich foods boost a brain chemical called *serotonin,* which helps regulate moods and sleep. The problems don't start until bread is topped with butter or other calorie-dense toppings, or when quantity knows no limits. More on this in chapter 9.

There is one additional way that carb-rich foods might get us hooked, and this one relates specifically to bagels, bread, cookies, and cake—anything made of wheat. Researchers have found that the wheat protein, called *gluten,* breaks apart during the digestive process into compounds that have a variety of mild opiate effects. They can slow down your digestion, just as mild narcotics do, and their effects can be blocked by the same drugs that block the effects of narcotics (e.g., naloxone).[5,6] So far as we know, these wheat-derived opiates work within the intestinal tract and do not seem to pass into the blood-stream. However, some researchers have speculated that druglike compounds released from wheat (or from cheese or other foods, as we will see in chapter 4) may be the trigger that causes psychiatric symp-toms in susceptible individuals.[7] It would not be surprising if researchers were to find that wheat-derived opiates actually can affect the brain, either directly, by passing into the bloodstream, or indirectly, by causing the release of various hormones from the digestive tract. Stay tuned.

Is It Good to Break a Sugar Habit?

So, are carbohydrates—and sugar, in particular—a biochemical bless-ing or a calorie-dense curse? Well, that depends. Carbohydrates them-selves are not fattening. Despite their repeated condemnation in the popular press, scientific studies clearly show that carbohydrate-rich foods eaten in normal quantities have virtually no effect on body weight. A baked potato has only about 150 calories, a piece of bread about 70. It's not easy to gain weight with numbers like that. However, there are a few problems you need to look out for.

Toppings and Hidden Fat

First, what is going on that potato? It might start out with 150 calories, but a tablespoon of butter adds another 100, a dollop of sour cream another 25, and a sprinkle of bacon bits adds 25 more. Pretty soon, the potato is nothing but a vehicle for fatty toppings that have at least as many calories as the potato itself.

Same for bread. Start with a piece of whole wheat bread, with 70 calories. Melt an ounce of American cheese over the top, and you're suddenly up to 180 calories. Blame the carbs if you want, but it's the toppings that will really fatten you up.

Far more treacherous are the fats you don't see. Take popcorn, for example. Air-popped, there are all of 61 calories in a two-cup serving. But cooked by the usual oily method, that innocent popcorn is encum-bered with nearly double the calorie load—108, to be exact.

Snack pastries are far worse. There are a 15 grams of fat baked into a pack of Ho-Ho's or Zingers. And while the label calls them vegetable oils, they are hydrogenated oils, also called *trans* fats, which are as bad as butter or lard for your arteries and general health.

Quantity

Now, let's say you don't go near the fatty toppings. You could still gain weight from carbs, but you have to work at it. Because carbohydrates are modest in calories, most people fill up before they get very far. And even when you overdo it a bit, many of the calories in carbohydrates are either stored as *glycogen*—the high-energy molecules your muscles use for power and endurance—or are lost as body heat and are not turned to fat at all. It is no easy biochemical task to convert a piece of bread into human fat, and studies of controlled overfeeding show very little effect from even hefty amounts. Nonetheless, if you take in more calories than you burn, you will gain weight.

Sugar

If it's sugar itself you choose, rather than complex carbohydrates like pasta or beans, the calories can come fast and furious, especially as serving sizes have gone out of bounds. And this is where those who criticize carbohydrates make a good point: Sugar is concentrated calories. A typical soda now holds twenty ounces and packs 250 calories of pure sugar. Those calories don't displace food—they *add* to whatever else you are eating. In contrast, 250 calories of rice—which is a bit more than a cup, would cause you to compensate by eating less of everything else. So, next time you reach for a soda, remember that you could have a glass of water instead. A cup of rice or three slices of bread have fewer calories than a typical soda.

Despite these potential problems, carbs are not the enemy. Populations whose dietary staples are rich in carbohydrate—rice, noodles, beans, or split peas, for example—tend to be considerably slimmer than those who make meat and cheese their dietary mainstays.

You may also wish to pay attention to how sugar affects your mood. Many people find that, although they crave sugar and it may even have a calming effect, over the long run it makes them irritable and depressed. Some women report that, if they give in to premenstrual sugar cravings they will pay for it with worsening spirits.

You might want to see if this is true for you. If you have moody episodes, take a look at what you were eating during the 48 hours prior, and see if getting off sugar helps restore your moods to a better equilibrium. You may wish to jot down what you've eaten each day in a notebook. When you note down sugary foods, you'll want to include *anything* with a fair amount of sugar in it—even juices. At the end of each day, rate your overall mood and note any times when your fuse seemed shorter than normal. Separate the premenstrual week from the other three weeks of the month, as food-induced mood changes might be accentuated at that time.

If sweet or starchy snacks have taken over your life, the answer is not to avoid them, but to be selective, keeping an eye on fat content and the *glycemic index,* a number that shows how quickly carbs release their natural sugars into the bloodstream. We will go into detail on this in chapter 7. Briefly, the glycemic index (GI) of various foods was calculated by feeding them to volunteers and then drawing blood samples at regular intervals. Some foods break apart into sugars very rapidly, others much more slowly, and the faster any given food releases its sugars into the bloodstream, the higher its glycemic index.

For now, all you need to know is that the main high-GI foods are white bread, big baking potatoes, most cold breakfast cereals, and sugar itself. Better choices include pumpernickel and rye bread, which have lower GI values, as do new potatoes, yams, and sweet potatoes. Beans, green leafy vegetables, pasta, and most fruits have very low GI values. Going low-GI lets you eat carb-rich foods without fear.

The Sugar Pushers

The Sugar Association is an industry group of sixteen sugar companies, one of which I got to know as a child growing up in Fargo, North Dakota. When the wind was right, Crystal Sugar's sugar beet processing plant sent its distinctive odor over my childhood home.

> ⇥ Many people find that, although sugar may have a calming effect, over the long run it makes them irritable and depressed. Some women report that, if they give into premenstrual sugar cravings, they will pay for it with worsening spirits.

The Sugar Association is eager to point out that Americans don't really eat as much sugar as they might think—only about 40 grams (about 10 teaspoons) per day. Not very much, is it? Well, that's just cane and beet sugar. Plenty more comes in the form of corn syrup—which you'll find in a great many foods—as well as honey and other sweeteners. Next time you're in line at a convenience store, pick up any snack pastry. Or look at a typical 20-ounce soda bottle. You'll find more than 60 grams of sugar lurking inside.

Food companies don't rely on sugar alone to keep you hooked. In the case of sodas, companies have long added other chemicals to keep you coming back. Coca-Cola's story began in 1886, when Atlanta pharmacist John Pemberton mixed up a caramel-colored liquid as a cure for headaches. It was sold at Jacobs' Pharmacy for five cents a glass and was soon advertised as "The Ideal Brain Tonic." Indeed it was. It was a mixture of cocaine and kola nut extracts. Eventually, the company replaced cocaine with caffeine, but it still qualifies as a "brain tonic," as any college student who has overindulged the night before will tell you. A 20-ounce bottle of Coke has 58 milligrams of caffeine, and a Diet Coke about 78, slightly less than a typical cup of coffee.

Is the company concerned that kids might get hooked on caffeine? Quite the opposite. Take a look at what the Coca-Cola Company recently posted on its Web site under the category "Myths and Rumors":

"Caffeine is not addictive. Caffeine has had a long history in the food supply, consumed as long ago as 2700 B.C. Scientific evaluation of caffeine's physiological effects, in light of the criteria for drug dependence, clearly shows that caffeine is not similar to the use of drugs of abuse or dependence. It is true that some symptoms of withdrawal can be experienced by some people if caffeine consumption is stopped abruptly. When done gradually over a reasonable time period, most people do not even experience these symptoms. More importantly, the amount of caffeine in typical soft drinks is minimal. The amount in most cola beverages is about one third of the caffeine in the same amount of coffee and one half of the amount found in tea."*

Caffeine is not addictive? This is what your mother used to call "a lie." There is no question that caffeine is addictive. And dedicated caffeine users are very familiar with the symptoms, like headaches, that

---

*http://www2.coca-cola.com/contactus/myths_rumors/ingredients_addictive.html (accessed August 13, 2002)

they experience when they stop using it. None of these symptoms is especially serious, of course, and, ounce for ounce, there is indeed less caffeine in Coke than in coffee. But that's a bit like saying there is less alcohol in wine than in hard liquor. Users of all these products adjust their serving sizes accordingly in order to get the brain effect they seek.

Meanwhile, serving sizes of sugary foods have been carefully and deliberately pushed upward. When I was a child, sodas came in 6-ounce bottles and were only consumed at picnics or other unusual settings. As 12-ounce cans gradually took over, they seemed a bit much to some people, who had trouble finishing them. Many people were frustrated that they could not put stoppers on cans as they could on bottles. Eventually, 12 ounces grew to 16 and then 20. And it is safe to say that not many people save half for the next day.

Down the hatch it goes. Fast-food restaurants and movie theaters serve sodas and virtually no other beverages. This is partly marketing— the supersizing phenomenon that extracts slightly more money from your pocket than smaller servings would—and partly addiction. People acclimating to any addictive substance gradually zero in on their daily dose and then stay there, whether it's a pack of cigarettes, a beer or two at dinner, or 20 ounces of Dr. Pepper in the morning.

You can break loose, of course. And you'll very likely feel much better and be glad you left the sugar habit behind. So, even though your infant sweet tooth might make you coo and gurgle a bit when your old friend sugar walks in the room, you will have finally broken the seduction.

The Bottom Line

- Sugar can be addicting. It triggers the release of opiates in the brain, an effect you can spot even in newborn babies. The primary problem with sugar is that it is concentrated in calories.

- When people feel hooked on "carbohydrate," they are really hooked on foods that release sugars rapidly into the blood (e.g., cookies or potatoes), rather than on carbohydrates that release sugars slowly (e.g., beans, fruit, or pasta). The primary health issue with these foods is not their ability to release sugar, but their fatty toppings or ingredients: butter on toast, sour cream on potatoes, margarine whipped into cookies, etc.

- If you're ready to get that white powder out of your life, the steps in part II will cut your cravings, and the menu and recipe section will give you plenty of healthy choices.

3

Give Me Chocolate or Give Me Death: The Chocolate Seduction

C hocolate is an affair. It's decadent, it's sinful, and—let's face it— for many, many people, it's simply irresistible. We crave it, dream about it, and ultimately savor it, all the while knowing no good will come from it.

Why such passion about chocolate? After all, it is a gooey bean extract, not a romantic dream come true. Researchers have tried to nail down the chemistry behind the attraction—and so have chocolate manufacturers, hoping to sustain the affair as long as possible. It's clear that the secret is not simply chocolate's sugary taste. After all, a dedicated chocoholic would never be satisfied with a box of plain Domino sugar. It is also not merely a source of some vital nutrient, like magnesium, as some have suggested. The fact is, there is quite a lot of magnesium in figs, tofu, and spinach, too, but you don't hear of people craving them very often.

The truth is that chocolate is, in essence, an addicting drug. It targets the same spot on your brain as heroin or morphine. As we saw in the Introduction, the opiate blocker naloxone dramatically reduces chocolate's attractiveness. When University of Michigan researchers infused the opiate blocker into volunteers' bloodstreams and then pre-

➤ Researchers found that blocking chocolate's opiate effect cut snacking on Snickers and M&Ms in half, and Oreo snacking fell by 90 percent.

sented them with a tray of snack foods, naloxone did not change their taste for popcorn—it was as popular as ever. Same for breadsticks and crackers, suggesting that an opiate rush is not what anyone is looking for from those foods. But everything was different when it came to the chocolate items on the tray. Blocking chocolate's opiate effect with naloxone cut snacking on Snickers and M&Ms in half, and Oreo snacking fell by 90 percent. In other words, chocolate's sweet taste and creamy texture are pleasant, but its real attraction depends on its effect on your brain. When that brain effect is taken away, chocolate is no longer the kind of food anyone would crave.[1]

Don't panic. Yes, chocolate acts like a drug, but this does not mean that you're going to knock over a convenience store to get your fix. Chocolate does not stimulate opiate receptors to anywhere near the degree that narcotics do. But it does affect the brain, and that is important to remember. Taste, smell, and "mouth feel" are all nice, but it's what happens inside your brain that keeps you coming back.

Jennifer, a thirty-four-year-old bank vice president, adored it. She had come to our office for an interview about joining a diet study, and before long the conversation turned to chocolate. She was worried that it was adding more calories to her diet than she could afford. Her favorite was a small chocolate bar imported from England that had tiny bits of nuts and fruit in it. But she was happy with virtually any kind of chocolate. And it seemed to call out especially loudly at certain times. She had an especially insistent taste for chocolate when she was fatigued or, for some reason, after she had eaten something spicy. And it virtually screamed out at her during the two or three days before her period. Her friends knew the feeling all too well, too. They had all experienced it, and they knew there was no reason to argue with it.

This compulsive quality was what bothered Jennifer the most. She was a dedicated label reader, and she knew how many calories there were in a chocolate bar, but there didn't seem to be any way to keep it from ending up in her stomach, and she found that disconcerting. After all, she had managed her education, her career, her finances—and her bank's and customers' money—but she couldn't handle this darn little drug in a shiny wrapper. As she gradually gained weight over the years, she wanted to get a handle on her chocolate cravings.

Well, she was not alone. The opiate effects hidden in a chocolate bar work their magic on millions and millions of people. Before we come back to Jennifer's situation, allow me to describe in a few paragraphs what chocolate actually does inside your brain. Its chemical actions go beyond its opiate effect.

Chocolate also contains caffeine, although not nearly as much as coffee or tea. A 1.5-ounce Kit Kat has 5 milligrams of caffeine, a 1.4-ounce Nestle Crunch bar about 10. For comparison, a serving of tea has 36 milligrams of caffeine, and you would have to eat an entire cup of chocolate chips to get as much caffeine as in a typical cup of coffee (100 milligrams).[2]

Chocolate is far richer in a related chemical, called *theobromine* (literally, "food of the gods"). Theobromine is a stimulant similar to caffeine in both its chemical structure and its "upper" effect, although it is much milder. If you have a dog you may have heard of theobromine—it is the reason chocolate can be poisonous to your canine friend. Dogs cannot readily break down and eliminate theobromine, which can damage their hearts, kidneys, and nervous systems. All chocolate products have hefty amounts of theobromine.

Chocolate also contains *phenylethylamine,* or PEA, an amphetamine-like chemical (although only about one-tenth as much as is found in cheddar cheese or salami[3,4]). It also harbors traces of compounds similar to THC, the active ingredient in marijuana.

What's this about chocolate being like marijuana? Here's what scientists have discovered: Brain cells normally produce a chemical called *anandamide,* which is related to marijuana's active ingredient, tetrahydrocannabinol, or THC. Certain chemicals in chocolate apparently delay the breakdown of anandamide in the brain, so that its pleasant brain effects persist a bit longer than normal.[5]

So the bottom line is, chocolate is not just a single drug-like compound—it's basically the whole drugstore: traces of mild opiates, caffeine, amphetamine-like components, and the equivalent of a slight whiff of marijuana, all wrapped into a smooth, sweet taste. Medical researchers have accepted its addictive potential for decades. In a 1999 study, researchers compared chocolate addicts to people who weren't especially hooked on it, and showed that the reaction is physically noticeable. The researchers gave them pictures of chocolate to look at, and then bowls filled with Cadbury chocolates. Chocoholics really do show a quickening of the pulse and start salivating when they smell, taste, or even see a picture of chocolate, and these reactions are much stronger than for other people. Just to be objective, the researchers also tested their responses to automobile magazines, which elicited no big reaction in either group.[6]

Quite apart from any chemical effects chocolate has, some researchers have suggested that its smell, taste, and texture alone would make it addicting. It certainly is possible for sensory experiences to be so overwhelming that they hook some people, as is the case for compulsive gambling in people with the low-D_2 gene. Their reactions to the sudden shifts of risk, unexpected wins, and crushing losses are dramatically different from those of other people. Similarly, chocolate presents a sensory mixture that is unlike that of any other food. As we'll see shortly, the mere *taste* of sugar touching the tongue appears to send a signal to the brain that triggers a virtually instant opiate effect, and chocolate very likely does the same, in addition to the effects of its chemical cornucopia.

No single component of chocolate—cocoa powder, cocoa butter, or sugar—quells cravings the way chocolate itself can.[7] This, of course, does not discount a physical basis for chocolate addiction. Just as smokers *ought* to be satisfied with a nicotine patch but generally are not, once they have become accustomed to the feeling of inhaling tobacco smoke, chocolate lovers come to associate all the sensations of chocolate with the subtle and pleasant feelings it provides, and no chocoholic would be satisfied with simply smelling and tasting chocolate. When you want it, you want to practically *inhale* it.

But Does It Make You Happy?

Does chocolate really make us feel better? Well, sort of. A study of self-described chocolate addicts found that they felt a definite sense of contentment after eating chocolate. But their pleasure was tainted by a big dose of guilt, something occasional chocolate eaters do not experience.

Jennifer felt this acutely. Although she thoroughly savored each bite, and it did seem to make her feel good, about halfway through a chocolate bar she started to feel a sense of regret, and she sometimes threw the rest away. And she then started to calculate how much exercise it would take to burn off the calories she had just eaten.

She also experienced something else that this research study had shown: Her cravings were not driven primarily by hunger. Yes, hunger could make them worse, but she also binged on chocolate when she was full, which turns out to be a very common experience.[8]

What is Chocolate, Really?

Despite the passions aroused by chocolate, including an often-pointed finger of blame as our waistlines expand into unexplored regions, chocolate could well plead innocent. Seductive, it may be, but it is not the Devil. Here is the truth about this botanical black gold:

Chocolate comes from the beans of the cacao tree. In prehistoric Central America, Aztecs turned these beans into a drink called *chocolatl,* meaning "warm liquid." Montezuma, living in what was eventually to become Mexico, was particularly keen on chocolatl and served it to the early Spanish explorers. Christopher Columbus had already brought cocoa beans back to Spain, but their bitter flavor made them a tough sell in Europe, and King Ferdinand and Queen Isabella saw no commercial potential. It was not until a bit of added vanilla and cinnamon made the drink a hit.

Solid chocolate as we know it today did not exist until the mid-nineteenth century. That was when chocolatiers made a key discovery. They found that, if they extracted cocoa butter from the beans, they ended up with cocoa powder, so useful in baking. More importantly, if they added extra cocoa butter to the beans, they produced a creamy chocolate that goes perfectly in a candy wrapper and has been a hit ever since. It is surprising to imagine that the buttery, dark brown concoction we now know as chocolate candy did not exist until the mid-1800s, but the truth is that chocolate is a strictly modern product.

Today, making chocolate means cultivating the delicate cacao trees and cracking open their bean pods to reveal a couple of dozen cream-colored beans, which are then fermented, dried, roasted, and crushed to produce chocolate liquor, from which cocoa butter can be extracted. White chocolate is made from cocoa butter, milk solids, sugar, and vanilla.

The world's most serious aficionados are the members of France's Le Club des Croqueurs de Chocolat (*croqueurs* means "crunchers"), which meets four times a year to rate the latest entrants to the market of brown ambrosia. If you'd like to join, you'd better be patient— membership is limited to one hundred and fifty people, and someone has to die or resign to give you a space. You'll need to study up, too, because the interview includes questions like, "If you were to buy chocolate in a supermarket, what would you look for on the label?" (The answer is not the price tag or sell-by date. The *croqueurs* want to hear that you'll scan the label for a cocoa percentage of 60 percent or better and the country of origin of the beans.) If you've made it that far, they'll try to zing you with "What does *criollo* mean to you?" The answer is not "It really burns when you spill it on a cut," or "We keep it under the sink." Rather, it's a type of cocoa tree in Central and South America that produces the very best chocolate. If you'd like a bigger taste of the Le Club des Croqueurs de Chocolat, check out www. croqueurschocolat.com.

Is It Good to Break a Chocolate Habit?

If your chocolate "habit" means the occasional candy bar, there is little reason to worry. It is not terribly likely to pack on the pounds. But if it is more than occasional it could spell trouble. For starters, it may con- tribute more fat than you can afford. A typical chocolate bar is a roughly fifty-fifty mixture of fat and sugar, with about 200 calories and 10–15 grams of fat, which is, well, plenty.

Chocolate can do more than fatten you up. Along with dairy prod- ucts, red wine, meat, and a few other foods, chocolate is a common migraine trigger.* It can also affect your mood in a not-so-helpful way. Some women find that it aggravates irritability in the premenstrual week, which is, unfortunately, exactly when you'll crave chocolate most. Its effects differ from one person to the next, so you'll want to pay attention to what it does to *your* mood.

---

*Other common migraine triggers include eggs, citrus fruits, wheat, nuts, tomatoes, onions, corn, apples, and bananas. For details on how foods contribute to migraines, see my book *Foods That Fight Pain* (Harmony Books, 1998).

The Chocolate Pushers

Every five years, representatives of the Chocolate Manufacturers Association make an absurd trek. They march into government hearings in Washington, D.C., where a federal panel is redrafting the *Dietary Guidelines for Americans,* the blueprint for a healthy diet that we looked at earlier. The chocolate industry joins the Sugar Association, Salt Institute, and every other healthy and unhealthy food lobby to make a case that all these foods should be included in the diet.

The Chocolate Manufacturers Association has nine members, including Hershey, M&M/Mars, Nestlè, and other lesser-known brands, which, all together, control 95 percent of the chocolate production in the U.S., which is worth billions of dollars every year. Now, compared to the dairy and meat industries the chocolate lobby is minuscule. It has yet to convince the government to include a chocolate group in the Food Guide Pyramid or to feature chocolate in school lunches. Still, the Chocolate Manufacturers Association issues reassuring press releases, such as "Chocolate Supplies are Ample" and "Chocolate Contains 'Healthy' Antioxidants." The only major controversy the industry has stumbled into is a dispute over exploitive child labor practices in West Africa. The problem is serious, involving thousands of children in slavelike conditions. The industry has begun to address the problem, but it is far from being solved.

Industry scientists have dedicated a great deal of effort to finding exactly the right ingredient balance to keep you coming back. It turns out that when sugar and fat are just about a fifty-fifty mixture, chocolate reaches its point of maximal irresistibility. However, the mix has to be adjusted slightly, depending on the customer. Taste scientists have found that small children prefer tastes that are a bit too sweet for adults. Overweight people tend to choose higher-fat foods, while thinner people really do follow a bit of Jack Sprat's lead. Men go more for higher-protein, high-fat, salty foods (steaks, burgers, and the like), while women tend toward sugar-fat mixtures, like doughnuts, ice cream, and, of course, chocolate.[9]

The candy industry takes all this into account in order to capture as much of the market as it can. For the high-sugar market, M&M/Mars makes 3 Musketeers, which packs 40 grams of sugar in a single bar, with about twice as many sugar calories as fat calories. For the high-fat

◄ When a chocolate bar is made with a fifty-fifty mixture of sugar and fat, chocolate reaches its point of maximal irresistibility.

market, Twix and M&Ms Peanut variety have more fat calories than sugar calories. And the company markets Milky Way and Snickers for those whose tastes lie in between.

A Word about Medications

Just as industry scientists are working to keep you hooked on chocolate, health researchers are trying to find ways to free you. Some have turned to medications to knock out chocolate cravings, and, to a degree, they work. As we saw earlier, naloxone blocks cravings, reducing the tendency to binge, and cuts food consumption overall. The more enticing the food—that is, the stronger its effect on the brain's pleasure center—the more naloxone blocks the binge. But it is not the only drug to have this effect:

Bupropion (Wellbutrin) is an antidepressant that reduces chocolate cravings for some people. A fifty-six-year-old woman, for example, had chocolate cravings nearly all her life and was eating up to two pounds of chocolate per day when, having lapsed into depression, her doctor put her on bupropion to raise her spirits. Almost immediately, her chocolate cravings ceased. Chocolate simply had no appeal. In just the first month of treatment, she lost seven pounds. The benefit is not simply due to the drug's salutary effect on mood. It knocks out cravings, even when you're feeling fine. Perhaps bupropion works because it is chemically similar to phenylethylamine (PEA), which, as we saw earlier, is an amphetamine-like compound found in chocolate, cheese, and sausage.[10]

Topiramate (Topamax) is used to treat seizures. After researchers found that the drug also seemed to reduce appetites and even caused weight loss, they tested it in people with serious binge-eating problems to see if it might help. It does. After a few months of treatment, the average participant had lost about twenty-five pounds.[11]

A note of serious caution, however. All drugs have side effects. Naloxone can cause liver problems, and topiramate can cause glaucoma. In contrast, the side effects of diet changes are all positive—weight loss, reduced cholesterol, lower blood pressure, and others.

Most people can get into a better relationship with chocolate without medications. If you need to, you can make a clean break of it, or perhaps you'll simply turn a destructive preoccupation into a more platonic relationship. Part II gives you the steps that will take you there.

The Bottom Line

- Chocolate addiction is real. Health researchers have identified a surprising number of natural compounds that contribute to chocolate's subtle, pleasant brain effects. However, its taste alone triggers opiate effects in the brain. The same drugs that block the effects of heroin and morphine also knock out chocolate's appeal.

- Yes, chocolate really is as high in fat and sugar as you may have feared. But chefs have discovered tricks that keep the flavor while trimming the fat, as we'll see in the menu and recipe section.

- If you're looking to get a grip on your cravings, the steps in part II were designed with you in mind. If you're a young woman, you'll notice that the desire for chocolate can change with your monthly cycle, and a diet adjustment easily balances the hormones responsible for these cravings, as we'll see in chapter 9.

4

Opiates on a Cracker: The Cheese Seduction

What do you think of when you think of cheese? Do you conjure up a picture of hot pizza with gooey mozzarella dribbling from each slice? Or do you think of a baguette and goat cheese? Brie and a glass of wine? Do most of your meals have some form of cheese or another included? If you answered yes, you are like a great many other people. And chances are, you've been struggling with your weight, too.

Cheese may get 70 percent of its calories from nothing but waist-augmenting milkfat and have, pound for pound, more cholesterol than a steak, but it is also one of the foods health-conscious people have the most trouble leaving behind. Some people describe it as vividly as alcoholics remembering their last drink. What is it about cheese?

That's what Jo, one of our research volunteers, asked. As a child, she didn't especially care for it. But she began eating the occasional grilled cheese sandwich in high school, and bit-by-bit, cheese crept onto her plate: pizza, salad sprinkles, cheesy lasagne, and sometimes slices straight out of the pack. She was especially fond of cheese melted over toast, heated in her toaster oven just to the point where it almost started to burn in spots. It was quick to make, it tasted good, and it filled her up.

Her weight began to be a problem in her late teens and, as the years went by, things gradually escalated. When she arrived at our office our dietitian gave her a scale and asked her to weigh and record everything she ate. A week later she returned with her list, which read like a cheese advertisement: She had a grilled cheese sandwich for lunch, with 18 grams of fat, and stopped at Pizza Hut for dinner, where two pizza slices packed in another 20 grams. She also had a late-evening snack of Brie and crackers, with another 15 fat grams. That was 53 fat grams from cheese alone in a single day.

But, seeing the problem was not the same as solving it. As she contemplated life without cheese, she made a list of all the things she might let go first. Her boyfriend, her stereo, her car—she could live without them if she had to. Ditto for french fries, bread, fruits, and vegetables. Chocolate was a tough one, but the truth is, even it did not deliver the satisfaction she got from cheese.

Is Cheese a Drug?

Cheese's attraction is not mainly due to taste or smell, at least not at first. After all, no one ever marketed a perfume, air freshener, or incense that smelled of old socks. Like beer or cigarettes, cheese's taste can even be a bit off-putting at first. Its real lure may be hidden in its mother lode of opiates—dozens of them—whose effects have been surprising scientists in recent years. The smell and taste are secondary. Scientist speculate that, in the same way that people come to associate the taste of an alcoholic drink with the pleasant relaxation that soon follows, we associate the taste of cheese with what really counts, which is what is happening in our brains.

In 1981, Eli Hazum and his colleagues at Wellcome Research Laboratories in Research Triangle Park, N.C., reported a remarkable discovery. Analyzing samples of cow's milk, they found traces of a chemical that looked very much like morphine.[1] They put it to one chemical test after another. Finally they arrived at the conclusion that, in fact, it *is* morphine. There is not a lot of it. But indeed morphine has been found in both cow's milk and human milk.

Morphine, of course, is an opiate and is highly addictive. So how did it get into milk? At first the researchers theorized that it must have come from the cows' diets. After all, morphine used in hospitals comes

⇨ The opiates in milk may be responsible for the calming effect of nursing in infants—and perhaps for the addictive qualities of cheese.

from poppies and is also produced naturally by a few other plants that the cows might have been eating. But it turns out that cows actually produce it within their bodies, just as poppies do. Traces of morphine, along with codeine and other opiates, are apparently produced in cows' livers and can end up in their milk.[2]

But that was only the beginning, as other researchers soon found. Cow's milk—or the milk of any other species, for that matter—contains a protein, called *casein,* that breaks apart during digestion to release a whole host of opiates, called *casomorphins.*[3] A cup of cow's milk contains about six grams of casein. Skim milk contains a bit more, and casein is concentrated in the production of cheese.

A one-ounce slice of cheese holds about 5 grams of casein, and each one of those grams holds millions of individual casein molecules. If you examined one of these molecules under a powerful microscope, it would look like a long chain of beads (the "beads" are *amino acids*—simple building blocks that combine to make up all the proteins in your body). When you drink a glass of milk or eat a slice of cheese, stomach acid and intestinal bacteria snip the casein molecular chains into casomorphins of various lengths. One of them, a short string made up of just five amino acids, has about one-tenth the pain-killing potency of morphine.[4]

What are they doing there? It appears that the opiates from mother's milk produce a calming effect on the infant and, in fact, may be responsible for a good measure of the mother-infant bond. No, it's not all lullabies and cooing. Psychological bonds always have a physical underpinning. Like it or not, mother's milk has a druglike effect on the baby's brain that ensures that the baby will bond with Mom and continue to nurse and get the nutrients all babies need. Like heroin or codeine, casomorphins slow intestinal movements and have a decided antidiarrheal effect. The opiate effect may be why adults often find that cheese can be constipating, just as opiate painkillers are.*

---

*Cow's milk is actually quite different from human milk. Cow's milk is loaded with casein, which gives milk curds their white color, and very low in *whey,* the protein that remains in the watery portion after milk curdles. Human breast milk is the opposite: low in casein and high in whey.[5]

It is an open question to what extent dairy opiates can enter an adult's bloodstream.[6,7] Until the 1990s, researchers thought that these protein fragments were too large to pass through the intestinal wall into the blood, except in infants, whose immature digestive tracts are not very selective about what passes through. They theorized that milk opiates mainly acted within the digestive tract and that they signaled comfort or relief to the brain indirectly, through the hormones traveling from the intestinal tract to the brain.[8]

But French researchers fed skim milk and yogurt to volunteers and found that, sure enough, at least some casein fragments do pass into the bloodstream. They reach their peak about forty minutes after eating.[9] Other researchers found that, if a breastfeeding woman includes dairy products in her diet, cow proteins actually pass from her digestive tract into her bloodstream and then *into her own breast milk* in large enough amounts to irritate her baby's stomach, causing colic.[10]

Other fascinating—and disturbing—findings have emerged. Human milk contains casein, too, albeit less than in cow's milk and in a slightly different form. In studies of women who had recently given birth, Swedish researchers found that opiates from breast milk sometimes pass from the breast into a woman's own bloodstream and then into the brain.[11-13] Some women with very high levels of these opiates in their blood—opiates that came originally from the casein in their own breast milk—have developed postpartum psychosis. It had long been suspected that this syndrome of confusion, hallucinations, and delusions (symptoms that go beyond the mood changes of postpartum depression, a more common disorder) is not simply due to the stresses of childbirth, the arrival of maternal responsibilities, or the loss of youthful innocence. The fact is, something is poisoning the brain. The Swedish researchers suggested that that "something" might be an opiate released from casein in mother's milk. The point is, casein is as much a drug as a nutrient, and it is a primary ingredient in all milk products, but especially in cheese.

Cheese contains far more casein than is found in milk from either cows or humans. And it holds other druglike compounds as well. It contains an amphetamine-like chemical PEA, phenylethylamine, that we looked at earlier, which is also found in chocolate and sausage.[14] And there are many hormones and other compounds in cheese and other dairy products whose functions are not yet understood. Researchers are gradually tearing them apart and trying to understand their biological effects, including their contribution to the cheese craving that is so common.*

Is It Good to Break a Dairy Habit?

Let's say you're stuck on cheese. The question is, does it really matter? The answer is a resounding yes. To see why, you don't have to go much further than the bathroom scale. Our volunteer, Jo, decided that, in the interests of science, she could set aside cheese for a limited time. And, of all the diet changes she made, this single step had, by far the biggest effect on the tally of fat grams she kept. And it also made a big difference in her weight. Even without exercising or limiting her calorie intake or meal size, she saw the pounds melt away slowly but surely—on average, about a pound per week, week after week after week.

Here is your payoff when you break the seduction:

Trimming the Pounds and Cutting Your Cholesterol

The whole point of the cheese-making process is to concentrate fat and protein (that is, casein), while squeezing out water and lactose sugar. Not surprisingly, a typical 2-ounce serving has at least 15 grams of fat and about 200 calories—before it even touches your sandwich. When you set the cheese aside you've spared yourself all that fat and all those calories.

Unfortunately, Americans are going in the opposite direction. Dairy industry figures show that annual cheese consumption in the U.S. doubled from fifteen pounds per person in 1975 to thirty pounds in 1999, as I mentioned earlier. That works out to 14,400 milligrams of cholesterol and 4.5 kilos of fat—that's ten pounds of dairy fat from cheese alone—for every single person in America. If just one of those pounds of fat lingered on your waistline, adding an extra pound to your weight

---

*One recent review identified the following hormones and related natural chemicals in cow's milk: prolactin, somatostatin, melatonin, oxytocin, growth hormone, leuteinizing hormone-releasing hormone, thyrotropin-releasing hormone, thyroid-stimulating hormone, vasoactive intestinal peptide, calcitonin, parathyroid hormone, corticosteroids, estrogens, progesterone, insulin, epidermal growth factor, insulin-like growth factor, erythropoietin, bombesin, neurotensin, motilin, and cholecystokinin.[15]

◄⧸ Cheese consumption in the U.S. doubled from fifteen pounds per person per year in 1975 to thirty pounds in 1999. That works out to 14,400 milligrams of cholesterol and 4.5 kilos of fat for every single person in America.

year after year, you could explain nearly the entire weight problem the country is experiencing—that is, the average American is now gaining about 1.5 pounds per year, and our collective cheese fetish may be a big part of the explanation. If you're looking for a simple way to trim your waistline, breaking a love affair with cheese can help enormously.

When you've broken the cheese seduction, you've not only freed yourself from a lot of fat, you've stepped away from the worst kind of fat. Most of the fat in cheese is *saturated*, the kind that tends to increase your cholesterol level and raise your risk of artery blockages and heart problems.

In case you're getting fat and cholesterol mixed up, they are actually two entirely different things. Fat is what you find under chicken skin or marbled through a piece of beef. It also what makes milk thick and cheese smooth. Cholesterol, however, comes in tiny particles packed into the cell membranes of all animal tissues. In meat, most cholesterol is actually in the lean portion. Cheese has cholesterol, too, in hefty amounts. There are about 50–60 milligrams of cholesterol in a 2-ounce serving of cheddar or mozzarella. Ounce for ounce, that's as much as you'll find in steak or ground beef. So, when you find other ways to top a sandwich or prepare a casserole (see the recipe section), you'll do your body a huge favor.

Help for Arthritis and Headaches

If you have arthritis or migraines, side-stepping cheese and other dairy products might be just the prescription you need. In 1985, a British medical journal reported a case of an eight-year-old girl with juvenile rheumatoid arthritis whose cause was a mystery until she stopped eating dairy products. The condition cleared up completely.[16] But even a small amount of milk was enough to trigger her symptoms. At the time, cases of arthritis caused by foods were thought to be rare. But systematic studies have shown that anywhere from 20 to 60 percent of typical rheumatoid arthritis cases are linked to diet, and dairy products appear to be the most common trigger.* The problem in this case is not dairy fat—and it is not necessarily an allergy in the usual sense of the word. The symptoms are apparently a reaction to dairy proteins, so the payoff comes from avoiding both nonfat and full-fat versions.

Skipping dairy proteins can help migraines, too. Cheese is a notorious migraine trigger.† And some people are allergic to dairy products, which can mean digestive problems, worsening asthma, or other symptoms. If you thought you had to put up with pain or other symptoms, breaking the cheese seduction might bring you a very pleasant surprise.

Preventing Prostate Cancer

Researchers have set about trying to see what might reduce the risk of various forms of cancer, and it turns out that, in addition to increasing vegetables and fruits and pumping up the fiber in their diets, men can take another good step by avoiding dairy products. Although this finding was unexpected and is obviously surprising, at least sixteen studies have shown it to be true. Among them are two recent and very large Harvard studies that showed that men who generally avoid dairy products have about a 30 percent reduction in their risk of prostate cancer, compared to those who consume them often.[17,18]

The reason, apparently, is that dairy consumption increases the amount of a substance in the blood called *insulin-like growth factor-I* (IGF-I), which is an aggressive promoter of cancer cell growth.[19,20] Recent studies have linked higher IGF-I levels not only to prostate cancer, but also to breast cancer.[21,22]

A second explanation relates to vitamin D. This vitamin is actually a hormone that helps your body absorb calcium from the digestive tract and also has the job of protecting the prostate against cancer. Vitamin D is normally produced by sunlight hitting the skin, and it can also come from the diet. However, these forms of the vitamin are inactive precursors. In order to function, they must pass to the liver and kidneys to be activated by a slight change in their molecular structure.

*Other common arthritis triggers identified in research studies include corn, meats, wheat, eggs, citrus fruits, potatoes, tomatoes, nuts, and coffee. For more details, see Barnard ND, *Foods That Fight Pain* (New York: Harmony Books, 1998).
†See Barnard, *Foods That Fight Pain.*

And this is where dairy products become a problem. As their calcium floods into the bloodstream, it apparently signals the body that, since there is plenty of calcium in the system already, the body does not need to activate vitamin D to try to absorb any more. The result is a substantial drop in the amount of activated vitamin D in the blood. With less vitamin D in the blood, the risk of prostate cancer climbs. Of course, milk often contains some added vitamin D, but it is in the inactive precursor form, and dairy consumption actually suppresses vitamin D activation in the body.[17] In addition, diets rich in animal fat, whether from dairy products or other sources, tend to increase the body's production of testosterone, which is linked to prostate cancer risk.[23]

Cutting Sodium

Cheese is loaded with sodium that comes from the cow's milk it is made from and the additional salt used in the cheese-making process. Two ounces of cheddar cheese contains about 350 milligrams of sodium. Two ounces of Velveeta have more than 800 milligrams, and a cup of low-fat cottage cheese has more than 900 milligrams. Sodium's effect on blood pressure is well known, but more troubling is its role in osteoporosis. Sodium encourages the passage of calcium through the kidneys where it is then lost in the urine. When you set cheese aside, you skip one of the biggest sources of sodium in the diet.

Calcium? Yes, But . . .

What about the calcium in cheese? Well, you do need a certain amount of calcium for building bones, and calcium has other functions in the body, too. But you do not need dairy products for calcium, as has been amply demonstrated in Japan, China, parts of Africa, and elsewhere where they are not traditionally used. Bone development is perfectly normal, and bone breaks caused by osteoporosis—the thinning of the bones with age—are actually much rarer than in the U.S. and Europe. The fact is, there is plenty of calcium in green vegetables, beans, fortified juices, and many other foods.

Researchers at Pennsylvania State University found that, in girls in their peak bone-building years—ages twelve to eighteen—getting extra calcium made no difference at all in bone growth.[24] It is a bit like dumping extra bricks at a construction site, hoping that they will become part of the building. They won't. What did make a difference in bone growth, by the way, was exercise. Exercising teens had clearly better bone development than their more sedentary classmates.

Similarly, Harvard researchers found that, in a twelve-year study of nearly 78,000 women, dairy calcium didn't help bone strength at all. Those who got the most calcium from dairy sources actually had nearly double the hip fracture rates, compared to those who got little or no dairy calcium.[25] Advertisers have tried to capitalize on the myth that dairy products—or calcium in general—prevents bone breaks, but scientific studies have clearly shown that greatly increasing your intake of calcium—from dairy products or any other food—does little or nothing for the bones.

Other factors do make an important difference, however. Exercise is key. And vitamin D—from sunlight or vitamin supplements—also helps keep bones strong. Fruits and vegetables provide vitamin C to build your bones' inner collagen matrix. And it is important to understand that osteoporosis is not a condition of inadequate calcium intake, for the most part. Rather, it is a condition of overly rapid calcium loss. It is accelerated by sodium (salt) and animal protein in the diet, smoking, and other factors. But adding extra calcium, either from dairy products or supplements, is largely ineffective at preventing or slowing it.

So, you can feel good about breaking the cheese seduction. You'll say good-bye to a lot of fat and calories, and you'll do your body many other favors in the bargain.

The Dairy Pushers

If cheese and other dairy products present so many health problems, why have they profited from a healthy image for so long? First of all, government programs promoting dairy use began in the early 1900s, long before researchers had taken a serious look at their health effects. Today, hundreds of millions of dollars are pumped yearly into advertising campaigns designed to maintain dairy's image.

In the United States, the dairy industry is intertwined with the federal government in a peculiar relationship. Milk producers and processors pay a portion of their sales revenues into a fund. The Secretary of Agriculture appoints the thirty-six-member Dairy Board and the twenty-member Fluid Milk Board to spend this two-hundred million-dollar kitty, commissioning advertising campaigns, fast-food promotions, and other schemes through an organization called Dairy Management, Inc.

The *USDA Report to Congress on the Dairy Promotion Programs* for the year 2000 described how the government and industry worked with Wendy's, Pizza Hut, Shoney's, Denny's, and Bennigan's fast-food chains to make sure that cheese was prominently displayed in menu items. It details the USDA/dairy industry program to launch Wendy's Cheddar Lover's Bacon Cheeseburger, which singlehandedly pushed 2.25 million pounds of cheese during the promotion period—that works out to 380 tons of fat and 1.2 tons of pure cholesterol in the cheese alone. And, yes, this was an officially sanctioned U.S. government program designed for no purpose other than to push Americans to fatten the industry's wallet.

In 1996, cheese was not a required ingredient in Subway sandwiches. So Dairy Management, Inc., signed a contract with Subway, committing $58,000 to help the restaurant chain promote cheese and include it as a required ingredient in two new sandwiches, the Chicken Cordon Blue and Honey Pepper Melt, anticipating the sale of an extra 70,000 pounds of cheese.

Dairy Management, Inc., also worked with Pizza Hut to promote the "Ultimate Cheese Pizza"—with an entire pound of cheese per pizza—selling five million pounds of it during a six-week promotion in 2000. Burger King jumped in, aiming to push cheese in its chicken and beef sandwiches, and the industry has worked out financial relationships with many other restaurant and grocery chains.

The dairy industry weighs heavily on nutrition policies in the United States. The eleven-person panel that drew up the Dietary Guidelines for Americans 2000—the blueprint for all federal nutrition programs—included six members with financial ties to the dairy, meat, and egg indusries. In addition, the panel kept most of its records from

> ❧ The U.S. Department of Agriculture worked with Wendy's to launch the Cheddar Lover's Bacon Cheeseburger, which singlehandedly pushed 2.25 million pounds of cheese—containing 380 tons of fat and 1.2 tons of pure cholesterol—during the promotion period alone.

public view during its deliberations. Because we believed that this closed-door process violated federal law, my organization, the Physicians Committee for Responsible Medicine, sued the Departments of Agriculture and Health and Human Services in federal court. The court agreed with us and ruled that the panel erred in not opening its workings to public scrutiny.

Dairy industry market analysts are well aware that some people get hooked on cheese. In fact, they have separated cheese buyers into cheese "cravers" and cheese "enhancers." "Cravers" don't stand on ceremony. They eat it straight out of the package or off the block. For them, life without cheese is basically not worth living. Cheese "enhancers" use cheese as an ingredient, sprinkling it on pizza or using it in recipes.

At a "Cheese Forum" held December 5, 2000, Dick Cooper, the Vice President of Cheese Marketing for Dairy Management, Inc., showed slide after slide documenting the escalating cheese consumption in the U.S., and proudly credited the industry's marketing schemes. One slide asked the question, "What do we want our marketing program to do?" and then gave the answer: "trigger the cheese craving." He then detailed the industry's plans for pushing cheese in grocery chains, food services, and fast-food restaurants. He concluded with a cartoon of a playground slide with a large spider web woven to trap children as they reached the bottom. The caption had one spider saying to another, "If we pull this off, we'll eat like kings."

The Bottom Line

- Many people get hooked on cheese. Like other dairy products, cheese contains casein, a protein that breaks apart during digestion to form opiates, called casomorphins. What makes cheese different—and presumably more addicting—is that it has much more casein than is found in milk, ice cream, butter, or other dairy products.

- It is hard to find a more fattening food. Typical cheeses derive about 70 percent of their calories from fat, mostly artery-clogging saturated fat and, ounce for ounce, have more cholesterol than a steak.

- If you were hoping for some redeeming health benefits, the fact is, large, well-conducted research studies have shown that cheese and other dairy products do not build strong bones, nor do they slow osteoporosis.

- Government-sponsored programs aim to keep you hooked. They have worked with Wendy's, Pizza Hut, Subway, and other restaurant chains to add more and more cheese to menu items, intentionally trying to "trigger the cheese craving." They have managed to boost America's annual cheese consumption from fifteen pounds per person in 1975 to thirty pounds in 1999.

- If you'd like to break free, part II will show you how to get started. And the recipe section will give you a great many tips on how to get all the taste with none of the regrets.

5

The Sizzle:
The Meat Seduction

The sizzle of a steak can be the quintessence of allure. Burgers on the grill, roast chicken, a tantalizing holiday turkey, a fish filet smothered in tartar sauce—for many people, they are more mouth-watering than just about anything else. They may hold enough cholesterol to sink a ship, health organizations might plead with us for moderation, and cartoonists may mock our meat habit—"You want chemotherapy with that?" the butcher asks—but even so, it's hard to pry the steak knife from our meaty fists.

Most health authorities encourage people to limit how much meat they eat—or skip it entirely—and for good reason. More life-threatening illnesses have been linked to meat-based diets than to just about any other factor in our lifestyle or environment. Cancer, heart disease, diabetes, kidney problems, obesity, food-borne infections, and many other conditions are much more common among meat-eaters than among those who give meat a wide berth.[1] And research teams have come a long way toward explaining why animal protein, animal fat, and cholesterol lead to these problems.

Meat aficionados have resisted such concerns, floating semi-scientific arguments favoring flesh-heavy diets, such as the Atkins Diet. Their arguments have not held up very well, as we will see. But the fact remains that once people get hooked on meat, they want to stay hooked. As we saw in the first chapter, fast-food chains pushing burgers and fried chicken in Asia found an almost immediate following, despite the fact that the arrival of Western eating habits brought weight problems, heart disease, and cancer rates that were previously unknown.

I recently took a plane from Los Angeles back home to Washington, D.C. As the lunch cart arrived, the man and woman seated next to me chose beef over the pasta dish. As the conversation turned to food, it was clear she was worried about him. He had had a stent put in his heart to prop open a coronary artery. But he hadn't changed his diet—in fact, his doctor had not offered any diet advice at all—and a recurrence of heart problems loomed before them. He did not exercise. Although they were both in their sixties, this was a fairly recent marriage, and she was afraid that her beau was not taking care of himself.

He had heard the arguments about cutting back on meat and was quite willing to believe that a diet change would help him. But he couldn't imagine a meatless meal being satisfying. Nonalcoholic beer or decaffeinated coffee might be tolerable. But life without good food just wasn't worth living.

However, a coast-to-coast flight lasts a good five hours. And that's more than enough time to think things through a bit more. Before we get back to this couple, let's take a look at what is really at the heart of the matter.

Is Meat Addicting?

Many children don't take to meat right off. As infants and toddlers begin to taste solid foods, they like fruit and rice cereal instantly. But they often resist meat, as if Mom had offered them a beer or a cigarette. Before long, however, they will become habituated to it, and it can then develop into a very persistent habit. An April 2000 survey of 1,244 adults revealed that about one in four Americans wouldn't give up meat for a week even if they were paid a thousand dollars to do it. People from Asian and Hispanic backgrounds were more willing to accept the hypothetical offer (fewer than 10 percent turned it down), presumably because meatless choices are major parts of their traditional cuisines. But black and white Americans were more reluctant, with 24 percent of whites and 29 percent of blacks absolutely unwilling to swap meat for cash. Cholesterol, fat, salmonella, *E. coli,* Mad Cow disease, and foot-and-mouth disease may come and go in the public's mind, yet meat eating goes on.

Why such enthusiasm over meat? After all, nature designed animals' muscle tissues to help them move their legs, flap their wings, or wiggle their tails, not as a nutritional supplement.

Well, for starters, an attraction to any fatty food makes some biological sense. Fat happens to be the most calorie-dense part of any food we eat (fat has nine calories in every gram, compared to only four for carbohydrate or protein.) Presumably, as our species evolved, those people who knew a calorie when they saw one—that is, those who were attracted to fattier foods—would be more likely to survive in times of scarcity. If that taste for fat leads us to the occasional nut, seed, or olive, no harm is done. But nature never figured that this same attraction would lead us to prefer hamburgers, fried chicken, and other dangerously fatty, high-cholesterol foods. When you look at what meat is made of, anywhere from about 20 to 70 percent of its calories come from pure fat.

The taste for meat may be similar to the taste for french fries, onion rings, or anything else with a lot of fat in it—that is, it is due to evolutionary pressures leading us to prefer high-calorie foods. And there is also a role for the simple force of habit. Scientists believe that, once we get used to fatty foods as a result of their being on our plate day after day, we come to prefer them and tend to seek them out.

But there may be another side to the meat habit. Scientific tests suggest that meat may have subtle druglike qualities, just as sugar and chocolate do. When researchers use the drug naloxone to block opiate receptors in volunteers, meat loses some of its appeal. Researchers in Edinburgh, Scotland, found that blocking meat's opiate effect cut the appetite for ham by 10 percent, knocked out the desire for salami by about 25 percent, and cut tuna consumption by nearly half.[2] They found much the same thing for cheese, by the way, which will not surprise you, considering cheese's cocktail of opiates we looked at in the previous chapter.

What appears to be happening is that, as meat touches your tongue, opiates are released in the brain, rewarding you—rightly or wrongly—for your calorie-dense food choice and propelling you toward making it a habit.

And scientists are examining another part of the addiction puzzle. It turns out that meat stimulates a surprisingly strong release of insulin, just as a cookie or bread does, a fact that surprised nutrition researchers. In turn, insulin is involved in the release of dopamine between brain cells. Dopamine, as you'll recall from chapter 1, is the ultimate feel-good chemical turned on by every single drug of abuse—opiates, nicotine, cocaine, alcohol, amphetamines, and everything else. Dopamine is what powers the brain's pleasure center.

Now, the fact that meat stimulates insulin release is foreign to people who think of insulin as relating only to carbohydrates. The idea is that carbohydrates—sugary or starchy foods—break apart into natural sugar molecules during the process of digestion, and, as these sugar molecules pass into the bloodstream they spark the release of insulin, the hormone that escorts sugar into the cells of the body. True enough. But protein stimulates insulin release, too. In research studies, researchers feed various foods to volunteers, and then take blood samples every fifteen minutes over the next two hours. Meat causes a distinct, sometimes surprising, insulin spike. In fact, beef and cheese cause a bigger insulin release than pasta, and fish produces a bigger insulin release than popcorn.[3]

Researchers are only beginning to unravel the interplay between insulin and addictions. They have been intrigued by occasional case studies of patients who require insulin to treat diabetes surreptitiously upping their doses, and evidence that insulin function is altered in opiate addicts. Stay tuned.

The good news is that, once a meat habit has been decidedly broken for a few weeks it fades from memory surprisingly easily. Both in our study of Dr. Dean Ornish's heart patients and in our later studies, including a study of women aiming to lose weight, few people reported any continuing desire for meat once they had left the habit behind. They could have it if they wanted, but it no longer controlled them. Many described it the way reformed smokers think of tobacco—as something they were glad to be rid of.

Meanwhile, back at 37,000 feet, my fellow air passengers asked about how people actually break a meat habit. "I just don't think I

> Beef and cheese cause a bigger insulin release than pasta, and fish produces a bigger insulin release than popcorn.

could do it," he said. "It's hard to imagine." I reassured him: "You shouldn't do it—that is, not at first. The first step, before you take anything out of your diet, is to bring in new foods. There are probably plenty of meals you like already that have no meat in them at all." We thought through our list: spaghetti with tomato sauce and fresh basil, vegetable stew, split pea soup. Chili could be made without meat and still be very tasty. All the vegetable curry dishes are great. Mexican food—bean burritos with spicy salsa. They had not yet tasted a veggie burger, but took it on faith that they might be up to snuff. Mushroom gravy might go well on a baked potato.

"Take your time and find the ones you really like," I said. "Once you have plenty of good choices picked out and your kitchen shelves are stocked with healthy things to eat, then it's time to make the break. But the trick is to do it for just three weeks." The idea is that, if you set meat aside for three weeks, your tastes change. In the same way as people switching from whole milk to nonfat milk quickly come to prefer the nonfat variety—and can no longer stomach full-fat brands—when you lighten your whole diet, the same process occurs. It takes only about three weeks. If you do it really well and don't cheat, your taste buds learn a new set of preferences. After three weeks you can decide whether to stick with it or not.

By the time we landed they were intrigued at the possibilities. He might just be able to tackle this heart problem after all. And the new menu was starting to sound pretty good. They could gain energy, get in shape, knock off a few pounds, and really enjoy their lives together.

Is It Good to Break a Meat Habit?

We've all heard hints that we might live longer or be a bit healthier if we set meat aside. It's true. When you step away from the meat counter you do yourself a huge favor.

Preventing—and Reversing—Heart Disease

Perhaps the best-known advantage of breaking a meat habit is what it does for your heart. In 1990, Dr. Dean Ornish sparked a revolution in cardiology when he showed that a vegetarian diet, along with other healthy lifestyle changes, actually reopened blocked arteries in 82 per-

Fat and Cholesterol: Meat vs. Plant Foods

	Fat*	Cholesterol		Fat*	Cholesterol
Atlantic Salmon†	40	70	Apple	6	0
Beef, round bottom, lean	28	78	Beans, navy	3	0
Chicken white meat, skinless	23	85	Broccoli	12	0
Pork loin, lean	41	81	Lentils	3	0
Shrimp, raw	15	151	Orange	2	0
Tuna, white	21	42	Rice, brown	8	0

*Based on percentage of calories
†Meat servings are 3.5 ounces

cent of his research participants—without surgery and even without cholesterol-lowering drugs.[4]

Heart disease typically starts with fat and cholesterol from meat and other animal products, which increase the amount of cholesterol in the bloodstream. Cholesterol particles then invade the artery wall, causing the formation of small bumps, called *plaques*, which strangle the flow of blood to the heart muscle. But setting aside animal products and keeping the fat content low in the foods you eat stops this process in its tracks.

Now, chicken-and-fish diets are not low enough in fat or cholesterol to do what vegetarian diets can. Take a look at the numbers: The leanest beef is about 28 percent fat, as a percentage of calories. The leanest chicken is not much different, at about 23 percent fat. Fish vary, but all have cholesterol and more fat than is found in typical beans, vegetables, grains, and fruits, virtually all of which are well under 10 percent fat. So, while white-meat diets lower cholesterol levels by only about 5 percent,[5] meatless diets have three to four times more cholesterol-lowering power, allowing the arteries to the heart to reopen.

Easy Weight Loss

Not only did Dr. Ornish's patients reopen blocked arteries, they also lost weight—more than twenty pounds, on average, over the first year.

PCRM's studies of meatless diets have shown the same thing.[6] While some people have tried to lose weight by leaving off their plates *everything other than meat*—using the Atkins Diet and similar approaches that ban bread, potatoes, pasta, beans, and every other shred of carbohydrate—an equally effective and far healthier method uses exactly the opposite approach, emphasizing grains, vegetables, fruits, and beans. Because meat and other fatty foods are, by far, the most concentrated source of calories, when they are off your plate your calorie intake naturally falls. So, even when people have about as many carb-rich foods as their appetites call for, the average weight loss is about one pound per week, week after week after week, even if they don't count calories or limit portion size. More on this in a moment.

Preventing Alzheimer's Disease

Recent studies have suggested that choosing foods that drive your cholesterol down might do more than prevent a heart attack. It might also cut your risk for Alzheimer's disease. People who keep a low cholesterol level are at significantly less risk of the cognitive impairment as they age.[7]

And researchers have gone a step further and zeroed in on an amino acid—that is, a protein building block—that comes primarily from the breakdown of animal proteins. It is called *homocysteine,* and it appears to increase the risk of Alzheimer's disease.[8] Cutting the amount of homocysteine in your bloodstream appears to cut the risk of the disease, and it is wonderfully easy to do. The keys are (1) to get your protein from plant sources, rather than animal sources, and (2) to have plenty of the vitamins that break homocysteine down—folic acid and vitamin B_6 (from beans, vegetables, and fruits) and vitamin B_{12} (from fortified foods or supplements.)

Preventing Cancer

Breaking a meat habit cuts your overall cancer risk by about 40 percent.[9] Your risk of colon cancer drops by about two-thirds, according to Harvard University studies including tens of thousands of women and men.[10,11]

In their search for the smoking gun linking meat to cancer, scientists have discovered cancer-causing chemicals, called *heterocyclic*

> ◈ As meat is cooked, cancer-causing chemicals, called *heterocyclic amines*, form within the meat tissues.

amines that form as meat is cooked. And the issue does not stop at *red* meat. While these carcinogens are often present in well-done beef, they have turned up in far higher levels in grilled chicken, as well as in fish.[12] The good news is that meatless meals—whether it's pasta marinara, vegetable curry, spinach lasagne, or anything else—are generally free of these problem compounds and are rich in nutrients that protect against cancer.

Preventing Osteoporosis

When you get your protein from plant sources instead of animal products, your bones breathe a sigh of relief. Here's why: Animal proteins are high in what are called *sulfur-containing amino acids*.[13] These acidic protein-building blocks tend to leach calcium from the bones, and that calcium passes through the kidneys and into the urine.[14,15] Plant proteins are far more healthful. While still containing all the essential amino acids you need for building and repairing body tissues, they are far lower in sulfur-containing amino acids, and they help protect your bones.

A Cleaner Food Supply

Many people have turned from red meat to fish, encouraged by reports that fish contains "good fats." However, those "good fats" are just as fattening as any other kind of fat, as the native populations of Arctic regions have demonstrated. People chowing down on salmon are likely to store a fair amount of "good fats" all around their middles and up and down their thighs.

Perhaps worst of all, fish is by far the most contaminated food. As environmental experts monitor chemical contamination in fish, they routinely issue advisories, such as one from Virginia's Department of Environmental Quality, which recently pointed out that catfish and carp had PCBs up to 3,212 parts per billion, more than five times the allowable limit. PCBs, or polychlorinated biphenyls, are chemicals that were used in electrical equipment, hydraulic fluid, and carbonless carbon paper. They linger in waterways and, like mercury and other contaminants, flow through fish gills, lodge in fish muscle tissues, and routinely show up in governmental tests. Because fish migrate and water currents spread chemicals from place to place, such contamination is now ubiquitous. Air currents carry mercury from power plants and waste incinerators to water sheds hundreds or even thousands of miles away, and the metal ends up in tuna and other fish as a matter of routine.

When it comes to thinking about healthy foods, many of us tend to focus on one problem at a time. When news reports carry alerts about chemical contaminants, we switch from fish to chicken or beef. When salmonella and E. coli hit the headlines, we quit eating chicken and beef and rush back to fish. Happily, there are plenty of healthful foods that skip all these problems. More on this in part III.

Meat Strikes Back: The Atkins Diet

On July 7, 2002, *The New York Times Magazine* published a huge cover photo of a greasy T-bone steak. The cover story, entitled "What if Fat Doesn't Make You Fat?" rose to the defense of steaks, chops, and fried chicken, while striking out at the scientists and public health officials who counsel against fatty, meaty diets. Meat doesn't make you fat, the article wanted readers to believe. It might even do the opposite. Wrapped up as the Atkins Diet, meat was offered as the centerpiece of a weight-loss plan that, the article went on, had now gained a sort of scientific respectability.

Apparently, the article was exactly the signal a meat-hungry nation was waiting for. Many people were all too glad to accept the idea that meat could actually help them lose weight, just as they had hoped for fen-phen, amphetamines, cabbage soup, ab-trainers, and just about every other dangerous or useless would-be remedy. The media went crazy with the story. Every newspaper in the country ran headlines saying beef and pork might be healthy after all, and evening talk shows had serious-sounding debates on the subject. Office water-cooler conversations pondered the "real truth" about meat, as if tens of thousands of scientific journal pages linking meat to illness were suddenly and miraculously erased, exonerating meat once and for all.

Because I imagine some readers have gone a little way down this same road, we should take a bit of time to understand a few things about the meaty, high-protein diets that win on-again, off-again popularity.

First, here is the idea behind high-protein diets: The human body naturally gets its energy from carbohydrate—the starchy part of beans, vegetables, potatoes, bread, and so forth. During digestion, carbohydrates break up into sugar molecules that power your brain and other organs. The Atkins Diet and other high-protein, very-low-carbohydrate diets operate on the theory that if you cut out carbohydrate—which is 50–60 percent of what people normally eat in a day—your body will have no choice but to burn fat. That's true enough, provided cutting carbs means that you take in fewer calories than before. If you don't, it doesn't work at all.

Despite occasional accounts of dramatic weight loss, the results most people actually achieve with high-protein diets are not much different than with any other weight-reduction diet. On average, they lose about a pound per week.[16] This is about the same as is seen with any other low-calorie diet, or with low-fat, vegetarian diets.[17] And, for many people the diet is tolerable only for so long. Sooner or later you will return to a normal calorie intake. All the lost weight returns, and you are right back where you started.

Almost. Unfortunately, while you were on the high-protein diet you consumed astronomical amounts of fat, protein, and cholesterol. Needless to say, that has doctors worried about the risk of colon cancer, heart disease, kidney damage, and osteoporosis, among other problems.

The August 2002 issue of the *American Journal of Kidney Diseases* reported what happened when ten healthy individuals were put on a low-carbohydrate, high-protein diet for six weeks under controlled conditions. They found exactly what they feared—urinary calcium losses increased 55 percent, showing that the risks of bone loss, kidney stones, and kidney damage are not simply theoretical.[18]

Some high-protein diet advocates have gone to great lengths to try to make these problems disappear. When diet-book author Robert Atkins himself had a cardiac arrest at breakfast in 2002, news reports dutifully parroted the high-protein school's suggestion that fat in his diet had nothing to do with the unfortunate event.

Meaty diets are also based on several nutritional myths. The first, which was the basis of *The New York Times Magazine* article, was that fatty foods must not be fattening, because fat intake supposedly fell during the 1980s, just as America's obesity epidemic began. Ergo, fatty foods are not the culprit. The notion was that Americans had suddenly begun to shun fatty foods and had turned instead to fat-free cookies and low-fat foods of all kinds, so these new-fangled defatted foods must be to blame.

The truth, however, is clear from food surveys conducted by the National Center for Health Statistics. During the period from 1980 to 1991, daily per capita fat intake did not drop one iota. The number of trips to the golden arches and KFC did not dwindle in the least. While the American public added sodas and other sugary and starchy foods to the diet, forcing the percentage of calories from fat to decline slightly, the actual amount of fat in the American diet held steady as a rock.

The second myth was that people who eat the most carbohydrates tend to gain the most weight. In fact, the reverse is true. Many people throughout Asia consume large amounts of carbohydrate in the form of rice, noodles, and vegetables and generally have lower body weights than Americans—including Asian Americans—who eat large amounts of meat, dairy products, and fried foods. Similarly, vegetarians who generally follow diets rich in carbohydrates typically have significantly lower body weights than omnivores. Of course, it is true that when people cut carbohydrate or anything else from their diets and do not replace the lost calories with other foods they are likely to lose some weight. But carbohydrates are clearly not the cause of the weight problems of the Western world.

The bottom line is that, no matter how you slice it, meaty diets are bad news for your health.

The Meat Pushers

In the 1890s, my grandfather moved from Kentucky to southern Illinois, where he set up a small farm. He raised cattle, horses, and the occasional sheep or goat, and grew corn and soybeans to feed them. He passed the farm on to his children and grandchildren. Over time, that small farm grew. A great many pounds of beef have been raised at Barnard Stock Farms. And in recent years the farming business has changed beyond recognition. Across America and the rest of the world, farms have coalesced into huge agribusinesses.

When I was a boy visiting my farming relatives in southern Illinois, one of my uncles was complaining about government welfare programs. A big waste of tax money, he felt. His brother Lloyd, a minister, gently reminded him that he never seemed to complain when farmers got *their* government checks. What he meant, of course, was that farmers have been the recipients of enormous government programs.

They certainly have. In the 2001–2002 school year, the federal government bought up more than $200 million worth of beef, aiming to shore up farm profits. The beef ends up in school lunches and other programs. And, on September 9, 2002, Secretary of Agriculture Ann Veneman announced another purchase, this one for $30 million worth of pork, which soon ended up on school lunch trays. It's not that our government imagined that America's ever-fatter children needed more burgers or pork chops. Rather, school lunch purchases and other massive food-buying programs are designed to put dollars into farmers' pockets. They pay scant attention to the foods children really need for health.

Federally managed programs run meat advertising, just as they do for dairy products. "Beef, it's what's for dinner," "Pork, the other white meat," and other common slogans are government programs. In turn, farming organizations are generous donors to political campaigns, making sure that nothing changes.

The meat industry has kept as tight a rein on government nutrition guidelines. When the USDA released its "Eating Right Pyramid" in 1991, cattlemen took umbrage at the design. Meat was suddenly less prominent than vegetables, fruits, and grains. So a battalion of angry farmers stormed over to the office of the Secretary of Agriculture, who promptly agreed to send the Pyramid back to the drawing board. However, even the meat industry's influence was not sufficient to make meat trump vegetables and fruits for long, and the Pyramid was re-released more or less unchanged the following year.

The meat industry has done its best to control not only what goes

⇥ In the 2001–2002 school year, the federal government bought up more than $200 million worth of beef for school lunches and other purposes.

into your mouth, but also what you think about good nutrition. It has been a loyal backer of the American Dietetic Association, sponsoring informational materials, dinners, and convention meetings. It has played the same game with the American Medical Association. When the AMA released its "videoclinic" on what doctors need to know about cholesterol, its sponsors were none other than the National Livestock and Meat Board, Beef Board, and Pork Board.

Enough of the bad news. The good news is that supermarkets now carry an enormous range of products that substitute for meat, from soy hot dogs and veggie burgers to faux Canadian bacon and ground beef substitutes. And a great many foods provide protein, iron, and other nutrients without fat and cholesterol, as we will see in the menu and recipe section.

It is indeed possible to break the meat habit and reap enormous health benefits, as Dean Ornish, M.D., proved in his research, and as I've seen, not only in our research participants, but even in my own family. When my father—who grew up with tremendous respect for his hard-working family and the livestock business they had built over many decades—developed a taste for vegetarian foods, I knew that *anybody* can break a meat habit.

The Bottom Line

- Many people are hooked on meat. One in four Americans would not give it up for a single week—even if they were paid a thousand dollars to do so. The habit is aggressively spreading to other countries—especially in Asia—that traditionally had plant-based diets. In its wake, overweight, heart disease, cancer, diabetes, and other health problems have become epidemics.

- The biochemical reasons behind meat's ability to keep people hooked appear to be related to its high fat content, an apparent opiate effect, and perhaps its ability to spark the release of insulin.

- A switch from red to white meat does not help. Even without the skin, chicken has nearly as much cholesterol and fat as typical lean beef. While some people imagine that the fats in fish are "good" fats, anywhere from 15 to 30 percent of fish fat turns out to be nothing but artery-clogging saturated fat, and fish is easily one of the most chemically contaminated foods people eat.

• Breaking a meat habit brings a huge payoff. In research studies, people who choose meatless foods lose weight very easily. Their cholesterol levels fall, often dramatically, and diabetes, hypertension, and other health problems typically improve or even disappear.

• The U.S. government collaborates with industry to aggressively advertise meat products. When meat prices fall, the government buys up millions of dollars worth and puts it into school lunches and other programs.

• If you're ready to break free, part II will get you started. There are so many enormously tasty replacements, as you'll see in the menu and recipe section, you'll wish you'd made the switch long ago.

Part II

Seven Steps to Physical Resilience: The Keys to a Craving-Free Body

I f sugar, chocolate, cheese, meat, or other food habits have seduced your taste buds a bit too strongly and flirtation has turned into a love-hate relationship, the following chapters will help you change things. Wishing the seduction away is a waste of time. It is stronger than you are. The key is to regain physical strength and balance, so that you are no longer so vulnerable.

If your blood sugar is falling precipitously, your body will insist on food—and junk food fits the bill perfectly, as far as your appetite is concerned. If you have been dieting, you have almost certainly impaired your appetite-controlling hormone, *leptin*. If you are a young woman in your premenstrual week, hormone swings will accentuate cravings and destroy your resolve. And anyone—man or woman, young or old— who is fatigued or stressed will be drawn to the refrigerator in search of the calming opiate effects of foods. These factors are mysterious to most people who, not surprisingly, cannot understand why certain foods are so irresistible.

When your system is in balance, you can still have a not-so-healthy food if you want it. But you will be less likely to make that kind of choice. There are seven keys:

1. Start with a Healthy Breakfast
2. Choose Foods That Hold Your Blood Sugar Steady
3. Boost Appetite-Taming Leptin
4. Break Craving Cycles
5. Get Regular Exercise and Rest
6. Call in the Reinforcements
7. Use Extra Motivators if You Need Them

After you've looked through these simple steps you'll find all the tools for improving your diet in part III, with plenty of healthy and tasty foods to help you on your way. And once you see how good you feel when you're finally in charge of what you eat, the momentum will carry you right along into a new world of healthy eating.

6

Step 1: Start with a Healthy Breakfast

Professional golfers often say that the most important shot they'll hit in any tournament is not the soaring approach shot that clears the water hazard and lands lightly on the green, the surgically precise chip shot that comes within inches of the cup, or even the final putt for victory. The most important shot of the day is the very first one. Because, if the game starts well—you strike the ball cleanly and powerfully and it lands where you want it to—you're infused with confidence that will carry you along.

Nutritionists know that the most important meal of the day is breakfast. The reason is not just that you're famished from having had nothing to eat for eight, ten, or twelve hours, nor that you need to power up for physical and mental stamina; the fact is, just as a golf pro sets the tone for the entire round as he or she steps up to the first tee, you set the tone for your entire day with your first bites of food.

If you take in healthy foods, their proteins repair your body tissues, healthy carbohydrates give you energy, traces of fat play biochemical roles inside your cells, and vitamins and minerals turn on the metabolic processes that allow you to think, move, and carry out the activities of the day. You are providing nutrition, not only to keep your body running strong all morning long, but to keep your brain sharp, to keep your emotions calm, and—just as importantly—to keep your appetite quiet.

If your day begins with a rush out the door on an empty stomach your body will rebel. An hour or two later it will not only demand to be fed, it will overreact, miscalculating how much food you actually need.

You can also run into trouble if you eat the wrong kind of breakfast. Some foods can cause your blood sugar to spike upward, only to come crashing down later on, throwing you back into gnawing hunger and putting snacks firmly on your radar screen.

But, if you start your day with a healthy, craving-blocking breakfast you will be rewarded throughout the rest of the day. Snack machines, candy displays, doughnut shops, hot dog stands, and almost everything else will be less tempting.

Sarah was a busy executive at a credit card company. She knew she wasn't eating the right things, but she wasn't sure what to do about it. Every day she arrived at work with a resolve to eat properly. She would control her portions, cut down on fat, and steer clear of sugar. But her willpower didn't last till noon. Nearly every day hunger started its attack around midmorning, and it left her vulnerable to the lure of junk food. Her coworkers seemed to be forever offering her doughnuts and other gooey pastries, or leaving them around the office. Sooner or later she would give in, taking in more fat and calories than she wanted to think about. Every day she aimed not to let it happen, and almost every day some variant of this pattern played itself out.

The fact is, her problems did not start when she walked in the door to her office. They started as soon as she got out of bed. She had no time for breakfast, and she was not entirely sure which foods she would have chosen if she had. Sometimes she picked up a cup of coffee on her way to work, but that was about it. With her blood sugar bottoming out and hunger becoming more and more insistent, there was simply no way she could steel herself against the parade of food in her office.

At our office, Sarah and I planned out several different breakfast choices, each of which took minimal preparation time, and, over the next few weeks, she tested out how she felt physically after each one. Three of them were clear winners. They were quick, satisfying, and, most importantly, blocked hunger for hours. So, even though the junk food still arrived more or less every day in the office, it didn't call to her so strongly. As the day unfolded she found it easy to control temptation, and that turned out to be the single biggest factor in her successful weight loss over the next several months.

What were these magical breakfasts? I'll show you—but first, let's lay out the rules.

First, be sure to *have* breakfast. Even though some people skip breakfast in hopes of cutting down on calories, missing the first meal of the day propels them into overeating later on. This pattern starts in childhood. Kids who skip breakfast are generally the heaviest and most out of shape.[1] But it also happens in adults. If you miss breakfast, you'll overcompensate at lunch and in snacks during the day, and your overall calorie intake will end up higher than if you had eaten when you first dragged yourself out of bed. Having a healthy breakfast regulates your appetite.

It also reduces stress. Researchers have found measurable reductions in stress hormone levels when people have breakfast, compared to when they skip it.[2] In other words, breakfast makes you calmer. And you are better insulated against the kinds of snacking that stress and anxiety can trigger. Having breakfast also boosts your concentration. Students who have breakfast every day score better on tests, compared to those who arrive at school hungry.[3]

Second, fiber-rich foods are essential. Most people's breakfasts do more harm than good—a plate of bacon and eggs can easily pack more fat and cholesterol than all their other meals put together. Others have breakfasts that are little more than white toast or a bagel, which is not sufficient to block hunger later in the day.

What each of these diet patterns is lacking is fiber. It's what makes foods filling without being fattening. The word itself simply means plant roughage: the brown covering of a grain of brown rice, the chewy part of oats, or the skin of an apple. Fiber gives foods crunch. It makes them substantial. It gives them staying power.

To appreciate fiber, look at a few numbers: For comparison, let's take a generous-sized tablespoonful (about 15 grams) of any sort of fat or oil. That spoon of grease has about 135 calories. If we have some carbohydrate or protein weighing the same amount, it would pack only about 60 calories. *But that same amount of fiber has essentially no calories at all.* It fills you up at least as well as do fatty or high-protein foods, but you'll never see it on the scale.

A bowl of old-fashioned oatmeal, a half cantaloupe, some toasted pumpernickel bread—these are foods that give you loads of fiber.

> ◄ After the high-fiber breakfast, the volunteers snacked 75 percent less than after the bacon-and-eggs breakfast. And they continued to eat much less as the day went on—987 calories less, to be exact.

There is no fiber in eggs, bacon, sausage, yogurt, or any other animal-derived product. They aren't plants, and only plant foods have fiber.

Researchers in England showed how powerful the anti-snacking effect of a fiber-rich breakfast can be.[4] They compared different breakfasts, each of which had exactly the same calorie content. Two of them—a typical bacon-and-eggs breakfast with toast and grilled tomato, and a breakfast of croissants with margarine and jam—were high in fat and low in fiber. Although both were reasonably satisfying at the time, neither of these breakfasts had any staying power. The volunteers got hungry well before lunch. After the bacon-and-eggs breakfast especially, volunteers ended up dipping into mid-morning snacks. They also took fairly hefty portions at lunchtime, and a similar pattern was evident after eating croissants.

But the researchers also tested a breakfast of bran cereal with sliced banana and toast. It had a full 19 grams of fiber, and the difference on the volunteers' appetites was dramatic. Even though all the breakfasts were identical in calories, the bran cereal breakfast had much more staying power. After the high-fiber breakfast, the volunteers snacked 75 percent less than after the bacon-and-eggs breakfast. And they continued to eat much less as the day went on—987 calories less, to be exact, than when they had started their day with bacon and eggs. The high-fiber breakfast filled them up, kept them satisfied, and gave them energy. The researchers also measured alertness and found that it was much better after a low-fat, high-fiber meal than after the fatty meals.

In the Introduction we took a quick look at a similar study, this one in Boston, in which doctors gave boys different kinds of breakfasts.[5] After a breakfast of regular oatmeal the children snacked much less—about 35 percent less—than after a breakfast of instant oatmeal. Now, the two kinds of oatmeal had exactly the same calorie content; the difference was fiber. In instant oatmeal, fiber is broken up so that it cooks rapidly. It also digests rapidly, releasing natural sugars into the bloodstream a bit too quickly. The result is a quick rise and fall of blood sugar and an equally quick return of hunger.

Leaving the oatmeal intact gave the breakfast staying power. Natural fiber allows it to digest slowly, avoiding the rapid change in blood sugar and giving you natural resistance to snacking for hours after breakfast.

So, have a big bowl of oatmeal for breakfast. And if you are still eating instant, try the old-fashioned variety. It still cooks fast enough that it will not delay you on your way out the door. A couple of cooking tips, however: first, measure it as you prepare it. Good cooks can eyeball quantities for most other ingredients, but they seem to always get it wrong with oatmeal, making it too watery or too thick. Take a coffee cup, and scoop one cup of oatmeal into a saucepan, followed by two cups of cold water (Mixing the ingredients before heating makes the oatmeal smooth and creamy, while adding oats to already boiling water makes it flaky and a bit too chewy.) Bring it to a boil, then let it simmer on very low heat for a few minutes, and it's ready. You've just made enough for a generous bowlful. No need to add milk, sugar, or anything, although some people prefer it with fruit, cinnamon, and so forth.

Oats isn't the only blood-sugar stabilizing food. As we'll see in more detail in the next chapter, fruits and beans have the same effect, and some foods from these groups have managed to elbow their way onto the breakfast menu. More on this below.

Don't be too shy about quantity. If you find yourself getting hungry an hour or two after breakfast, it's a sure sign you've been a bit too miserly with portions.

Third, choose *healthy* protein sources. Some years ago the French government exhorted its citizenry to have more substantial breakfasts. It seemed that baguettes and croissants were not holding people until lunch, and their attention spans were starting to flag. The solution, of course, was not to turn to an American-style breakfast—French waistlines are Americanizing all too rapidly as it is, and bacon, sausage, and Egg McMuffins are the last things they need—but to eat healthier and more substantial foods. Low-protein, fiber-depleted breakfasts, such as bagels or white toast, don't have much staying power.

First of all, these sorts of "white-bread" breakfasts cause a blood sugar spike, as we've seen. That leads to a premature blood sugar *drop*, and that can leave you out of sorts and hungry enough to give in to whatever snacks drift by. More substantial, higher-fiber foods, like oatmeal, prevent this problem.

Also, foods such as bagels that release large amounts of sugar into the blood tend to increase the amount of serotonin in the brain, which is why people with seasonal depression tend to crave sugary or starchy foods. Serotonin is a chemical involved in regulating moods and sleep. As starchy foods produce a little extra serotonin, some people feel better, but others feel sleepy or on edge. So while some people feel fine with a high-carb, low-protein breakfast, others feel drained.

Here is the key: A little extra plant protein blocks that serotonin boost and prevents sluggishness. Notice the recommendation for *plant* proteins. Most North American and European breakfasts are quite a ways off the mark. As a child growing up in the Midwest, I had no idea what a healthy breakfast really was. Eggs were everyday fare. Bacon and sausage were commonplace. Yes, we got protein. But we ate enough cholesterol and fat to cause heart attacks, and, in fact, that is exactly what happened to all too many people. My grandfather died of a heart attack while still a fairly young man. Many other relatives have had other diet-related complications.

One easy way to rehabilitate standard breakfast fare is to try the new veggie sausage and bacon products that health-food stores carry and many regular groceries now stock, too. They have plenty of protein— but it is plant-derived protein, so it is not linked to the health problems of animal proteins—and generally have surprisingly little fat and no cholesterol. They come in a huge variety, so try several and see which ones you like, favoring those lowest in fat.

When it comes to replacing eggs, you'll love the scrambled tofu recipe on page XXX. If you are harboring any of the tofu phobia that first greeted the arrival of this versatile Asian product, it is only because you have not had it prepared in the right way. If you have it twice, I guarantee you will love it.

When it comes to finding healthy, high-protein foods, it pays to take a look around the world. Most other countries have several healthy breakfast choices. While visiting Mexico's Yucatan Peninsula many years ago, I noticed that, while American tourists breakfasted on sausage and eggs, the locals ate black beans with toast or tortillas. Odd thing, I thought—beans for breakfast. But nutritionally it cannot be beat. Beans are loaded with healthy protein, are very low in fat, and have no cholesterol at all. And that touch of breakfast salsa certainly opens your eyes in the morning, too.

Later, while visiting London, I noticed a similar phenomenon.

> ◈ When it comes to finding healthy, high-protein foods, it pays to take a look around the world. Most other countries have several healthy breakfast choices.

Beans on toast was a common choice. In Australia, the same breakfast fare didn't raise an eyebrow at all. And a friend from the Middle East told me that hummus, made from chickpeas, was a common breakfast food.

How is it, I wondered, that nearly every other country has found ways to turn various bean dishes into hearty breakfast fare, while North Americans still find the custom totally alien?

Well, things are changing even here. Breakfast burritos are becoming more and more popular. See the recipe on page 216. If you've never had one, break out of your old routine and try a truly healthy breakfast. Take a look at the recipe section, and experiment to your heart's content.

So, what were Sarah's favorites? She loved the Breakfast Scrambler, also on page 216, and the Breakfast Burrito. They are both very hearty and substantial and surprisingly quick. And, although she didn't think she could take to oatmeal, cinnamon and raisins did the trick for her, and she has come to really love a big bowl of it.

What really counts is that she not only feels better physically, she also feels better emotionally. The plant protein in the Breakfast Scrambler, burrito, or, for that matter, even oatmeal—about eight grams in a big, piping-hot bowl—balances the starchy part of these foods that might leave her feeling out of sorts if she had just had a bagel or some white toast. And these foods are loaded with fiber-rich ingredients to block hunger all morning.

Having gotten a grip on her cravings and bringing her weight under control, her self-esteem has gotten a huge boost. And that has motivated her to want to continue with a healthy diet, get regular exercise, and look after herself. She looks much more confident and in charge.

Her transformation depended on starting each day on the right foot. In the following chapters we'll look at the next steps toward breaking the food seduction.

7

Step 2: Choose Foods That Hold Your Blood Sugar Steady

A new suitor singing below your balcony is much less appealing if a devoted lover is already waiting in your boudoir. And a cookie is less seductive if your blood sugar is already up where it should be.

A steady blood sugar helps you avoid falling prey to impulse eating. When you choose foods that hold blood sugar nice and steady, you keep hunger in check.

It's easy to go wrong. Take the case of Manuel, for example. He was a forty-four-year-old lawyer who had developed a weight problem in his early thirties. He had been very fit and health-conscious as a teenager in Colombia and, in fact, had been an avid soccer player. But things started getting away from him in law school, and especially once he started working in a busy law firm. Arriving at my office, he told me his problem was simply being "a middle-aged man with a teenager's appetite." Snacks were his undoing, he felt. In the middle of every afternoon, he found himself heading for the candy machine, and he usually returned with more than one treat—a Snickers bar and some peanuts, or M&Ms and a bag of potato chips—and often a soda. As an adolescent, he seemed to be able to burn off any extra calories he took in, but those days were apparently long gone.

To his surprise, I asked him to stop focusing on his snacks and to look at what he ate at his regular mealtimes, especially lunchtime, the meal before his snack attacks kicked in. He was very "good" at lunch, he said, and never overdid it. He often had nothing more than yogurt and a bagel—a habit he had adopted from his wife. And that added up to less than 400 calories. Sometimes the office ordered pizza, but he usually had only two slices. The problems started at three o'clock or so, he felt, because that was when the cravings kicked in.

I suggested to Manuel that his lunch choices set him up for hunger later in the afternoon. A yogurt and bagel or two pizza slices are just too low in calories to touch his hunger and too low in fiber to fill him up. At the same time, what these foods provide is mostly sugar—or, to be more exact, ingredients that pass sugar into the blood stream. The predictable result is a midafternoon binge. Here are the details:

- First, Manuel undoubtedly burned well over 2,000 calories per day. There is no way a 400-calorie lunch could stop his appetite for long.
- Second, to make things worse, there is no fiber at all in yogurt and very little in a bagel. That means that they will not be very filling. Ditto for pizza: made of white flour, pepperoni, and cheese, there is virtually no fiber to be found.
- Third, most common yogurts are loaded with sugar, which comes both from the lactose in milk and from added sugar. And the white-flour bagels he was keen on were basically nothing but refined starch. The cheese pizzas were, similarly, just white flour topped with a dairy product.

As a teenager he had eaten very differently. He usually had beans and rice with a side of vegetables, and that seemed to hold him all afternoon. A look at these foods shows they are loaded with fiber and would easily stabilize his blood sugar through the afternoon snacking "window."

So Manuel's problem didn't start with the candy machine. It started with a lunch that propelled him into snacking.

Let's take a look at how to check your own choices to see if they will protect you from snacking later on. There are three very simple principles to keeping your blood sugar steady: You have to eat *enough,* you need plenty of appetite-taming fiber, and you need low-glycemicindex (GI) foods. Don't get nervous about this technical-sounding last point. Each of these is really a snap, as I'll show you.

You Must Eat *Enough*

When it comes to sizing up your lunch—or foods you eat at any other time of day—it goes without saying that you need to eat an adequate quantity, just as we saw for breakfast in the previous chapter.

Many people, like Manuel, are convinced that there is some sort of virtue in allowing hunger pangs to continue. There isn't. Hunger leads to binges.

Eating enough doesn't mean stuffing yourself. And it doesn't mean you can't cut back a bit if you feel you've been overdoing it lately. What it means is that you cannot skip meals or eat tiny diet-sized portions and expect to keep hunger at bay in the hours that follow.

You may find that it helps to eat at more or less the same time every day. If you get off track, especially if you delay a meal, you may find you overdo it when you do sit down to eat.

Beyond the simple guideline of being sure you're eating enough, keeping a steady blood sugar really means only two things. First, your foods must be generous with fiber, and second, they must have a nice, low glycemic index. These are very simple concepts (I hesitate to say they are a "piece of cake!"), and you can easily put them to work.

Go High-Fiber

Fiber is what fills you up, as we saw briefly in the previous chapter. At the risk of belaboring a point, there are a few more things you need to know about putting this humble part of foods to work. Researchers have found that you can cut your calorie intake by a full 10 percent just by adding an extra 14 grams of fiber each day.[1] Over the long run, that can really help trim excess pounds.

Researchers looked at the eating habits of a large group of people living in Alabama, California, Illinois, and Minnesota. They all followed typical American diets, more or less, but some got more fiber than others. The difference wasn't huge: about 10 grams of fiber per day for

> ☞ Researchers have found that an extra 14 grams of fiber in your diet each day cuts your calorie intake by a full 10 percent.

those at the lower end, compared to about 20 for those who got the most fiber. But, even within that range, fiber made a noticeable difference on the scale. Those whose diets were richer in fiber weighed *eight pounds less,* on average, than those who got less fiber.[2]

Now, the truth is, you can do far better than that. It's easy to get 30, 40, 50, or more grams of fiber a day. Where do you find it? Simple. There are four kinds of foods that have plenty of healthy fiber: beans, vegetables, fruits, and whole grains, in that order. The more of these foods you build into your diet, the better off you are. For example, if you have chicken soup, it doesn't have much fiber (about 1.5 grams, coming from the noodles and vegetable bits). That shouldn't be surprising. Chickens are not plants, so they don't have any plant roughage. But, instead, choose a hearty bowl of split pea soup, which has 5 grams. Lentil soup has about 6, and black bean soup has about 17.

Here's a second example: If you were to have a meat taco, you wouldn't get any fiber from the meat filling and less than 1 gram from the tortilla shell. But make that a bean burrito and you'll get 12 grams, because beans are loaded with appetite-taming fiber. Likewise, cream sauce or oil on your pasta doesn't have a speck of fiber, but have a chunky marinara sauce and you'll get an easy 3 grams. If your dessert is ice cream, you'll strike out again in the fiber department, but an apple, pear, or bowl of strawberries will each give you 3 to 4 grams.

So, in a nutshell, beans, vegetables, fruits, and whole grains give you the fiber you need to keep hunger at arm's length. There is no fiber in meat, dairy products, eggs, or oils, and only a little in refined grain products (e.g., white bread).

If you aim to control your appetite, you'll want to look at how much fiber is in the foods you eat. The Quick Fiber Check on page 88 will help you size up how you're doing now. Aim for 40 grams a day, and your body will thank you many times over.

QUICK FIBER CHECK

The Quick Fiber Check is a handy little tool. Using its simple scoring concept, which takes only a minute or two to learn, you'll automatically be able to estimate the fiber content of virtually everything in the grocery store.

To check your own meals, write down everything you eat or drink for one full day on the form on page 89. Next to each food, jot in its fiber score, using the following guide:

Beans: For each one-half-cup serving of beans or lentils or any food that includes about this amount of beans or lentils as an ingredient, mark 7. One cup of soy milk or one-half cup of tofu rates 3.

Vegetables: For each one-cup serving of vegetables, mark 4. An exception is lettuce, for which one cup scores 2. A potato with skin scores 4; without the skin, it scores 2.

Fruit: For each medium piece of fruit (e.g., apple, orange, banana, one cup of apple sauce, a banana smoothie), mark 3. For one cup of juice, mark 1.

Grains: For each piece of white bread, bagel, or equivalent, score 1. Whole grain breads score 2. One cup of cooked pasta scores 2. One cup of rice scores 1 for white and 3 for brown. One cup of cooked oatmeal scores 4. Score 3 for typical ready-to-eat cereals, 1 for highly processed and colored cereals, and 8 for bran, or check package information.

Meat, poultry, or fish: Score 0. Animal products do not contain fiber.

Eggs or dairy products: Score 0.

Sodas, water: Score 0.

Interpreting Your Quick Fiber Check Score

Less than 20: You need more fiber in your diet. As it is, your appetite will be hard to control, and you may have occasional constipation.

Boosting fiber will help tame your appetite and can cut your risk of many health problems.

20–39: You are doing better than most people in Western countries, but as you bring more fiber into your diet, you will find that it makes foods more satisfying and cuts your calorie intake a bit.

40 or more: Congratulations. You have plenty of healthy fiber in your diet. It tames your appetite and helps keep you healthy. Fiber also reduces your risk of cancer, heart disease, diabetes, and digestive problems.

QUICK FIBER CHECK

Food (only one food or ingredient per line):   **Fiber**

_____   _____

_____   _____

_____   _____

_____   _____

_____   _____

_____   _____

_____   _____

_____   _____

_____   _____

_____   _____

_____   _____

_____   _____

_____   _____

_____   _____

_____   _____

_____   _____

_____   _____

Total   _____

Using the Glycemic Index

Okay, so you're eating enough food, and you're going high-fiber, so it's easy to fill up with relatively little in the way of calories. But there is a third point you need to know about, particularly if you've been battling a weight problem. Within the world of high-fiber foods, some do a better job of keeping your blood sugar steady than others.

Let's go back to our breakfast table for a minute and compare a bowl of oatmeal, on the one hand, with a wheat cereal on the other. Yes, they're both better than bacon and eggs—by a long shot. And they both have about the same amount of fiber. But these two cereals have different effects on your body, as researchers have demonstrated. In one four-week study, researchers gave men whole wheat cereal (Weetabix) for breakfast, along with whole wheat bread. Then, for another four weeks, they switched to a muesli made of oats, apple, and a bit of fruit sugar (fructose), along with pumpernickel bread.

The researchers then checked the men's blood sugars and there was a surprisingly big difference between the two breakfasts. The oat-based breakfast stabilized blood sugar much more effectively than did the wheat-based breakfast.[3] And a more stable blood sugar means that your appetite stays under control. Now, wheat or corn cereals taste great and have no cholesterol and little fat. You really cannot fault them. But they don't have oats' power to stabilize blood sugars, and that's what counts when it comes to keeping your hunger in check.[4,5]

Scientists rate how quickly foods release their natural sugars into the bloodstream using a number called the glycemic index, or GI. As we saw briefly in chapter 2, foods with a low glycemic index release their natural sugars slowly over a long period of time. That's handy; it means that hunger will not return too soon. When you eat a typical low-GI food, it acts as a constant source of energy, providing you natural sugars, minute by minute, on an ongoing basis. It will not let your blood sugar climb too high, and if your blood sugar doesn't zoom up to a peak it will not be able to crash. High-GI foods are just the opposite. They release their sugars quickly, prompting a return of appetite and more snacking later in the day.

One caveat: The GI value of foods is a matter of continuing scientific study, and it clearly matters more for some people than others. If you have been slim all your life and have no trouble with your weight,

GI values are not especially important for you. Almost certainly, your body handles sugars very efficiently and never lets your blood sugar get too far out of line. You'll want to pay more attention to fiber content. If, on the other hand, you've struggled with your weight for some time, those added pounds have probably made your blood sugar harder to control, because extra weight makes your body tissues more resistant to insulin, the hormone that controls your blood sugar. This is especially true if diabetes runs in your family. You'll want to be sure to go high-fiber and low-GI with the foods you eat.

Among low-GI foods, beans again win out and green vegetables score very well, too. Most fruits have low GIs, but there are a few notable exceptions, as we'll see. Grains vary dramatically—some are low, others are high, and we'll soon learn which are which. Candy, honey, and white bread are examples of high-GI foods.

What is it about some foods that make them release sugars slowly and steadily, while others send sugar into your bloodstream almost explosively? If you could examine any carbohydrate-rich food—a bean, a carrot, or a bit of pasta, for example—under a powerful microscope, you would find that, for some, the carbohydrate molecules are long and straight, and are stacked up in an orderly way, like a dense pile of wood. When you eat them, it takes time for digestive enzymes to break up these densely packed molecules. These slow-digesting foods will not perturb your blood sugar very much.

Beans, peas, and lentils are in this low-GI category. Many types of rice are, too. In this case, fiber is not the issue. It all has to do with the arrangement of the carbohydrate molecules.

On the other hand, high-GI starches are built from molecules that are branched, like piles of small twigs. Enzymes quickly break them apart, releasing all their sugars into the blood at more or less the same time.

Typical wheat breads—even whole wheat bread—are in this quick-release category, as are bagels. In contrast, rye and pumpernickel release their sugars much more slowly. Again, it's not fiber that does the trick. It is a question of how the carbohydrate molecules are aligned.

So, to keep your blood sugar steady, don't avoid breads. Just be selective about which ones you choose. The same is true for potatoes. Baking potatoes have a high GI and release their sugars quickly, while sweet potatoes and yams have much lower GI values.

> ⌐ᴥ Typical wheat breads—even whole wheat bread—release their natural sugars into the bloodstream quickly, while rye and pumpernickel do so much more slowly. So... don't avoid breads. Just be selective... The same is true for potatoes. Baking potatoes release their sugars quickly, while sweet potatoes and yams do so more slowly.

Choosing low-GI foods protects you against a tendency toward snacking later in the day. Here are easy tips to picking out healthy, low-GI foods:

- Legumes—that is, beans and anything like a bean (lentils and peas, for example)—are GI champions.
- Green leafy vegetables are fine.
- Nearly all fruits are fine, despite their sweet taste. Pineapple and watermelon are exceptions, with somewhat higher GI values.
- The high-GI group mainly means sugar itself, white bread, wheat cereals, and large baking potatoes.
- For potatoes, choose new potatoes, sweet potatoes, and yams.
- For breads, favor pumpernickel and rye.
- Pasta has a much lower GI than bread, even though both are made from flour.
- Early fruit has a lower GI than ripe fruit.

So now you can see what was wrong with Manuel's lunch choices. As a boy, his favorite beans and rice gave him plenty of fiber (mainly from the beans), plus a nice, low GI to keep hunger at bay for hours. But the foods he ate at work were too miserly with calories and too low in fiber, and they couldn't give him a slow, steady release of natural sugars to quiet his appetite.

Happily, there are many choices beyond beans and rice. Although some people deny themselves pasta because it is high in carbohydrate, the fact is, it has a stunningly low GI and is quite low in calories, unless you use a greasy topping. Most vegetables and fruits do the same. These simple, basic foods are the keys to keeping a steady blood sugar.

But what about the foods we really crave—cookies, angel food cake, and doughnuts? As you'll notice in the GI chart below, they all have one thing in common: They spike your blood sugar.

THE APPETITE-TAMING POWER OF COMMON FOODS

For fiber, aim for 40 grams or more per day. And use the glycemic index to spot foods that release their natural sugars slowly and keep your blood sugar steady. Lower GI values are preferred; values over 90 are generally considered high.

	Fiber (g)	GI*
Fruits		
Apple (1, medium)	2.4	57
Apple juice (1 cup)	0.2	57
Banana (1, medium)	2.7	69
Grapefruit (½, medium)	1.4	36
Grapes (1 cup)	0.9	62
Mango (1, medium)	3.7	73
Olive (1, medium)	0.1	—
Orange (1, medium)	3.1	69
Orange juice (1 cup)	0.5	81
Peach (1, medium)	1.7	40
Pear (1, medium)	4.0	53
Pineapple (1 cup)	1.9	84
Watermelon (1 cup)	0.8	103
Grain Products		
Angel food cake (1 oz.)	0.4	95
Bagel (1)	1.6	103
Barley, pearled (1 cup)	6.0	37
Bread, white (1 slice)	0.6	100
Bread, whole meal (1 slice)	1.9	99
Bread, rye (1 slice)	1.9	83
Bread, pumpernickel (1 slice)	2.1	72
Bulgur wheat (1 cup)	8.2	65
Cereal, All-Bran (1 cup)	20.0	54
Cereal, Cheerios (1 cup)	3.0	106
Cereal, corn flakes (1 cup)	0.0	130

	Fiber (g)	GI*
Grain Products (continued)		
Cereal, oatmeal (1 cup, cooked)	4.0	87
Corn chips (1 oz.)	1.4	60
Popcorn, air-popped (1 oz.)	4.2	79
Spaghetti (1 cup)	2.4	55
Spaghetti, al dente (1 cup)	2.4	50
Rice, white (1 cup, cooked)	0.6	85
Rice, brown (1 cup, cooked)	3.5	72
Rice, parboiled (1 cup, cooked)	0.6	68
Legumes		
Baked beans (vegetarian, ½ cup)	6.4	69
Black beans (½ cup)	7.5	43
Black-eyed peas (½ cup)	4.2	59
Chickpeas (½ cup)	5.3	54
Kidney beans (½ cup)	6.6	42
Lentils (½ cup)	7.8	41
Lima beans (½ cup)	6.6	46
Navy beans (½ cup)	5.8	54
Peas (½ cup)	3.5	56
Peanuts (1 oz., dry roasted)	2.3	26
Pinto beans (½ cup)	7.4	64
Soybeans (½ cup)	5.2	25
Soy milk (1 cup)	3.0	57
Vegetables		
Asparagus (1 cup, boiled)	2.8	—
Broccoli (1 cup, boiled)	4.6	—
Carrots (1 cup, boiled)	2.6	58
Carrots (1 cup, raw)	3.8	23
Potato, baked	4.8	121
Potato, new	3.6	81
Potato chips (1 oz.)	1.3	77
Spinach (1 cup, boiled)	4.4	—
Sweet potato (1, baked)	3.4	77
Yam (½ cup, baked)	2.7	73

	Fiber (g)	GI*
Sweets		
Jelly beans (1 oz.)	0.0	114
Life Savers (2 pieces)	0.0	100
Chocolate (0.5 oz.)	1.0	70
Honey (1 tablespoon)	0.0	104
Sugar (sucrose, 1 teaspoon)	0.0	92
Meats, Dairy Products, and Eggs		
Beef, trimmed round (3.5 oz.)	0.0	—
Chicken breast, half, skinless	0.0	—
Egg, boiled	0.0	—
Halibut (3 oz.)	0.0	—
Ice cream (½ cup)	0.0	87
Ice milk (½ cup)	0.0	—
Milk (1 cup)	0.0	38
Pork, lean sirloin (3.5 oz.)	0.0	—
Salmon (3 oz.)	0.0	—
Tuna salad (½ cup)	0.0	—
Turkey frankfurter	0.0	—

*The GI uses white bread as reference value of 100. When multiple data sources apply, results have been averaged.

SOURCES: J. A. T. Pennington, *Bowes and Church's Food Values of Portions Commonly Used* (Philadelphia: Lippincott-Raven, 1998); the University of Sydney GI Web Site (http://www.glycemicindex.com); and Foster-Powell K, Holt SHA, Brand-Miller JC. International table of glycemic index and glycemic load. *American Journal of Clinical Nutrition* 2002;76:5–56.

Improving Your Body's Ability to Handle Sugar

Now we know how to select foods that release sugars slowly to tame cravings. But let's go a step further. It may surprise you to know that you can actually change your body's response to *any* food so that you are better able to handle whatever sugars it might contain. In other words, even though candy and cookies will cause anybody's blood sugar to spike a bit, you can actually adjust your metabolism so that your body can handle the sugar much more efficiently, preventing some of the spike.

⇥ Cutting fat from your meals improves what is called *insulin sensitivity,* meaning that you don't need much insulin in order to efficiently escort sugar into the cells of the body.

Marjorie was one of our research volunteers. In a laboratory test, we asked her to drink a syrup containing 75 grams of pure sugar. Taking blood samples over the next two hours, we saw what happened to her blood sugar. As you can see in the graph below, it peaked at about thirty minutes, then quickly cascaded downward. That's a pretty typical pattern. If your blood sugar falls too precipitously you may be set up for another binge, which is your body's way of bringing your blood sugar back up again.

Here's the problem: Insulin is the hormone that escorts sugar from your bloodstream into the cells of the body. It is like a doorman who turns the knob on the door to each cell, helps sugar go inside, and then closes the door. Now, while insulin is busily storing sugar in cells, it slows down fat burning. Biologically, this makes sense, because if you've just taken in food there's no need to be burning off fat for energy. If your insulin is working efficiently, it quickly stores the sugars coming from whatever foods you've eaten and then goes away, so fat-burning can resume.

But everything changes when you eat fatty foods, or when you gain a significant amount of weight. Insulin can't work in an oil slick. When there is too much fat in the bloodstream, insulin's hand slips on the knob. Unable to open the door to the cells, insulin lets sugar build up in the blood. Your body responds by making more and more insulin, and eventually it will get the sugar into the cells. But meanwhile that large amount of insulin traveling in the bloodstream has been slowing down your fat burning.

The answer is to get that grease out of the diet. Research shows that reducing fat, especially the *saturated fat* that is common in chicken, beef, fish (yes, anywhere from 15 to 30 percent of fish "oil" is nothing but saturated fat), dairy products, eggs, and tropical oils, like palm or coconut oil, has a tremendous effect on your body's ability to handle sugar. Cutting fat from your meals improves what is called *insulin sensitivity,* meaning that insulin efficiently escorts sugar into the cells of the body.[5] It does its job and gets out of the way. Boosting fiber helps, too.

With our guidance, Marjorie adjusted her diet to scrupulously cut fat and boost fiber. A few weeks later we repeated the test. She again drank exactly the same sugar solution, but the changes in her blood sugar were very different. Because the low-fat diet had tuned up her insulin, the blood-sugar rise was more muted, the peak was lower, and the fall was gentler than before. In the ensuing weeks, not only was her blood sugar stabilized, but she found that cravings were much less insistent. With a simple diet adjustment, you can do precisely the same thing—dramatically changing your body's blood-sugar response to any food. In our clinical studies, we have found that simple diet changes alone boost insulin sensitivity by an average of 24 percent, and it can increase even more if you also exercise.

So there you have it. Keeping a rock-steady blood sugar is no big challenge. It just means (1) eating enough food, (2) knowing where the fiber is and being sure to take advantage of it, and (3) taking a tip from

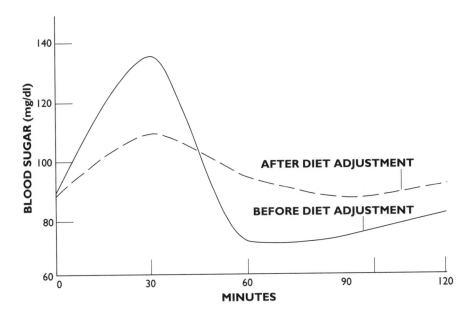

CHOOSING FOODS THAT STEADY YOUR BLOOD SUGAR

the GI chart. If your day has started with a healthy breakfast and continues with foods that keep your blood sugar steady, you're well on your way to knocking out cravings.

But you're not quite there yet. There are still some pitfalls you'll want to avoid, especially changes in the hormones that control hunger, which we'll tackle in the next two chapters.

8

Step 3: Boost Appetite-Taming Leptin

Your body has an appetite-taming hormone that can help you resist the seduction of unhealthy foods. It's called leptin. While it is critically important for controlling your appetite, and it is remarkably easy to boost this natural craving-busting chemical, almost no one other than laboratory scientists knows how to do it. In this chapter I'll show you how. We'll see how this appetite control switch works and how to use foods to augment its anticraving power.

There are, in fact, several different chemical substances your brain cells use to control your appetite. Brain cells use these substances to communicate with each other about how many calories you've taken in, the balance of carbohydrate and protein in your meals, and what sorts of nutrients you might need. Leptin is one of the key signals, and its job is to regulate the strength of your appetite and the speed at which your body burns calories.

Leptin had fifteen minutes of fame back in July 1995. Nearly every newspaper in America and much of the rest of the world ran headlines announcing what looked like a long-awaited answer to weight problems: fat mice injected with this magical hormone slimmed down nearly overnight. Eager dieters scanned the surprising news reports for any evidence that leptin might work in humans and, more importantly, for word on where they could pick some up. Drug companies went crazy, too, hoping to cash in on a weight-loss miracle.

To their disappointment, leptin treatments in humans failed miserably. In fact, it turned out that, unlike mice, overweight people have a considerable amount of leptin in their blood already, and adding more does virtually nothing. Leptin promptly slipped from the public's weight-loss consciousness and was forgotten, just like steam cabinets, vibrating belts, and cabbage soup.

However, leptin is critically important. Let me show you what can happen when leptin isn't working right: In 1997, British scientists reported the case of a child born with a rare genetic abnormality that meant she could not make any leptin at all. Although she was a normal, healthy baby at birth, it soon became apparent that she was preoccupied with food, as if her appetite had no turn-off switch, as indeed it did not. She cried inconsolably unless she was eating. As a growing child, she spent her days trying to filch food when no one was looking. It was her sole preoccupation. By the time she was six she needed liposuction of her legs in order to be able to walk. By age nine she weighed 208 pounds. Her cousin, born with the same abnormality, weighed 64 pounds at just two years of age.[1]

Later, doctors treated her with leptin injections, replacing what nature had neglected to give her. Her appetite gradually came under control, and she lost interest in between-meal snacks. Over the next year, she lost 36 pounds.[2]

Chances are you have leptin in your bloodstream, but the leptin you have is not working right and needs a serious tune-up. Perhaps you have noticed that your appetite doesn't seem to be adjusted quite right. That was the case for Louise, a young woman who volunteered for a research study in our office. She told us how, one day it suddenly hit her how much her appetite had changed over the years. As a youngster she had a pretty normal relationship with food. She generally became hungry shortly before each meal, and the empty feeling in her stomach was promptly cured by eating. After meals, she completely forgot about food until the next mealtime drew near.

In her late teens, however, things began to change. It started when her older brother made an off-handed comment that led her to be self-conscious about her weight. She spent more and more time looking at herself in the mirror and began to read about various diets.

She bought a canned nutritional supplement that was supposed to take the place of meals, and for two weeks she had almost nothing else. Most days she ate no breakfast other than the canned drink and barely had any lunch at all. She played with her dinner, mostly avoiding it. All this left her very hungry, but she was determined to lose weight. And indeed she lost more than five pounds over a period of a few weeks.

As time went on, however, she noticed that her appetite went a little haywire, sometimes getting a bit out of control, and she regained the weight she had lost. Over the years she tried several other diets, and each one seemed to disrupt her appetite more and more, to the point where she had nearly forgotten what it was like to have a normal appetite cycle. Eventually, she abandoned diets altogether, feeling that none of them really worked very well.

As a result of all these diet disruptions, she had very little semblance of a normal appetite cycle. She never felt terribly hungry—perhaps because she always ate something before hunger really kicked in. And, oddly enough, she never felt entirely full, even after meals. Even when she had eaten more than enough at mealtime, she could still make room for dessert, and often went back to the refrigerator, looking for something to eat when she wasn't the least bit hungry. What had happened to her normal cycle of hunger and fullness? It was time to see if we could help her get back on track.

Is Your Appetite Shut-Off Switch Working?

Let's take a minute to understand leptin a bit more, and then we'll see how Louise fared. Here is what you need to know: Leptin is made by fat cells, and its name comes from the Greek *leptos,* which means "thin." When your fat cells sense that there is more than enough nourishment coming into the body they release leptin into the blood. It has two jobs: First, it travels to your brain to reduce your appetite; second, along the way it boosts your metabolism—that is, it encourages the cells of your body to burn calories more quickly. So, as you can see, it has earned its name as the "thin" hormone.

Unfortunately, dieting derails leptin. If you go on a typical low-calorie diet, your body misinterprets the diet as starvation. After all, you're not eating, so you must be starving or, at the very least, neglecting yourself. So your fat cells quickly slow down their leptin production so that your appetite can increase again. Now, a big appetite is the last thing you want, of course. But your body unleashes your appetite to bring your eating back up to what it considers normal. Within a few days of beginning a diet, leptin drops to half its previous level.[3]

It comes as no surprise, then, that your appetite can go haywire. If you intentionally cut calories, your leptin level plummets and you'll find yourself tempted by foods that would never have attracted you otherwise. If you are not careful, you could soon be bingeing out of control.

This was exactly Louise's experience. After she had been dieting for a couple of weeks her appetite control was shot. She found herself bingeing, something she had never done before.

An even more common way we interfere with leptin is to eat high-fat foods, as was graphically shown in the Pimas, an indigenous population in the southwest U.S. and Mexico. Pimas living south of the border have more or less continued their traditional diet of corn, beans, and other simple, very low-fat plant foods, and they have generally remained healthy. However, Pimas in the U.S. have had a very different experience. They have been the "beneficiaries" of federal food assistance programs, meaning that cheese, meat, and other fatty fare have invaded, followed by epidemics of obesity, diabetes, hypertension, and other health problems. Checking blood samples, researchers found that Pimas in Mexico eating a healthy, low-fat diet have retained more leptin in their blood per unit of body weight, while their northern cousins on fattier diets have lower leptin levels.

The researchers believe that the low-fat, plant-based traditional diet helps keep leptin levels up, while fatty foods suppress leptin.[4] So, rice, beans, vegetables, fruits, and anything else that is pretty close to fat-free will give you a little leptin boost, while pork loin, meatloaf, and cheese pizza are likely to reduce leptin.

Low-fat foods don't just tend to increase the amount of leptin in your blood, they also boost its ability to work. The reason is that leptin has to attach to cells and influence their inner machinery in order to do its job. Low-fat diets boost leptin's ability to do that, making each molecule of leptin work more efficiently.[5,6]

> ❧ Low-fat foods don't just tend to increase the amount of leptin in your blood, they also boost its ability to work.

Boosting Leptin

In case you are wondering how much leptin is in your blood now, your doctor can easily check it. The problem is, he or she is not likely to know what to do with the result. The amount of leptin in one's blood varies enormously from one person to the next—and from one blood draw to the next, reflecting the changes in your daily diet—and doctors are not yet sure what should be considered normal. And as we've seen, leptin's effectiveness varies, depending on how well you're cutting fat from your diet. Even so, you can go ahead and maximize leptin's appetite-cutting effect. Here's how:

First, use the Rule of Ten

While many dieters imagine they are being especially "good" when they skip a meal or eat minuscule portions, the fact is, they are shooting themselves squarely in the foot. As we have seen, when you skip a meal, or eat less than you need, your body reduces the amount of leptin in your blood and your appetite can rebound out of control.

In order to make sure you're getting enough calories to keep leptin working well, use the Rule of Ten: simply take your ideal body weight and multiply it by ten. This gives you the number of calories you must eat each day *as a minimum*. For example, if your ideal body weight is one hundred and fifty pounds, you must eat at least 1,500 calories each day. If you eat fewer calories than this you risk disabling your leptin system.

Louise said that her ideal body weight was about one hundred and thirty pounds. So that meant her calorie minimum was 1,300. Now, as I emphasized to her, she could, and almost certainly should, have more calories than this, but she should not go below this number.

If you are a somewhat bigger person and your ideal body weight is, say, two hundred pounds, what is your calorie minimum? That's right—

⇥ To keep leptin working well, use the Rule of Ten: Simply take your ideal body weight and multiply it by ten. This gives you the number of calories you must eat each day *as a minimum*.

you'll need at least 2,000 calories each day in order to keep your appetite control working normally.

Keep in mind that these are minimums. You will need more food than this, particularly if you are at all physically active.

I understand that what I have just told you contradicts what nearly every dieter has been led to believe. They are all too eager to starve themselves, but the fact is, you have to eat to keep leptin—and your appetite—under control. Cutting back drastically on calorie intake is a prescription for disaster.

Do you remember the Biosphere experiment? Four men and four women in Arizona sealed themselves for two years into a huge capsule called "Biosphere 2," to experience life in an entirely self-contained environment. As fate would have it, their food supply ran a bit short and they ended up with pretty meager fare. Well, you can imagine what happened. The average participant lost about twenty pounds and their leptin levels, of course, plummeted. When the experiment was over and they were able to return to normal eating patterns they promptly put all that weight back on within six months. But even then their ability to burn calories had not recovered. Their bodies had adapted to a low-food intake by lowering their metabolisms, and they stayed that way over the long run.[7] The moral of the story is clear: If you cut back on calories in an effort to lose weight you'll impair your leptin system and slow down your metabolism for the long haul.

Don't do it. Use the Rule of Ten to keep your leptin level up, your appetite down, and your calorie-burning machinery running smoothly.

Second, use low-fat foods to boost leptin's power

You may not live with Pimas in the remote mountainous regions of Mexico, but there is no reason you can't make your leptin work as well as theirs does. If you were looking for yet another reason to steer clear of greasy burgers, salmon cakes, and french fries, preserving leptin's appetite-controlling effect is an important one. Chapter 13 shows how to cut the fat and boost the foods that keep leptin going strong.

You'll find ways to boost leptin with almost everything you eat. When you have a salad, you'll do better with the low-fat dressing than the regular variety, and better still with the fat-free balsamic vinaigrette or a drizzle of lemon juice. When you're thinking about soup, minestrone will reward you much more than clam chowder, because it is much lower in fat. And a chunky vegetable chili or bean chili will do you better than chili con carne. If you top your pasta with a light marinara instead of alfredo sauce you're building your advantage even more, and if your dessert is fresh fruit instead of cheesecake, you score again. All these foods trim away fat, allowing leptin to work more effectively.

Third, exercise makes your body respond better to leptin

In a Harvard study of 268 health professionals, men who exercised regularly had dramatically increased leptin sensitivity.[8] What this means is that exercise makes whatever leptin you have work that much more strongly.

Now, before you go out to buy a new sweat suit and jogging shoes, I should tell you that you do not need to run a marathon. A half-hour brisk walk or jog each day is about all you need. It has marked effect on leptin. Chapter 10 will get you started.

The cells of your body are happy to produce leptin for you all day long. In turn, it takes the edge off your appetite and gives your metabolism a boost. To keep leptin working its best, the keys are to use the Rule of Ten to spare you from low-calorie diets, go low-fat, and bring regular physical activity into your routine. Your body will do the rest.

As you can see, this is remarkably easy to do—and that was certainly Louise's experience. She had already sworn off very low-calorie diets. And with a little menu advice she found it easy to cut the fat from her diet. She brought in exercise gradually, and quite enjoyed it. She not only lost weight in a healthy way, she was able to keep it off. And, unlike every diet experience she had ever had, she actually felt healthy and balanced, able to re-experience the normal feelings of hunger and fullness and regaining control over her appetite.

As you do this let me encourage you to be patient with yourself. If your appetite control has been severely disrupted it will take a little time to get it back—but you will.

It is odd to imagine that the first rule for weight loss is to avoid dieting—that is, avoid old-fashioned calorie-counting diets—but that is clearly the soundest advice. You'll be much more in charge of your appetite day after day. In the next chapter we'll take a look at times when cravings tend to fly out of control, and how to predict those times and knock them out.

9

Step 4: Break Craving Cycles

Seductions occur on a cycle. Passionate tangos start late at night, not at 9 A.M., and fireside cuddles happen in January, not August. Food cravings have their cycles, too. Some hit every twenty-four hours or so, usually in the evening. Others, especially chocolate cravings, arrive on a monthly hormonal cycle. There are powerful yearly cycles, too. The keys for breaking out of these patterns may surprise you. Willpower plays virtually no role at all, while timing and biology matter a lot. Let's start with a look at the daily binge.

Breaking Out of a Daily Cycle

Eric was a forty-five-year-old man whose weight had gradually inched upward over the past fifteen years or so. His mother was Korean and had been quite slim all her life. However, Eric took after Dad, who was from Wisconsin and had a classic "apple" shape, with a fair amount of extra weight around his middle, most of which came on in midlife. Eric had been quite athletic as a teenager, participating in baseball and track, and had no problem burning up whatever he ate until he hit about thirty. Since then, his midsection had gradually expanded over and beyond his belt. He came to our offices for help.

I asked about his current diet, and he described a fairly normal Midwestern menu. I then asked him to note down everything he ate—and when he ate it—for the next three days, using a food scale and the diet record form you'll see in chapter 14. A few days later he came back to the office with the form dutifully filled out.

Looking at his diet record, there were clearly some ways to improve what he was eating. But what was even more noticeable was *when* he ate. In fact, his eating schedule was a classic pattern seen in people battling weight problems: everything was shifted toward evening. He ate surprisingly little in the morning, and considerably *more* later in the day. People who maintain healthy weight tend to space their meals out fairly evenly throughout the day, but overweight people very often skew everything toward nighttime.[1]

I asked Eric about this pattern. He took a deep breath and said, "Well, I knew it. I didn't want to admit it, but—well, I'm fine during the day. You'd be proud of me; I eat almost nothing." He took another deep breath. "At night it's a different story. It seems like I basically have no control." The truth is, he was actually not a lot different from other people, but he then proceeded to beat himself up with a protracted dietary confession.

He called himself a foodaholic. He got home from work about 6:30 and nibbled on cheese as he made dinner. By the time his meal was ready, he had already gone through so much cheese that he had almost no appetite left—but he ate his normal dinner anyway. Afterward he ate various snacks, including chocolate ice cream, a rolled-up piece of bologna, or a bowl of cereal. But it was always in the evening. He ate very little breakfast and had no great excesses during the day at work. But as soon as he arrived home the binge seemed to kick in. It made no difference how full he was from dinner. The evening hours called him back to the refrigerator. He found himself inventing reasons to go to the store—he needed a lightbulb or a newspaper or some tape—when what he was really there for was a chocolate bar, some potato chips, or a soda. As he gained weight over the years, he saw no way out of the habits that seemed to have him locked in.

Many people fall into similar patterns. Evening is the most frequent binge time. But some people are hit by the bagel tray or candy machine as soon as they arrive at work. For others, it's a late-morning snack to knock out the hunger caused by an overly rushed breakfast. Some people lapse into binges in the midafternoon.

Maybe something like this has happened to you. You get home and have a reasonable dinner, but then you want something sweet. And, a bit later on, you want another snack that you know you don't really need. The next day the same thing happens again . . . and the next day, and the next. And eventually you start to *plan* for a binge, one that arrives predictably, day after day.

These habits are not cued by hunger, but by *time* and by our surroundings. In large measure, they are learned in the same way that walking into a movie theater triggers a desire for popcorn, or that early morning makes you want a glass of orange juice.

Breaking Your Schedule

As Eric told his story, he looked at me as if I were a priest taking confession. But, as I told him, it pays to set aside guilt. Instead, we aimed to look at his problem as a *physical* cycle repeating on a biological clock.

We first looked at having a more ample breakfast and keeping his blood sugar stable during the day, as you've seen in the previous chapters. But we went a step further, focusing not on the food, but on *time.*

I asked Eric to break up his evening schedule every night for three weeks to the extent he could, and we plotted out a plan to do that. First, he aimed to get home a bit earlier each day, so he wasn't so hungry. He was then going to change his clothes and leave the house. He might go for a jog with a friend and then to dinner at an inexpensive restaurant. Or he could go to a bookstore or lecture. The idea was just to break the routine, get him out of the rut he was in, limit the time he had at home, and focus his attention on something other than the refrigerator.

When he knew he would be eating at home, he prepared dinner in advance, so that it would require only a quick reheating, and he made sure to go to bed at a reasonable hour, rather than staying up watching television. He also cleared the contraband out of his refrigerator and took advantage of the other tips you'll read about in chapter 14 and elsewhere in this book.

Eric found what most other people find: breaking a habit can be a very quick process. In a few weeks, a new habit can solidly displace an old one, and he found he quite easily drifted away from his old routine. His thoughts about cheese and other snacks didn't entirely disappear during this time, but they were toned down and were replaced by something that he wanted more: As he lost weight he felt more and more fit, and he even developed a taste for healthier foods. He very much liked the way he felt.

After three weeks he stopped planning so many evening activities but still found it fairly easy to stay on his new, healthier path. The bad news, as he discovered several weeks later, is that the rut you were in waits patiently for your return. It is perilously easy to slip back in. This is especially true if the habit you've fallen into also involves drinking, since alcohol dissolves willpower. In Eric's case, though, if he did find himself sliding back into Snackville, he simply broke his schedule up again and made sure that he had plenty of healthy things on hand ready to eat. It also helped him to remember why he was doing this. He taped a hand-written note to his refrigerator that read, "Losing fifty pounds will taste so much better than junk food."

In fact, over time he actually did lose a bit more than fifty pounds, and the key, he felt, was being able to break his craving cycle. Here are tips for breaking out of your own:

- First, be sure to eat a healthy breakfast, make sure your meals are keeping your blood sugar steady—and eat an adequate *amount* of food, especially early in the day, using the guidelines in the previous chapters.

- Change the people and places in your life that tend to trigger your binges. If you're alone, arrange to be with someone else at the time binges would normally arrive. It doesn't have to be a close relationship—being at a lecture, a library, a religious service, or even walking on a busy street still counts. If binges hit you at home, be somewhere—anywhere—else.

- Break your schedule. You need a new pattern, not just with food, but with *time*. If you stay in the same schedule, your internal clock will wake up cravings, right on schedule. It does not matter how firm your resolve is at other times of day. You have to break out of your time of vulnerability.

- Plan for competing activities.

- Go to bed an hour earlier. Fatigue fuels cravings. Rest shores up resolve. And get regular exercise, so you sleep soundly and wake refreshed. More on this in chapter 10.

- Don't seduce *yourself*. If you're leaving little presents of the very foods you'd like to get away from lying around in your cupboards, that's a sign that you have not made up your mind for a change.

As you've seen, the main focus is not on food, but on *time*. If you plan for your time of vulnerability and break up the cues that lead to bingeing, you've got the best possible control over the problem.

Monthly Cycles and Hormone Swings

If you are a young woman in the week before your period, cravings can go through the ceiling. You have probably heard the common observation that women seem to love chocolate more than men do. Well, it is entirely explained by the amount of chocolate they consume in that week alone.

Those cravings aren't always so helpful, needless to say. Every chocolate bar that floats into your life brings another 200 calories that leap out as soon as you tear open the wrapper. Once in a while you can get away with it. But if it's a couple of chocolate hits a day, and it lasts a week or more out of every single month, you're talking serious calories.

The culprit in all of this is estrogen, the female sex hormone.* Men have a little estrogen, but not very much. Women prior to the age of menopause have quite a lot of it, and what seems to cause premenstrual cravings is a sudden drop in the amount of estrogen coursing through your bloodstream.

Let me give you the details at the risk of being slightly technical:

---

*The term *estrogen* actually refers to a group of related compounds, including estradiol, estrone, and others. For simplicity, I will refer to them all as *estrogen*.

During the first week or so after your last period has ended, your body starts making extra estrogen to prepare anew for the possibility that you might become pregnant. It starts to make a fresh inner lining of your uterus, just in case a tiny new baby might come drifting down a fallopian tube.

But pretty soon your body senses that you did not get pregnant this month after all. So, during the week before your period the amount of estrogen in your bloodstream quickly falls, the lining of the uterus is shed in menstrual flow, and the whole process starts over again the next month. Now, in that last week of your cycle, this sudden drop of estrogen triggers all manner of symptoms. You might feel bloated, your mood can change, and, of course, chocolate will sing out to you in a way unlike that at any other time of the month. You don't *want* it, you *need* it.

Using Foods To Control Estrogen

You can tame estrogen with rather simple diet changes, as my colleagues and I demonstrated in a recent research study.

One of our research participants, Valerie, joined the study because she had terrible PMS and menstrual cramps every single month. In the week before her period her mood went south, and food cravings flooded in. And as her period was about to start, cramps kicked in so badly that she needed heroic doses of ibuprofen just to get through the day at work. She had put up with these symptoms ever since adolescence, but they seemed to worsen in her late twenties.

Previous researchers had found that women who follow very low-fat diets have much lower levels of estrogen in their blood, compared to women who eat fattier foods. This observation was important because it explained, at least partly, why breast cancer is very rare in countries such as Japan, where diets are much lower in fat. In countries where fattier foods are the order of the day, women have higher levels of estrogen in their blood, and, in turn, that means a higher risk of cancer. Of course there are other contributors to cancer, but the fat-estrogen connection has intrigued researchers looking for ways to prevent it.

The key point here is that trimming the fat from our diets can reduce estrogen. I reasoned that we could use this fact not just to

➔❙ If we keep fat intake low, estrogen stays at a more modest level throughout the month. It won't ever climb too high—and there will be no big drop at the end of the month. That helps tame PMS, cramps—and cravings.

reduce cancer risk, but also to reduce the menstrual symptoms that hit every single month. That is, if we keep fat intake low, so that estrogen remains at a more modest level throughout the month, it won't ever climb too high and there will be no big drop at the end of the month. We ought to be able to reduce PMS, cramps—and cravings.

Thirty-three women joined our study investigating what diet could do for menstrual symptoms. In order to really reduce fat we eliminated animal products entirely, which, of course, eliminates all animal fat. We also asked participants to keep vegetable oils to an absolute minimum. The diet took a little getting used to, but within a week or two everyone found recipes they liked and had figured out what to order at restaurants.

Valerie was not especially hopeful that the diet would work, but medication didn't seem a good enough answer, and it didn't do a thing for her mood or her cravings. In the study she didn't have to count calories or fat grams, but she did have to choose lighter options: pasta marinara instead of meat sauce, a hummus sandwich instead of grilled cheese, bean chili instead of meat chili, and grilled vegetables instead of french fries. Her diet records showed that her fat intake dropped to about 10 percent of her calories, or about 20 fat grams per day, while her fiber intake shot up to about 50 grams.

Even though there was no limit on portions, she lost about ten pounds over the eight-week study.

But what really counted was the change in how she felt. As her period approached she had no mood changes at all, virtually no noticeable cravings, and, as she put it later, her period "just sort of sneaked up on me. Instead of my usual, really bad cramps on the first day, it just happened, with basically no pain at all."

The change was dramatic for many other participants, too. We reported our results in the journal *Obstetrics & Gynecology* in 2000.[2] The average duration of menstrual cramps dropped from four days to about two and a half. PMS symptoms, like water retention, bloating, and difficulty concentrating, improved—and many participants reported that cravings dropped, too.

That drop in cravings can be a wonderful gift. If you have felt like biology has simply taken over and you are powerless to control what you eat, you'll find that you really can tame hormone-driven cravings to a great degree.

Using Foods to Block Hormone Swings

There are actually two ways diet influences how much estrogen is in your blood. First, as we've seen, fat increases the amount of estrogen your body produces. When you cut the excess fat from your diet more or less completely, the amount of estrogen in your blood stays at a lower level all month long. And since it is apparently the sudden estrogen plunges from peaks to valleys that trigger cravings and other PMS symptoms, smoothing out the terrain makes a big difference.

Second, fiber helps reduce estrogen, too. Here's how: Your liver filters your blood every minute of the day. As it does so, it not only removes waste products, toxins of various kinds, and whatever else

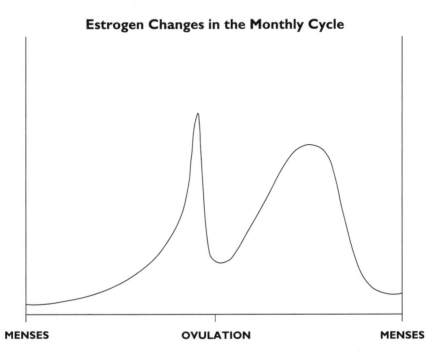

Estrogen Changes in the Monthly Cycle

MENSES   OVULATION   MENSES

might be floating along in your bloodstream, it also removes excess estrogens, sending them through a tiny tube, called the bile duct, into the intestinal tract. There, fiber soaks up this waste estrogen, just like a sponge soaking up water, and carries it out of the body.

If you have plenty of fiber in your diet, this estrogen-disposal system works pretty well. But, as you know by now, meats, dairy products, and eggs have no fiber at all. If you had eggs and bacon for breakfast, and yogurt and chicken breast for lunch, your body does not have enough fiber to do the job. So, the estrogen that your liver has carefully removed from your blood and sent into your intestinal tract actually ends up passing *back into your bloodstream*. The answer is to bring the vegetables, fruits, beans, and grains into your diet so their fiber can trap estrogen in the digestive tract and carry it away with the wastes.

The effect of a low-fat, plant-based diet is really quite profound, cutting estrogen levels nearly in half within a few weeks. There is still more than enough estrogen for fertility and for a normal cycle, but not so much so as to cause problems.

But getting this benefit requires making changes in your diet. Our research participants reported that the benefits of a low-fat, vegan diet were partially lost if they brought cheese or fried foods back onto the menu even occasionally. It also does not work if you change your diet for just the last week or so before your period. You have to follow the low-fat diet throughout the whole month. The idea is to stop estrogen from rising too high early in the month, so that it doesn't have so far to fall at the end of the month.

To try this, follow these steps:

- Begin the diet change on the first day of your monthly cycle (the first day of your period) and follow these guidelines through the entire month.

- Eliminate animal products and added vegetable oils. Use the recipes in this book, choosing those with the least fat.

- Be sure to go high-fiber, using the Quick Fiber Check on page 88 to help you.

- During the last week of the month pay attention to your cravings, PMS symptoms, and cramps. You will likely notice the benefits in the very first month, and you may also find that the effects become more and more pronounced with each new cycle.

You'll also probably lose weight. Valerie did—more than a pound per week—and that can be a big motivator for sticking with it.

Breaking Annual Cycles

Many people are locked into a yearly cycle. You'll start to notice it in the fall. Under the influence of holiday parties and cooler weather your appetite control begins to erode. You might feel a bit like a squirrel filling your cheeks for the cold days ahead.

Researchers at the National Institutes of Health in Bethesda, Maryland, nailed down the pattern exactly. They put 195 people on the scale at intervals throughout the year and found that *virtually all the weight people gain over the year occurs in the second half, especially from October through December.* As summer draws to a close our appetites increase and our weight ratchets upward.

Suddenly, at the stroke of midnight on New Year's Eve, we resolve to stop all this reveling and get back into shape. During the next few months we diet, start exercising, and manage to lose a little bit of the weight we've gained. Unfortunately, the overall trend is steadily upward. The NIH researchers found that the average person gained 1.7 pounds as the year drew to a close, and lost 0.2 pounds in the spring, for an annual increase of about a pound and a half. And when fall arrives again, the whole cycle starts over.[3]

This had happened to Eric, the man we met at the beginning of this chapter. He had a daily cycle that we helped him break, as we saw earlier. But he had a yearly cycle, too. It did not seem to relate much to parties, and he didn't actually start any new bad habits. It just seemed that his appetite was stronger in the fall. His portions always grew, and he found himself driven to back for seconds. "Every fall I start to notice that my clothes feel tighter," he said. "I can see my appetite is bigger." As the years went by, his weight gain was clearly strongest in the autumn and early winter.

The good news is that, if you can beat the autumnal weight gain, you've more or less got the whole year licked. So, what should you do?

Nearly All That Weight Adds On at Holiday Time*

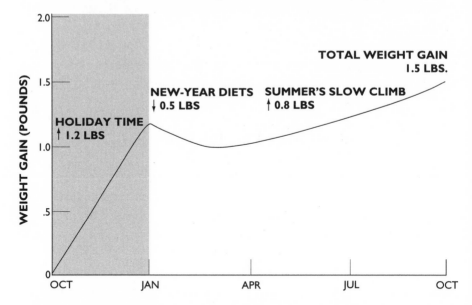

*Based on Vanovski JA, Vanovski SZ, Sovik KN, Nguyen TT, O'Neil PM, Sebring NG. A prospective study of holiday weight gain. *N Engl J Med* 2000;342:861–7.

First of all, don't slack off when it comes to exercise. Cooler weather often means that we're indoors, perilously close to the refrigerator, and far from bike trails, golf courses, the beach, or anywhere else where we might get a bit of physical activity. In the NIH study, *those who were the most physically active in the fall were least likely to gain weight.* This does not mean you have to sweat off the pounds; exercise also works simply by getting you away from food.

It also helps to be aware that holiday weight gain is essentially *permanent,* which puts snack trays in a whole different light. That cheese-on-a-toothpick or butter cookie is going to become part of you essentially forever. Maintaining normal eating habits during the holidays blocks that end-of-year weight spike. And if you actually improve your eating habits you can bend your weight graph into a whole new shape.

In a recent research study, we put a group of women on a low-fat, vegan diet in early January, when they were strongly motivated to knock off the pounds they had gained earlier. Needless to say, they lost weight in the ensuing months—about a pound per week over the first three months or so. But what was even more impressive was that those who stuck with the diet after this study period and through the follow-

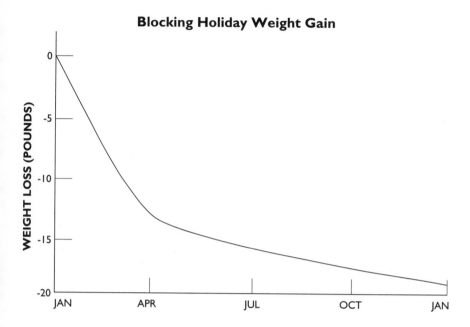

ing holiday season were *completely protected* from holiday weight gain. In fact, they continued to lose weight through the fall and into the following year.

Eric followed the diet recommendations you'll read about in chapter 13. He did not rush to take the weight off, and he had one fairly major slip while on vacation, and regained a few pounds. But he resolved not to let that happen again and, in fact, did not. As I mentioned above, he kept more than fifty pounds off with virtually no difficulty. He had beaten not only his daily cycle but his yearly one, too.

How to Beat Seasonal Depression

Winter brings another craving booster. As the days become shorter and shorter, low light levels can trigger depression, along with cravings that are muted during the warmer times of year. It is called Seasonal Affec-

 Those who stuck with the diet through the holiday season were *completely protected* from holiday weight gain.

tive Disorder (SAD), or winter depression. At the same time, you'll lose your normal energy and will have trouble getting out of bed. The pattern of increased appetite and increased sleep is different from what can happen in more typical cases of depression, in which people lose their appetites and suffer with insomnia. Seasonal depression hits most frequently in young women living at northern latitudes.

When the cravings hit you won't start looking for pickles or Belgian endive. What you'll crave are sweet or starchy foods. The reason is that high-carbohydrate foods naturally cause the brain to produce serotonin, a mood-controlling neurotransmitter, as we saw in chapter 2. This is the same brain chemical that is elevated by Prozac, Zoloft, and other common antidepressants. So, although some people feel more on edge with sugary or starchy foods, people with winter depression find that these foods cause a natural mood boost and make them feel better.

Now, there is nothing wrong with using foods to cope with winter blues. But you'll want to be careful about which ones you choose. Cookies, cakes, and chocolate contain plenty of carbohydrate (which is not likely to cause much weight gain all by itself), but they also have enough butter, shortening, or other fats to add a lot of calories. In contrast, whole-grain bread, brown rice or rice cakes, pasta, and fruit provide healthful carbohydrate, which increases your natural serotonin production with very little fat—as long as you don't add it in the kitchen.

If you suffer from this problem there is another treatment you should be aware of. Winter depression—and the overeating that comes along with it—responds beautifully to daylight, especially if you can get a generous amount of it early in the morning. One of our study participants, Jean, tended to really dig into cookies and starchy foods during the late fall and winter months. Come spring, she could not lose the pounds she had gained during the preceding months, and her weight ratcheted up higher and higher. I suggested that she try a simple form of "light treatment," by taking a twenty-minute walk outdoors in the first morning light. This step alone cut her cravings dramatically and boosted her mood and energy level, in addition to burning off a few extra calories.

For more refractory cases, psychiatrists use special lights that provide what nature has neglected. Used daily, they set a new light cycle and gently bring mood, sleep, and appetite back to normal. Some lamp models can be set to a timer, gradually waking you in the morning and setting a healthy diurnal cycle. Although they are quite safe, they should be used under the supervision of an experienced psychiatrist, because light treatments at the wrong time of day can actually reset your biological clock in the wrong direction and worsen insomnia.

So, if you find yourself in an annual cycle of autumn weight gain that you can't quite lose in the spring, you'll want to follow these recommendations:

- Focus first on the type of food you eat, in order to insulate yourself from the foods that cause the problem. Low-fat, fiber-rich, vegan foods always are best for weight loss. Check the recipe section for plenty of healthy choices.

- Be sure to maintain your exercise routine, despite cooler weather and holiday schedules.

- If you're using sweet or starchy foods to cope with winter blues, you'll want to be very careful about their fat content.

- If you suspect winter depression, by all means consult a specialist, who may recommend light treatments or other therapies that can knock out the mood and appetite problems.

Getting Off the Merry-Go-Round

If a daily binge cycle has you in its grip, you'll want to use all the other steps in part II, but break up your schedule, too. If you're on a monthly cycle, you'll want to use foods to tame hormone ups-and-downs. And, if the problem is a yearly ratcheting up of your weight as your appetite grows in the fall and winter, you can tackle the problem by focusing mainly on the *type* of food you're eating, rather than the amount, by staying active, and by looking for signs of winter depression.

We have seen many, many people from all walks of life who feel absolutely stuck in a self-defeating cycle, and yet they easily get on the path to breaking free. You can, too.

10

Step 5: Exercise and Rest

Okay, so work or family obligations have got you completely stressed out. You're not sleeping well. You wake up tired, and drag through the day. And you haven't had any sort of physical activity in about as long as you can remember.

Now, what if someone offers you something absolutely delectable to eat? It is solid calories, loaded with fat and cholesterol, with absolutely no nutritionally redeeming value. What do you do? Well, needless to say, you jump right in. Your resistance is shot. Your ability to say no to temptation is long gone.

When you are aiming to start on a healthy path, exercise, rest, and sleep can make all the difference. When you're feeling fit and well-rested you are much more resilient in the face of temptation.

So, if you've lost track of what it means to be physically fit, if stress has you in its grip, or if you can't remember the last time you had a good night's sleep, let's fix things.

A New Way of Thinking About Exercise

First, let's erase everything you ever thought about exercise. Whether your image of exercise is slogging down the roadway at 6 A.M., sweating through one weight machine routine after another, pumping free weights, or self-consciously donning a fancy outfit for an aerobics class in search of a svelte physique, let's set all that aside for the moment. Yes, exercise burns calories. But there is a whole other side of exercise that is far more important. It might actually surprise you how few calories exercise actually burns. Next time you're at a gym, jump on the treadmill and run flat-out for a mile, or as close to it as you can. Then, as you catch your breath and mop your sweaty brow, push the little button that tells you how many calories you've burned. You'll discover it's all of about 100. There are more calories than that in just half a small order of McDonald's french fries, or thirty M&Ms, or half a 20-ounce bottle of Coke. In a few minutes of eating, you can take in all the calories you've burned, and then some.

The point is this: Exercise does indeed burn calories, but your body is so efficient at conserving energy that the calorie burn is actually pretty modest in any given workout. To get exercise's calorie-burning advantage, it has to be a regular part of your life, so that it adds up to something that really counts. And it has to be done *with* major changes in what you eat, not instead of them.

But exercise is not just a way to burn calories, it is much more than that. Exercise is like a giant reset button on your body. When you have a good workout several vitally important things happen: it blocks appetite swings, it resets your mood and your exercise-rest cycle so you can sleep properly—which strengthens you against cravings; and it puts you in a different relationship with your body.

If you're new to exercise, the first thing you'll discover is a curious effect on appetite. You'll find that you have much less desire to stuff yourself with food. Exercise demagnetizes your refrigerator. Although your body will naturally seek to replenish the energy it has used, exercise has a powerful antibinge effect. Partly, this is because, as we saw in chapter 8, exercise makes your body more sensitive to leptin's appetite-taming effect. But it also tires your muscles just enough to block the fidgetiness and restlessness that lead you to the refrigerator.

Exercise lifts moods. After a good workout, your body feels like more than a number on a scale. You can feel the work your muscles have done, the air in your lungs, and the heat in your skin. You feel better than you do on sedentary days. You are much more motivated to stick with healthier habits. You feel calmer and more resolved. And, of course, if your workout was vigorous enough, you'll get a bit of the natural endorphin effect that dissolves pain and anxiety and, at its extreme, brings on the "runner's high."

Exercise is also a powerful sleep aid. If your muscles are tired, they push you to sleep so they can get their overnight repair work done. If you are sedentary, your sleep will be more fitful.

Exercise also has another effect: it shows you your future. After a brisk walk, if you feel a bit of fatigue and you need to rest, well, this is how in the not-so-distant future you will feel *all the time.* You have just glimpsed your old age. If, however, you increase your stamina so that, after walking a longer distance or working out for a longer time, you feel energized rather than fatigued, then this is how you can expect to feel as the years go by.

But don't think the benefits of exercise are all in your head. Exercise tunes up your body from top to bottom.

Researchers at Laval University in Quebec found that just three weeks of exercise improved insulin sensitivity dramatically. This is important. In case you've forgotten what we covered in chapter 7, sometimes insulin falls down on the job of moving sugar from the bloodstream into your cells. When that happens, your body produces larger amounts of insulin in an effort to move sugar to where it belongs, and, in turn, that ever-larger amount of insulin seems to interfere with weight loss. But the good news is that exercise helps cure the problem. The Quebec researchers found that, after three weeks of exercise, peak after-meal insulin levels dropped by more than 20 percent.[1] Any kind of aerobic exercise does the job, whether it's walking, biking, running, dancing, an aerobics class, or any other.

So exercise does not just burn calories, it resets your appetite, your mood, your sleep cycle, and even your ability to handle sugars. So, how do we begin? We begin slowly. And we'll add big doses of fun and company. Let me show you what I mean:

Be Patient with Yourself

Start slow. This is not the Olympics. We are beginning a path that leads to health. If you have been sedentary for some time, are over forty, have gained a few extra pounds, or have any health condition, you are not ready for a vigorous workout.

See your doctor before you increase your physical activity. Your doctor will be especially interested in two things: your heart and your joints. Pushing too fast with an overly strenuous exercise program can spell disaster. Take it slow, and gradually increase your activity.

Having said that, don't be a wimp either. Sauntering along a park path can be delightful, but your body does not recognize it as exercise. So long as your doctor has given you the go-ahead to get your heart pumping, make sure you are quickening your pulse a bit.

A good starting point for most people is a half-hour walk per day, or, if it works better for your schedule, go three times a week for an hour. If your doctor has advised shorter walks than this, follow his or her advice. And to be sure it happens—put it on your schedule, just as you would a doctor's appointment, and don't let it slide.

From there you can increase your time and your vigor, and you can add other activities: biking, rollerblading, dancing, tennis, running, or whatever calls to you.

Make It Fun

If exercise machines seem like torture devices to you, go for a walk instead. Or join an aerobics class. You'll find them for all ages and all levels of ability. If it's fun, you'll stick with it.

One of our research volunteers, Brenda, has arthritis, and finds that swimming is exactly her cup of tea. In a water aerobics class, she stretches, then does a series of exercises with gradually increasing intensity. For the rest of the day she feels invigorated and more limber, with less pain in her joints.

> ⇥ Exercise does not just burn calories, it resets your appetite, your mood, your sleep cycle, and even your ability to handle sugars.

It might interest you to know that you don't have to do your exercise all in one bout. In a recent study, a research team asked a group of people to exercise for forty minutes a day. But they asked half of them to do it in one continuous bout and others to do it in ten-minute sessions four times a day, using a home treadmill. The people doing the shorter sessions lost weight just as well as those who did the single long exercise bout.[2] You can do much the same thing, either with a treadmill, as the research team used, or with a quick walk before work, at lunch, after work, and in the evening. It almost feels like you're not exercising at all, but your muscles know the difference. The key, though, is to schedule it and stick with it, so you don't keep pushing it aside. So exercise when you want and in the way you want.

Do it with Other People

You're not the Lone Ranger. Exercise with someone else. Not only do our friends distract us from whatever complaints our muscles may make, they also keep us from canceling our exercise sessions. It's easy to skip a daily walk if you're by yourself. But, if your exercise buddy is arriving in an hour you're going to do it. Two of our research participants made a pact to support each other as they exercised, but they lived nowhere near each other. So, the one on her stationary bicycle telephoned the other who was on her treadmill. Even over the telephone wire they could keep their resolve, support each other, and make the time go faster.

Letting Stress Go

When we're stressed by depression, loneliness, anger, or boredom, food offers quick and easy solace. In chapter 11 we will look at ways to shore up friendships and family relationships, which are—or should be—our number-one stress fighters. But there are other easy de-stressors anyone can use. Here are some you might try:

To relax your mind, start with your muscles. *Progressive relaxation* relaxes the muscles in a specific sequence, and when your body is relaxed your mind follows suit. These techniques are quick and easy and you can do them at any time—at work, at home, and even on the subway or bus. You'll feel more in charge of emotions and less likely to turn to the refrigerator for comfort. Many people prefer to do relaxation techniques in the morning before work and in the evening before dinner. Or you might use them after exercise, when your muscles are a bit tired.

Here's a simple, five-minute technique: Sit comfortably and close your eyes, if you can. (However, this method still works if you are seated at the head table of a thousand-seat banquet and can't close your eyes.) Focus your attention on your breathing and intentionally slow it down, like that of a person sleeping. Notice how air entering your nose makes a cooling sensation. Now, imagine that, as this cool air flows in, it gathers up your stress and carries it away as you exhale. As you breathe in, imagine the air flowing into your nose and up around your cheeks and forehead, carrying a cooling feeling throughout your face. As you breathe out the air carries away all the stress in the muscles of your face. Imagine the air actually touching each of these areas and carrying away stress, like lapping waves gently washing away sticks and pebbles.

Now, work your way down your body, a bit at a time. Breathe in and imagine the air flowing to the sides and back of your head. As you exhale, tension in these areas passes out, too. Breathe in again and imagine the cooling air relaxing your neck muscles. As you exhale, out goes the tension. Now imagine a breath of air passing to your shoulders, and, in turn, carrying tension away. Breathe slowly and calmly. Focus, in turn, on your upper arms, lower arms, and hands, and then your chest, abdomen, buttocks, thighs, calves, and feet. When you've finished, sit quietly for a minute or two before getting up. You'll notice a profound sense of relaxation that deepens each time you do it. The whole exercise can take just a few minutes, or longer, if you prefer.

A variation on this technique is to momentarily tighten each muscle group and then let it relax. This is especially useful for people with chronic tension, who have trouble spotting where their muscular tightness is. Just follow the same sequence, starting at the head. You'll gently tighten the muscles of your forehead, then let the tension go. Then do the same with your cheeks and jaw, then your neck, your shoulders, and so on. Just tighten them for an instant before letting all that tension go.

Andrew Weil, M.D., taught me what must be the fastest and easiest stress-reducing exercise ever devised. It is deceptively simple, but it really does work—apparently because it focuses your attention and slows down your breathing, causing a relaxation response as a reaction. Start by placing the tip of your tongue on the roof of your mouth, on the slight ridge about a half-inch behind your front teeth. Leave your tongue there through the entire exercise. Breathe in through your nose to a count of four. Then hold your breath for seven counts. Open your mouth slightly and exhale to a count of eight, letting your breath make a whooshing sound past your tongue and teeth.

Do this exercise four times at whatever pace is comfortable for you. You can do it anywhere—driving, walking, waiting for a meeting to start, or whenever—as many times a day as you like. You'll notice it takes the edge off your anxiety.

There are many other very easy stress-reducing techniques. Exercise, yoga, or meditation in the morning and evening can work wonders for restoring your equilibrium. For details, let me refer you to my previous book, *Foods That Fight Pain,* which applies these techniques, along with diet changes, to headaches and other day-to-day symptoms. You'll find they work beautifully for the anxieties that encourage cravings.

Getting a Good Night's Sleep

When it comes to beating stress, there's nothing like a good night's sleep. Unfortunately, many people don't get the rest they need. Mike was a fifty-six-year-old accountant who was gradually losing the battle of the bulge. He never slept well, and every morning he dragged into the office feeling more or less miserable. He drank a fair amount of coffee to get his brain in gear for the day. Unfortunately, morning coffee led to a midafternoon slump, which brought him back to the coffee pot. And the caffeine was not entirely out of his bloodstream by bedtime, so it ended up aggravating his sleep problems.

Chronically exhausted, he found his ability to resist junk food was nil. His main goal in life was just to get through the day, and even though snack trays or fatty lunches with clients ought to have set off his internal alarm bells, he found he just couldn't awaken that part of himself that was able to say no to these indulgences.

If you've gone through a patch of being unable to sleep well for days on end, you know it makes life feel as if it's not worth living. You have little interest in much of anything, much less sticking to any kind of diet. But it is indeed possible to turn things around. Here are the keys to a good night's sleep:

Steps That Help You Sleep:

- *Physical activity.* Sleep is not just for your mind—sleep is nature's way of resting your body, too. If your muscles are not tired because you are getting no exercise during the day, there is less physiological reason for sleep. So you'll want to tire your muscles a bit to trigger the sleep response. Go out for an evening walk, or use a stepper or treadmill at home. Or try exercises specifically aimed at large muscle groups, such as push-ups or squats. Once you feel the fatigue in your muscles, you'll know you are almost certain to sleep better.

- *Stretch and yawn.* Children stretch and yawn as their day draws to a close. While most of us think of these signs of tiredness as having no physical function, it is worth noticing that they help ready the body for sleep. Most animals, of course, do exactly the same thing as they prepare for slumber. Cats and dogs stretch out their legs and make a big yawn. When I was a medical student, my pet rat—a refugee from a laboratory—used to stick out her little white leg with a big yawn and then curl up to sleep.

  Many adults no longer go through these sleep preliminaries, either because they are not *physically* tired or because alcohol or caffeine has disrupted their normal physical rhythms. But if you intentionally bring them back you'll find you sleep better. Here's how: About a half hour before you go to bed, stretch out your arms the way you did as a child, and open your mouth to simulate a yawn. At first, you're just going through the motions, but you'll soon end up triggering a genuine deep muscle stretch and yawn. Do this four times before you go to bed and you'll notice a definite effect on sleep.

- *Nap during the day if you need to.* Many people imagine that daytime naps interfere with sleep. But scientists have studied this question, and just the opposite turns out to be true. People who nap during the day tend to be a bit less wired at bed-time and have an easier time sleeping.

- *Win the lottery.* Like it or not, worries intrude on sleep. Whether they relate to finances, family matters, job responsi-bilities, or personal problems, you're going to have continuing challenges with your sleep until the situation is resolved. So, while you're waiting for lottery winnings to escort you to some sunny, carefree spot, you'll want to do the best you can to follow the other tips listed here.

Things That Interfere with Sleep:

- *Caffeine.* Everyone knows that caffeine can disturb sleep, but what they may not realize is how persistent it actually is. Caf-feine is part of our national biochemistry—the average Amer-ican has two milligrams of it circulating in every liter of his or her blood plasma at any given time. And while a morning cup of coffee wakes us up and gets us going, coffee drinkers can also get irritable, sometimes so subtly they may be the last to notice. That cup of joe also worsens premenstrual symptoms. Unfortunately, many coffee drinkers find that their daily caf-feine habit does nothing more than cure their withdrawal after the previous day's hit.

    Caffeine should not be a source of worry if it is causing no problems. But if you're not sleeping well, be aware that the half-life of caffeine is about six hours, which means that, if you have a cup of coffee at 6 p.m., fully half its caffeine is still in your bloodstream at midnight. A quarter of it is still circu-lating in your body at 6 the next morning.

    Luckily, when you aim to set it aside, caffeine does not put up much of a fight. Decaffeinated coffees, teas, and colas are widely available and much more palatable than in years past. A gradual transition minimizes any withdrawal. Within a cou-ple of caffeine-free days, you'll be back to your old self. The biggest problem with breaking a caffeine habit is that you'll lose the drug that has kept you alert and feeling well in the face of the stresses of daily life. When caffeine is gone, you'll find that regular exercise and an adequate night's sleep make you feel more like yourself.

- *Alcohol.* Think alcohol makes you sleep soundly? Just the opposite. A few hours after you have a glass of wine or beer, alcohol converts to closely related chemicals, called *aldehydes.* Where alcohol had a calming effect, aldehydes are stimulants, accentuating anxieties and interfering with sleep. So the pleasant somnolence induced by an evening glass of wine can be replaced by the worries of the world arriving at 4 A.M. Alcohol can also lead to low blood sugar, which can further aggravate sleep problems. If you're looking for an extra reason to minimize your alcohol use, its biggest problem may be its effect on cancer risk. Even one drink per day, if it is every day, increases the risk of breast and colon cancer.[3]

- *High-protein foods.* That big bean burrito may be packed with protein, but have it for lunch, not dinner. When you have high-protein foods in the evening they can disrupt your brain's ability to produce serotonin, the mood-regulating chemical that also helps you sleep. Here's why: Serotonin is made from an amino acid (protein building block) called *tryptophan,* and, while many high-protein foods contain tryptophan, they contain even more of the other amino acids that compete with tryptophan for entry into the brain. So, the more turkey, chicken, beef, or eggs—or, for that matter, bean burritos—you eat, the less tryptophan gets into the brain and the less serotonin you make during the next few hours. Instead, let your dinner be a bit starchier, and the natural sugars that are released from it will stimulate more serotonin production in your brain, letting you sleep more soundly.

If you've been physically inactive and stressed and you find yourself tossing and turning during the night, you can break out of these patterns. When you get into a groove that includes regular exercise that's fun and sociable, along with times to decompress during the day, followed by a good night's sleep, you'll feel alive and well and will be much less likely to fall prey to dietary indiscretions.

11

Step 6: Call in the Reinforcements

Mary Ann, who we met at the beginning of this book, came into the research meeting with an announcement. Like our other volunteers, she had been struggling with her weight for about as long as she could remember. And one of the things that especially stuck in her mind was her church's bake sale, where volunteers made enough cakes, pies, cookies, and muffins to feed an army. Year after year she had helped out with the preparations and dutifully stored cases of butter—each weighing thirty-six pounds—in her refrigerator. One day, while lugging a case of butter out to her car and putting it in the trunk to bring to the church, it suddenly hit her: "This is exactly what I've been doing every day. Gaining weight is like carrying around a case of butter." She had set her sights on losing it. So she planned out her menus, using the guidelines you'll see in chapter 13. Week after week, she gradually lost weight. And on this particular day she said, "I got on the scale, and I want to let everybody know that *I've now lost an entire case of butter.*" The group burst into applause.

While many people find it tough to change eating habits, our volunteers are remarkably successful. One of the big reasons is that *they have each other.* Mary Ann got the enthusiastic support of the whole team, and her success felt like a victory for everybody. In the beginning phase of a study we all get together every week, sit around a table, and talk through our successes and failures. We look at the odd events that have occurred over the past week. We take stock of things as they are, and discuss how we will make them better. Each participant supports each other like a lifeguard helping a struggling swimmer.

What is it about the company of other people that is so important? Well, for one thing, sometimes we turn to food when what we really need is personal contact. So a key part of changing food habits is to give yourself a bit of what you are *really* looking for. No, you don't need a torrid affair to save you from chocolate. But the fact is, friendships, love, and even sexual attraction stimulate the same reward centers in the brain that addicting foods work on, as we saw in chapter 1. A personal connection is what your brain is looking for, whether it is a conversation, a friendly encounter, a romp with your dog, or simply being near someone else. When we're alone, there's no distraction from foods and no one to shore up our determination to succeed.

Your support network doesn't have to be big or elaborate, but it can really help you keep your resolve. If you are looking for a little support, let me offer a few suggestions, both for your personal life and at work.

Support in Your Personal Life

Some people fill their dance cards, so to speak, by joining clubs or religious groups. Organizations centered on activities other than eating— music, languages, athletics, art, and so forth—can build your social network, along with some healthy habits. Some people enjoy cultural groups, such as the Alliance Française or a Jewish community center. If you're a bit shy of such places, or worried about acceptance, you might do well with a class, or volunteer activity. Art galleries, libraries, nursing homes, animal shelters, and children's hospitals will be thrilled to have your help. Vegetarian societies combine social interaction with a commitment to healthy eating habits and will give you plenty of healthy food ideas to boot.

The husband of one our volunteers, Arthur, had a health problem of his own. He had gained a considerable amount of weight, which he blamed on snacking that kicked in more or less every day in the middle of the afternoon. It had started when he was working at a large

> ◀ Sometimes we turn to food, when what we really need is personal contact. So a key part of changing food habits is to give yourself a bit of what you are *really* looking for.

accounting firm in Washington, D.C. Potato chips and soda were his big thing, but it might also be a hot dog, a pack of nuts, or some other not-especially-healthy food that he ate to get through his long working hours. After retiring, he improved his diet quite a bit, but still got the munchies every day around two or three o'clock.

What cured him was not just some good dietary advice, but also a volunteer job. He took a position in the bookstore of a local art gallery. For one thing, eating was off-limits at the gallery, so there was no temptation, and very soon he found that he *had* to eat a proper lunch in order to get through the afternoon. But he also made many new friends with a wide range of interests and got invitations to unusual events (most of which did not serve food). He enlarged his social circle with people who were very different from the accountants working at the high-stress firm he had left behind. His life was enriched with friendships and activities that made the pleasures of junk food pale by comparison.

Arthur had managed to schedule volunteer activities for what would otherwise be his prime eating times. Now, your problem may not be afternoon snacking; perhaps you need an evening aerobics class to get you out of the house and into a group of friends at just the time your refrigerator was planning to ring you up. If you're uncomfortable at slick clubs where everyone seems to look amazingly fit in athletic clothes, you might feel more comfortable at a more down-to-earth YMCA, YWCA, or YM/YWHA. Women-only clubs are also available.

If overeating has become an issue for you, and you would like get together with other people coping with the same challenge, you may benefit from Overeaters Anonymous, a support group that meets in almost every city (call 1-505-891-2664, check your local white pages, or visit www.OvereatersAnonymous.org). Weight Watchers' support groups have also been very helpful for many people (and, for best results, you'll want to favor Weight Watcher's vegetarian menus.) To find a meeting near you, visit www.WeightWatchers.com, or call 1-800-651-6000.

Enlisting the Support of Family and Friends

When Cecilia joined one of our research studies she knew she was in for some major diet changes, and she welcomed them. The study cut out meat, dairy products, eggs, and fried foods, with the goal of seeing how a drastic cut in fat intake would affect hormone balance. She had had menstrual problems for many years, and she aimed to fix up her diet in order to conquer them. Her one worry was her husband—she had no idea how he would react to her diet change. A diet would clearly be a good thing for him, too, since he needed to lose some weight—but would he give her a hard time? Would she end up having to cook two different dinners? Would he eat out at restaurants, and she'd never see him again?

It turned out that her worries were needless. Rather than resist the diet changes, her husband joined in. Together they made vegetable stews, spinach lasagne, bean chili, and many other foods that lightened the menu considerably. And, while her hormones came into much better balance—bringing marked reductions in PMS, menstrual pain, and other hormone-related symptoms—*he* lost a substantial amount of weight. Her mother then decided to change her diet, and she lost weight, too.

Not everyone has such a happy story. Ella, another young woman in this same study, found her husband totally resistant. He made fun of her new diet and made it all but impossible for her. After two weeks she quit.

When family members are supportive they can be a tremendous shot in the arm. But, when they give you a hard time they can really slow you down. So, let's take a minute to understand their resistance and see our way around it.

When friends or family balk at your diet changes, it is usually either a sign that they are having trouble understanding the value of the changes you envision or that they fear that you'll push them to make the same switch when they don't feel the need for it.

They might subscribe to various nutritional myths that busily circulate in popular culture. For example, if you were going vegetarian and setting aside fatty foods, like french fries and chocolate bars, they might feel compelled to point out that they've heard that kids need lots of fat for brain development, that meat is the best source of protein, that a craving for chocolate is a sign of magnesium deficiency, or other common, but inaccurate, notions. Chapter 13 will help you deal with common nutrition questions. If you need additional nutritional details, you'll find many more in my previous books and at the Physicians Committee for Responsible Medicine's Web site, www.pcrm.org.

Don't feel daunted when family members resist a diet change. It is natural—and even beneficial—to be a bit cautious about changing your diet. Jane Goodall observed that the chimpanzees in Tanzania are true dietary conservatives. They maintain their eating habits with the same rigidity you'd find in any human culture, and they try to enforce their normal eating patterns in their families—and for good reason. Sticking to the tried-and-true prevents poisonings that could occur from being overly adventurous. If a baby chimp picks up a berry or shoot that is not part of the eating habits of the group, a mother or sister is likely to flick it away. These eating patterns have evolved into fairly rigid traditions. At Gombe, where Goodall recorded most of her observations, chimps eat the fruit of the oil nut palm, while their cousins at nearby Mahale avoid it completely. Table manners hold constant in chimpanzee cultures, too. The Mahale chimps crack open the strychnos fruit with their teeth, while the Gombe chimps open it against a stone.

Many people, too, are naturally shy about new foods and new ways of eating, even though they may come to prefer them later. So, when your reluctant spouse balks at a new dish, it helps you to recognize that this is nature's way of guarding against potential dangers. Just be glad you're not trying to teach your poor family how to break open a strychnos fruit.

Having said that, it pays to help your family to move toward healthy eating habits. If you prepare your family's meals, I would encourage you not to cook a healthy meal for yourself and a fatty, entirely unhealthy meal for your spouse or children, simply because they seem to demand these foods and you have not yet found the assertiveness to prepare healthy meals for everyone. If you're in this situation, let me encourage you to seize control of the kitchen. Put orange traffic cones outside the kitchen door if you need to. You are the only person qualified to enter. You can't control what anyone eats outside the house, but you can limit it there.

Several years ago, my mother had a high cholesterol level and decided to go vegetarian. Were she less assertive, she might have continued to cook meat for my father or visiting family members. But instead she made the healthiest possible foods for everyone—stews, soups, and casseroles that fit her diet and that others would like, too. Her decision to revamp the diet not only brought her cholesterol level down, it has been a boon to everyone's health.

Sometimes unhealthy food habits persist in families because food is used as an awkward expression of caring. A neighbor of mine continually pushed food on her overweight teenage children, including foods they did not want and that she did not eat herself. For years, she felt that if she were anything less than a twenty-four-hour catering service she would be not be conveying her love for them. Meanwhile, they felt that saying no would hurt Mom's feelings. Finally, one of the children developed a fairly serious digestive problem and they were forced to find healthier ways to express their feelings.

People who encourage bad habits in others are sometimes called "enablers," especially in the context of alcohol and drug abuse. The word applies just as well to those who bring home buckets of fried chicken and sausage pizza when you're trying to leave those foods behind. If family members seem to be sabotaging you in this way, you'll have to gently but firmly ask them to quit it. It is time to ask family members for help.

Asking for Help

To enlist the help of your family or friends, you might start by letting them know that you are reading this book. Point out parts of it that might interest them and let them know that you want to try the program I've recommended. Ideally, they will join you. The Kickstart Plan in chapter 14 lasts only three weeks, and your family is likely to benefit as much as you will. If they do not wish to try it with you, at the very least they must not get in your way. Ask them, politely but very clearly, not to offer you foods that you're avoiding and not to make any comments that are not supportive, even in good humor.

If family members are being less than helpful, often the cure is simply to find the right words. Let them know that they are the most important people in your life and that their encouragement will mean a lot to you. That includes helping you to avoid temptation and not encouraging you to eat any foods you're trying to set aside. You may be surprised how they will rally to support you, once asked.

It might help to reflect for a moment on what *you* can do for them. If one partner is trying to make a diet change and the other is trying to quit smoking, they can support each other by planning activities that distract them both.

One of our research volunteers asked for a doctor's note—which sounded a bit odd at the time—but it actually worked wonders. If you'd like to do the same, just photocopy this note, and give it to anyone you need to:

From the Desk of Neal D. Barnard, M.D.

_____ is making some dietary adjustments that are important for health. Starting a new way of eating can be difficult, and your support can make the difference between success and failure.

When people are trying to improve their diets, sometimes their companions, with the best of intentions, encourage them to have foods that are not on their regimen. Instead, you can help by taking the focus *off* food for the time being. This is a good time to be generally supportive and to avoid comments and jokes about food.

Thank you for your concern and participation.

Neal D. Barnard, M.D.

Support at Work

For some health-conscious people the office is a torture chamber. You're minding your own business, while cookies, brownies, and candy parade by. "Hey! Have you tried one of these?" they say, shoving a muffin under your nose. Or, "I'm going out for a double-latté-mocha-chocolate espresso and a croissant. Want anything?" Noontime brings invitations to share greasy burgers or a cholesterol-laden business lunch, followed by more junk food in the afternoon.

If your coworkers are continually offering you food, ask them to leave you out of the cookie-and-cake culture. Don't feel obliged to eat food out of politeness. The truth is, most people offering food really do not care if you eat it or not. They want to appear courteous, generous, or clever in the kitchen, or they might want to show they like you. So long as you tell them how wonderful they are and how appreciative you are, the food itself is irrelevant.

Be proactive. Bring your lunch, or plan in advance where you'll eat, so you are not at the mercy of others' suggestions. At an office party or potluck, you might want to bring some healthy items, or skip it for now.

Yvonne, one of our study participants, spoke of a friend who was always pushing food. The answer, she found, was not to confront her friend directly. Rather, she talked to him about another person they both knew "who is so helpful. He *never* pushes food and, in fact, tells me *not* to eat foods that are bad for me. That is just what I need." She found that her friend dropped the food-pushing routine and joined in encouraging her to stick to her resolve. A touch of diplomacy helped everyone save face.

Party Platters and Other Torture Devices

Many people fear parties. Or, rather, they fear caterers who have perfected the art of seduction with one tray after another of painfully attractive foods. You may be reluctant to shun the spread for fear of offending your host. But if you give in to the Marquis de Sade Catering Company you'll hate yourself in the morning. What to do? Here are some tricks for breaking party seductions:

Offer to bring a healthy dish

When I am invited to a party, I mention well in advance that I've changed my diet, and, to avoid giving the hosts any extra trouble, I offer to bring something, such as a bowl of cut exotic fruit, a low-fat guacamole with crackers, or some hummus (a Middle-Eastern chickpea pate that has become a popular party spread). The hosts invariably say, no, there will be plenty to eat. Whatever they were really thinking, at least they've gotten the idea that some guests will appreciate some lighter items, and it wasn't sprung on them at the last minute.

Bring a healthy gift

I often arrive with a packaged food gift in the same way many guests bring a bottle of wine. It might be a couple of interesting dips (e.g., a ranch dressing made with low-fat tofu, instead of dairy-rich versions), some exotic bread, or a small fruit basket. Health food stores now have hundreds of attractively packaged products that are perfect gifts.

Don't arrive hungry

Yvonne said, "I eat before going out with friends or to parties. If I'm not so hungry, it's easier for me to decline those foods I shouldn't eat at all."

When overzealous hosts push exactly the wrong foods, you'll find they will happily leave you alone if you already have something else in your hand. If you are mingling with guests, an appetizer plate filled with crudités or bread will help.

Repaying Their Kindness

Social support is a two-way street. Your family and friends can encourage you as you adopt a healthier diet, and, in turn, you will have a very positive effect on them. You will be a wonderful role model, showing the path to better health. You will know which recipes work and which do not, and which restaurant items really satisfy the taste buds. Chances are, you'll have learned plenty about nutrition and health, and *they* can benefit from this knowledge, too. It is a wonderful thing to see families or groups of friends all getting healthy together, and that, I hope, is what is in store for you.

12

Step 7: Use Extra Motivators

When you're faced with an overwhelmingly seductive food, it helps to remember why a change is important. This chapter presents an extra boost to keep you on track, based on the many benefits of changing the way you eat. Of course, different motivations matter to different people, depending on their ages, values, and backgrounds, and range from increased longevity and health improvements for your children to advantages for the environment.

I have a business associate, Kent, who is a classic example of a low-D_2 individual—the sort of person born with less than the normal number of dopamine receptors, as we saw in chapter 1. Like many people with this genetic trait, he feels chronically empty and gets hooked on everything that feels momentarily good. He used to smoke, drink in binges, and overeat high-calorie food. Despite having gained quite a bit of weight over the years, he just didn't have enough motivation to overcome his unhealthy eating habits. Even after getting married and the birth of two children, he still carried on risking his own health.

Finally, his doctor sat him down for a serious talk. He sternly pointed out that he was not only too overweight to play with his children, he was almost certain to have a heart attack—particularly considering that his family history riddled with heart problems. The doctor looked him in the eye and asked if he had a will. This stunned Kent. "What do you mean?" he asked. The doctor repeated his question: "Do you have a will?"

Kent was speechless in the face of what seemed a pretty nervy thing for a doctor to ask. But his doctor quietly explained that, in his medical opinion, the risk of serious health consequences and even premature death was too great to ignore. And the fact was that Kent clearly needed to be ready to spare his wife and family the difficulties that would come if he died without having prepared for it. Kent chuckled at what he took to be a joke, but the doctor looked dead serious.

Well, as Kent drove home, the message sank in. His father had, in fact, died of a sudden heart attack in his mid-forties, when Kent was just twelve years old. And he had to admit that he himself was not exactly a picture of health. By the time he pulled into his driveway he made a dramatic decision. First of all, he started seeing a psychiatrist for a brief course of treatment dealing with anxieties and stress that seemed to drive him toward overeating, drinking, and tobacco. Then, along with his wife, he consulted a dietitian for a better meal plan.

Over the next year he lost a considerable amount of weight, despite also quitting smoking. He relied fairly heavily on his doctor's and dietitian's support, calling them with one question or another every week or two. And he also managed to get "addicted" to something healthy: He joined an aerobics class that was down the block from his office. It started out slowly, but over about a year's time it got vigorous enough that he felt what he took to be a bit of "runner's high." He now works out every day (he is actually afraid to stop), and, surprisingly enough, aspires to one day become a fitness instructor himself. I have never seen such a behavioral transformation. The key was finding the right motivator.

What Really Matters to You?

Sometimes finding the right motivator is a bit of a challenge. Several years ago a community group outside New York City asked me to give a series of nutrition lectures at various schools. Dean Ornish had just made a huge splash with his research showing that a vegetarian diet, exercise, and stress management, could actually reverse heart disease, and my hosts were eager to convey this message as broadly as possible.

The first talk was at a college. The students listened politely to my lecture, although it was pretty clear that the dangers of cholesterol and saturated fat seemed pretty remote to this young and generally healthy group. The second lecture was for a high school crowd that was far more interested in acne creams and music videos than heart disease risk factors. So I decided to switch gears and talk about other reasons they might want to forego meat, figuring that they might find filthy slaughterhouse conditions and sloppy government inspections to be suitably "gross" and controversial, which they did.

But the third talk was at an elementary school. As I walked into the gymnasium the students were sitting on the floor, and teachers were busily reprimanding the rowdier kids. While I had long harbored the illusion that I was still in touch with my "inner child," I soon realized I had absolutely nothing to say to these kids. What could possibly motivate a grade-school child to think about diet? I couldn't spot any budding cardiologists in the group and couldn't recall a single storybook character who had ever had a cholesterol problem. In the end, all I could think to do was to ask the students how they felt about farm animals. "If you were a pig," I ventured, "would you rather be stuck in a huge indoor farm—in a stall where you could barely even turn around—or would you rather be out in the field with your families?" They reacted instantly. "With our families! With our families!" the kids yelled. And that was the way the talk went. I figured that, three decades hence, those who had decided to simply leave the pigs alone would certainly have healthier hearts and trimmer waistlines than the kids who decided to go ahead and eat them.

If you're looking for a bit of extra motivation, see which of the following points mean something to you. They are all linked to the advantages of breaking free from unhealthy eating habits.

- **Your family and friends will have a healthier you.** Adolescents take all too many risks—driving too fast, drinking too much, smoking cigarettes, taking drugs, and eating heaven-knows-what. But, about the time we get married and start having children, we come to realize that other people depend on us. Parents who risk cutting their own lives short with dangerous lifestyle habits are not doing their dependents any favors. But, by taking care of yourself you'll be around to help your family through the challenges that lie ahead.

- **You'll slim down.** By stepping away from calorie-dense foods, you'll have a much easier time trimming your waistline.

- **You'll cut your cancer risk.** If you ever wondered whether breaking a meat-and-cheese habit is worth it, studies of vegetarians show that you can expect to cut your cancer risk by a good 40 percent.[1]

- **You'll reverse heart disease.** In the classic research study conducted by Dean Ornish, M.D., 82 percent of individuals who switched to a low-fat, vegetarian diet, along with exercise and stress management, actually reversed their heart disease.[2] This is especially important, given that most people in Western countries have the beginnings of artery blockages before they finish high school.

- **You might even prevent back pain.** Studies show that blockages in the lumbar arteries are a major contributor to the vertebral disk problems that cause common lower-back pain (which is also why smokers have more backaches).[3] Simply put, if the vertebrae don't get the blood and oxygen they need they become more and more fragile. If they rupture, the result can be severe and chronic back pain. So the same diet that is good for your heart—opening your arteries and increasing blood flow—might be good for your back, too.

- **You'll stay young sexually.** Ordinary impotence, which is common in middle-aged and older men, is not caused by performance anxiety. It is caused by blocked arteries. In the same way that blockages in the arteries to the heart lead to heart attacks and blockages in the *carotid* arteries leading to the brain cause strokes, blockages in the arteries to the genitals lead to impotence.[4,5] That's right—a Philly Cheese Steak doesn't make you a better Romeo, but the veggie burger might just do the trick.

- **You can prevent diabetes, or even reverse it.** Research studies show that if you change your diet enough, type 2 diabetes improves or even disappears, and all the problems it causes—heart disease, blindness, kidney disease, and amputations—are much less likely to occur.[6] When you get the fat out of your diet, insulin works much more efficiently, enabling many people with diabetes to reduce their medications or get off them completely. If you have type 1 diabetes, you can minimize your insulin to the smallest possible dose.

- **You can reduce your blood pressure.** In research studies, a combination of diet changes and exercise can bring down blood pressure enough that most people can reduce or even stop their medications.[7] A note of caution: High blood pressure can be very dangerous, so let your doctor decide if and when the time is right to stop medication.

- **You can say good-bye to constipation.** Switching from a fiber-depleted diet loaded with sugar, chocolate, cheese, and meat to a menu filled with healthy vegetables, fruits, beans, and whole grains gives your digestive tract everything it needs to work properly. You can throw away the laxatives.

- **You might cut the risk of appendicitis.** The improved movement of intestinal contents caused by a healthy, high-fiber diet may be the reason vegetarians are much less likely to develop appendicitis. The condition usually starts with a bit of compacted stool (from a low-fiber diet) clogging the opening of the appendix.

- **Bye-bye hemorrhoids.** Famed cancer researcher Denis Burkitt, M.D., discovered that a high-fiber diet could do more than cut the risk of colon cancer, it could also prevent and possibly cure hemorrhoids, which are often the result of too much straining by constipated people.[8]

- **You'll be safer from food-borne illnesses.** Virtually all the bacteria that make headlines in food-poisoning cases originate in livestock feces. Traces of chicken manure and the bacteria they harbor taint, believe it or not, as many as two-thirds of chicken packages in the retail store. When you slice open the package at home, those bacteria dribble out—*alive*—along with the "chicken juice" that spills onto your countertop, ready to contaminate your kitchen sponge, utensils, and hands. Since plants do not have digestive tracts, fecal bacteria (e.g., salmonella, or E. coli O157:H7) only contaminate vegetables and fruits when they are tainted with manure (e.g., as a fertilizer) or when handlers have used poor hygiene.

- **You'll keep stronger bones.** People who stop eating meat tend to hold onto calcium more readily, as we saw on page 68. Animal protein leaches calcium from the bones and sends it through the kidneys, to be lost in the urine.[9]

- **You'll reduce menstrual symptoms.** Premenstrual symptoms and menstrual cramps are reduced in most women who break a meat-and-dairy habit, because your hormones come into significantly better balance.[10] And getting away from sugar can help stabilize PMS-related mood swings. For details, you may wish to consult my previous book, *Foods That Fight Pain* (Harmony Books, 1998).

- **You'll have more energy.** I don't know why it happens, but it does. When people break free from unhealthy foods they often notice a surge in their energy levels.

- **You'll be healthier in your old age.** Getting older doesn't have to mean losing your health. The illnesses that strike many older folks—diabetes, heart disease, cancer, arthritis, stroke, and even Alzheimer's disease—are linked to diet to a substantial degree. Breaking away from sugar, dairy, and meat is a powerful prescription.

- **You'll be more likely to *make it* to old age.** Living fast and dying young might make for a romantic James Dean movie, but it doesn't work out so well in real life. Vegetarians live years longer than their meat-eating counterparts.[11]

- **You'll find new and interesting tastes.** When I was a child growing up in North Dakota, dinner meant roast beef, potatoes, and corn. Or sometimes pork chops, potatoes, and corn. Or meat loaf, potatoes, and corn. That was about it. And we had two spices: salt and pepper. Breaking into healthier tastes also means much more interesting tastes: Italian pastas with plum tomatoes, exotic Indian curries, piquant Mexican dishes, Cuban black beans and rice, Mediterranean and Middle-Eastern foods, vegetable sushi, endless Chinese and Thai dishes, Ethiopian cuisine, and many more. Even without their health benefits, there would be no reason to step backward from such exquisite foods to the plain fare I grew up with.

- **You'll save money.** Just as cigarette smokers spend a small fortune on their habit, those packs of cheese, chocolate, and cookies can add up pretty fast, too.

- **You'll save *serious* money.** In 1995, my colleagues and I calculated that the direct medical costs attributable to meat consumption in the United States—for the excess cases of heart disease, cancer, hypertension, diabetes, food-borne illness, obesity, and appendicitis among meat-eaters, compared to vegetarians—reached $61 billion per year.[12] The current figures are unfortunately much higher, and show up in escalating insurance premiums, prescription drug costs, and Medicare outlays.

- **You'll help fight world hunger.** Environmentalist Frances Moore Lappé wrote, in *Diet for a Small Planet,* that acre after acre of usable land is cultivated for nothing but feed for the one hundred million cattle, billions of chickens, and millions upon millions of other livestock living in the barns and fields of North America. Breaking the spell that the meat and dairy industries have had over us for many decades would free up land for other uses, including feeding the world's hungry.

- **You'll be a real environmentalist.** If you live downwind from a hog farm for more than five minutes, you'll wish your neighbors had all gone vegetarian.

- **You'll be kind to animals.** U.S. Department of Agriculture figures show that Americans now eat, believe it or not, more than one million animals *every hour.* Breaking a meat habit changes a lot more than just what's on your plate.

- **You'll be kind to farm workers.** As we saw in chapter 3, a major issue in the chocolate industry is the heated debate over the conditions in which field workers live.

A great many people take care of their own health, not for themselves, but because they feel obliged to be healthy for their families, or they feel some responsibility toward the world they live in. By all means nurture those motivations and ultimately capitalize on them. Your coronary arteries and waistline don't care *why* you change your diet. But they're thrilled when you do.

Part III

Breaking Free: Falling in Love with Food—the Healthy Way

In the next three chapters we'll look at how to get started with a truly optimal diet—one that not only keeps you strong in the face of cravings, but that also helps you slim down and stay healthy.

We'll first look at some basic guidelines for healthy eating. Next, I'll show you a three-week plan that lets you jump in with confidence. And, finally, we'll look at how to make it work in real life—that is, how to eat healthfully and love it, whether we're at a top restaurant, a fast-food joint, or on the road.

13

Foods That Love You Back

I n the preceding chapters I have described how you can revamp
your diet to tone down cravings, starting with a healthy breakfast to
keep hunger at bay, using low-GI foods to hold your blood sugar
steady as the day goes on, avoiding the low-calorie or high-fat diets
that could destroy leptin's ability to rein in your appetite, and breaking
out of unhealthy craving cycles.

To see how these principles translate into actual meals, let's take a
look over the shoulders of Cynthia and Steven, whom we met in the
first chapter. As you might remember, her goal was to tame the chocolate seduction that hit every evening and that, over time, had made her
more and more shy of her bathroom scale. His goal was to cut his cholesterol, and that meant putting something on his plate that was healthier and lighter than the salmon, beef, poultry, cheese, and other
fat-filled foods he had become accustomed to.

First we'll look at the anticraving menu they chose, and then at the
basic keys to planning your own.

For breakfast, they decided to make a pot of old-fashioned oatmeal.
(If you do the same, let me encourage you *not* to follow the package
instructions. Instead, see page 81.) Cynthia topped hers with straw-

berries, but cinnamon and raisins would have gone well, too. Steve ate his plain.

Because I encouraged them to have something high in plant protein as a starter (see chapter 6), they chose veggie sausages. Steven quite liked "Smart Links," a vegan sausage made by LightLife Foods that, properly browned in a nonstick pan, has the taste of meaty sausage, with seven grams of protein per link, and none of the cholesterol or saturated fat of regular sausage (Health food stores and larger groceries stock innumerable other meatless sausages, bacon strips, and Canadian bacon, too.) For a high-protein starter they would also have done well with a serving of chickpeas, baked beans, tofu scrambler, or any of the others you'll find in the recipe section. They had also sliced open a cantaloupe, but were already full when it came time to eat it.

Their breakfast gave them a good start on the day. It let them skip the cholesterol, fat, and animal protein that are the curses of typical breakfast fare. It filled them up with healthy fiber, had no sugar at all, and had plenty of good, complex carbs to keep blood sugar on an even keel for hours.

As the morning went along they felt energetic and healthy and did not find their attention wandering toward snack foods at all. So far, so good.

For lunch Cynthia had split pea soup with a large salad. Steven was on the road with a coworker, and they stopped into a fast-food taco shop where he got a couple of bean burritos, minus the cheese. Nothing fancy, but it was all zero-cholesterol, low in fat, low-GI, and tasty.

The foods they had chosen were quick, easy, and familiar. And there was no question that they did the job. The combination of a good breakfast and low-GI foods at lunch blocked hunger and cravings all afternoon.

They were at home again for dinner, and started with lentil soup that they got from a can for simplicity. Then they had a salad of fresh greens with balsamic vinaigrette and cooked up some angel-hair pasta with a spicy *arabiata* sauce made from tomatoes and pepperoncinos (Italian hot red chilis). They were also tempted by a recipe for pasta *puttanesca,* made of tomatoes, garlic, red peppers, olives, capers, and parsley (named for Italian ladies of the night, who supposedly needed to be able to make dinner very quickly between clients, and who also often threw in anchovies, but you wouldn't, if you wanted it truly healthy and cholesterol-free). They also steamed, then lightly sautéed, some broccoli and asparagus on the side.

The dinner took all of about fifteen minutes to prepare and was absolutely delicious. It was hearty, and, if they happened to check the GI of lentils, pasta, or the other foods on their plates, they would have felt very proud of themselves.

Later on they went for a walk in the evening air. It wasn't intended to get their pulses racing, it was just a way to be together. And it had the added benefit of breaking into Cynthia's evening refrigerator-raiding time.

And that was their day. On other days, they had the kinds of foods you'll see in the recipe section and chapter 15, and they made sure they were well-stocked with fresh fruit for snacks and desserts. "What we're eating now appeals to me more than the heavy foods I used to eat," Cynthia said. "It just 'feels' healthier. And it's really helped us both. I've been steadily losing weight, and Steve's doctor is thrilled with his cholesterol readings."

This of course was very different from their previous routine, where dinner usually left them too tired to even think about an evening stroll, let alone any hope for losing weight or reducing Steve's cholesterol. Their new menu was just what the doctor ordered.

Basic Food Groups

Planning healthy meals is easier than you might have imagined. Let me give you the basics.

While the food industry would like you to plan your meals from the Chocolate Group, the Cheese Group, the Chicken Nuggets Group, and the Sugar Cookies Group, the truth is there are four *healthy* food groups that you should use. The *New Four Food Groups* were developed in 1991 to replace the old 1950s "four food groups," which included meat, dairy products, and grains, and relegated vegetables and fruits to a single group. The new groupings make for a diet that is richer in protective nutrients, like fiber and vitamins, while omitting cholesterol, animal fat, and other undesirables:

The Vegetable Group includes asparagus, broccoli, carrots, cauliflower, spinach, sweet potatoes, and endless other varieties. They are loaded with vitamins and with surprising amounts of calcium, iron, and other minerals. Be generous with green, yellow, and orange vegetables—they are cancer fighters. And green leafy vegetables (other than spinach) are great sources of calcium. When it comes to potatoes, favor sweet potatoes and yams.

The Fruit Group includes apples, bananas, blueberries, cherries, grapefruit, oranges, peaches, pears, and other fruits that are the treats of the produce department. They are loaded with vitamins and, despite their sweet taste, have very little effect on your blood sugar, with a few exceptions (e.g., watermelon and pineapple).

The Legume (Bean) Group includes high-protein, high-fiber foods. Beans, lentils, and peas are also loaded with calcium, iron, soluble fiber, and even traces of "good fats"—that is, omega-3 fatty acids. This group also includes the endless array of soy products, from tofu, tempeh, and miso, to veggie burgers, meatless hot dogs, and deli slices that look just like turkey, chicken, bologna, pepperoni, and Canadian bacon.

The Whole Grain Group includes brown rice, oatmeal, barley, whole-grain bread or pasta, corn, quinoa, and all their relatives that are loaded with complex carbs, fiber, and protein. Among wheat products, pasta has a lower GI than typical breads. And when choosing breads, pumpernickel and rye have a lower GI than white or wheat.

For a craving-busting diet that is also optimally healthy, you'll want to plan your meals using these four food groups, while omitting meats, dairy products, and eggs, and keeping added oils to a minimum. These foods are naturally low in fat and high in fiber, and most have low GI values.

On your plate they turn into a breakfast of old-fashioned oatmeal with cinnamon and raisins, a half cantaloupe, and whole-grain toast; a lunch of chunky vegetable chili, split pea or lentil soup, or a bean burrito with rice; and a dinner of pasta marinara, autumn stew, or veggie lasagne with plenty of fresh vegetables.

How many servings should you have from each group? Although I have provided some basic guidelines below, it's really up to you. Many people, including those who fashioned the Food Guide Pyramid, look to traditional Asian cuisine as a model, which means that your plate should be especially generous with whole grains, with slightly less emphasis on fruits and vegetables, and smaller amounts of other foods. That is fine. However, you might just as well emphasize vegetables and fruits, and also include bean dishes (in modest amounts if you are not used to them, because they are likely to cause some gassiness, at least at first.) Whole grains can then be used to fill up the rest of your plate.

The New Four Food Groups

The numbers of servings listed are suggestions only.

- **Vegetables:** 4 or more servings per day. A serving is 1 cup raw or ½ cup cooked.

- **Legumes** (beans, peas, and lentils): 3 servings per day. A serving is ½ cup cooked beans, 4 ounces of tofu or tempeh, or 8 ounces of soy milk.

- **Whole grains:** 8 servings per day. A serving is just ½ cup cooked grain, such as oatmeal or pasta, 1 ounce of dry cereal, or 1 slice of bread.

- **Fruits:** 3 or more servings per day. A serving is one small piece of fruit, ½ cup chopped fruit, or ½ cup cooked fruit or juice.

Add a daily multivitamin as a convenient source of vitamin B_{12} (unless you choose B_{12}-fortified products, such as Kellogg's Cornflakes, Product 19, Total Cereal, or fortified soy milks), and vitamin D if you rarely get exposure to sunlight.

As you've noticed, the recommended foods do not include meat, dairy products, eggs, or greasy fried foods. If you're unsure about the health reasons for setting these foods aside, let's encourage you to take another look at chapters 4 and 5.

Now, if you're imagining that a transition to healthier eating might be a pretty serious challenge, relax—we'll make it easy, and you'll be glad you did it.

You should also add a daily multivitamin. Any brand is fine. It will provide you vitamin B_{12}, which you need for healthy blood and healthy nerves, and which is not found in substantial amounts in foods that come from plant sources other than those, such as breakfast cereals or soy milk, that are vitamin-fortified. It also provides vitamin D, which normally comes from sunlight on your skin, but which many people miss because they are indoors most of the day. The *Journal of the American Medical Association* reported on June 16, 2002, that a daily multivitamin was a good idea for everyone, and I agree with this simple prescription. While meat-eaters might imagine they have complete nutrition without a multivitamin, they often run low in vitamin C, folic acid, beta-carotene, and other nutrients. Fortified foods can make up for all these problems, but a multivitamin is a simple way to be sure. Meat-eaters also generally run low in fiber, but multiple vitamins cannot make up for a fiber deficit (and, of course, a vitamin pill cannot remove the cholesterol, fat, or other undesirables found in animal products.)

The Transition to Healthy Eating

While the idea of breaking away from meats, cheese, and fatty foods changes the eating habits that are routine in North America and much of the rest of the world (let's face it, you are breaking the principal food addictions and unhealthy habits of our culture), we have found that it is certainly the healthiest diet and probably the easiest to follow over the long run.

In 2000, my colleagues and I published in the *American Journal of Cardiology* the greatest cholesterol-lowering of any diet trial ever reported in women under fifty, using this sort of diet for just five weeks.[1] Other studies by our research team, and others, have found this eating pattern to help people lose weight and to improve diabetes, hypertension, arthritis, digestive problems, and many other conditions.

Diets based on "moderation"—including small amounts of meat or cheese, as in the diets that are commonly used in attempts to control cholesterol, diabetes, blood pressure—include so many rules (no more than six ounces of meat per day, only one egg yolk per week, no more than 30 percent of calories from fat, 7 percent from saturated fat, etc., etc.) that they soon become tedious.

More importantly, they tease you with the very foods you're trying to limit, leading to the "appetizer effect." That is, let's say you have a little bit of cheese, on the theory that moderation in all things must be good. But that first bite triggers an opiate release, and soon you find yourself swept far beyond "moderation," to right back where you

⊰⊱ Some diets tease you with bits of cheese, chocolate, sugar, or meat—the very foods you're trying to limit.

started. This, of course, is exactly what many diets do: they prescribe just a few ounces of meat each day, an ounce or two of cheese, just a bite of chocolate, and no more than a tiny bit of sugar. Pretty soon you'll feel you're not on a diet, but on some sort of continuous tease.

Just as quitting smoking is easier than trying to limit yourself to one or two cigarettes per day, it is easier to simply skip cheese, meat, and other less-than-healthy foods than to continually tease yourself with them day after day. Yvonne, one of our research volunteers, said, "I find it easier to have none of the foods to which I'm addicted, rather than a little of them. For me, there's no such thing as two or three Twizzlers or jelly beans."

Another reason why it is easier to make major diet changes—even for a short period of time—than to tinker with minor adjustments is that *cravings feed off each other.* As fatty foods drive hormones out of control they accentuate cravings for chocolate or sugar. In turn, sugary foods cause your blood sugar to rise and fall abruptly, sparking other cravings. One food problem leads to another.

The principal challenge with any major diet change is that seductive foods are everywhere nowadays. At first you might feel like a person who is trying to quit smoking while surrounded by people constantly offering you cigarettes. But it soon becomes second nature, as we have seen over and over again in our studies. And the diet has rubbed off on our staff as well. In our Washington, D.C., office, most of our twenty or so staffers have seen the value of a low-fat, vegan diet, and they follow it themselves. And it shows. I recently escorted a group of visitors around our office, and they couldn't help but comment on how extraordinarily healthy and slim everyone was.

⊰⊱ Cravings feed off each other. As fatty foods drive hormones out of control, they accentuate cravings for chocolate or sugar. In turn, sugary foods cause your blood sugar to rise and fall abruptly, sparking other cravings. One food problem leads to another.

Let Your Tastes Change

Your taste buds have a memory of about three weeks, and you can exploit this fact as you change your diet. Did you ever switch from whole milk to skim? As I mentioned in chapter 5, at first the lower-fat versions seem watery and don't taste right. But, three weeks later what happens? Skim tastes totally normal. And if you were to try whole milk again it would seem too thick and fatty. In just a few weeks your preferences have turned completely around. This is not to suggest that skim milk is health food. Far from it—there are many health concerns about dairy products, as we saw in chapter 4. But this common example illustrates how easy it is to learn new tastes.

Now, when you lighten your *entire diet* you have the same whole-milk-to-skim experience, but to a much more profound degree. In research studies in which we have used very low-fat and vegetarian foods, at first some volunteers balk a bit. But within a week or two the lighter foods taste perfectly fine—often better than the heavier foods they have replaced. And then if our volunteers happen to taste their old unhealthy foods again, they find their desire for them is largely gone.

In the next chapter we'll use an easy, three-week time frame so you can do this yourself. There is no long-term commitment. You just follow, for three weeks, a diet that is as close to an optimal regimen as humanly possible, letting old, unhealthy habits drift away. After three weeks, if you like how you feel, you can stick with it.

The diet change can work wonders. Lisa, for example, was hooked on sugar. She was a telephone operator and got virtually no physical exercise. Her appetite was under control during the day, but every evening after work, cookies, cake, and candy bars all called out insistently. She was in her late thirties at the time and was at the point of deciding that food addiction was basically unconquerable. She also smoked about a half pack per day and was reluctant to stop for fear it would aggravate her weight problem, which had gradually increased over the years. Her self-esteem had taken a terrible beating—she no longer wanted to look at herself in the mirror—and it was just a matter of time before her physical health would start deteriorating, too.

Lisa and a friend saw a newspaper advertisement about one of our research studies. Lisa was excluded from the study itself because of her smoking. But we gave her some basic diet information, focusing especially on breakfast and lunch to make sure that she was adequately nourished, with a steady blood sugar that would help defeat evening cravings. She had not been very big on beans or vegetables, so she planned out some simple choices that she could picture herself eating: baked beans, lentil soup, black beans with rice and salsa, along with spinach salads, steamed broccoli with lemon, and asparagus.

Because she was obviously on a daily craving cycle, I suggested she might try to disrupt her normal schedule. She decided to exercise during the morning and switch to the evening shift at work for a month or so. She also made quite a study of vegetarian cookbooks, picking out simple recipes that met our guidelines. She checked out the local health food stores and filled her cupboards. She was determined to start each day with a really healthy breakfast and to stick to the good food groups we recommend.

Her initial burst of motivation lasted a couple of weeks, and by then she had lost a few pounds, and that motivated her to want to continue. Eventually she got back on the day shift, but she made it a point to not get started on the "sugar trip," as she put it. Over the next year or so she lost about sixty pounds and simply does not look like the same person.

Her friend, Elena, had an equally powerful experience. After we accepted her into the study, but before the study began, her father died of complications of diabetes. The experience bowled her over in many ways, one of which related to her own sense of risk. Her father's two sisters also had the disease and had had many problems as a result. One was on dialysis, due to kidney failure. She did not want to follow in their footsteps. Elena felt that life had just grabbed her by the scruff of the neck and given her a good shake.

She basically threw herself into the study. She had been a fairly enthusiastic meat eater up until that point, but she aimed to try something very different. She carefully planned out her menu for the week ahead, bought the foods she'd need, and did not stray from the diet. She lost weight steadily, about a pound per week or slightly more.

And what meant more to her than anything was the fact that her morning blood-sugar level, which we checked periodically, gradually descended from a borderline value of 120 mg/dl (over 125 is considered diabetic) to a totally healthy 82. She felt that she took control of her diet, her weight, her health, and her future.

What was most remarkable was that both Lisa and Elena had lost all desire to return to unhealthy foods. They felt in charge. For once in their lives, foods did not control them, and even the seductions at convenience stores and supermarkets held no sway. The foods that appealed most to them were those that kept them fit and healthy.

We have seen this phenomenon very frequently, but, each time, it is wonderful to see people gain a whole new level of strength and vitality. While the process of change does require an initial willingness to step into new and slightly unfamiliar waters, a new way of eating will repay your effort many times over.

Complete Nutrition

When you're changing your diet, especially when you're setting aside meat and dairy products, you're likely to wonder where you'll get your protein, calcium, iron, and so forth. It is actually quite easy. Let's take a quick look at nutrition in plant-based diets:

Protein

Protein is used for building and repairing body tissues. If you could look at a molecule of protein under a powerful microscope, you would see that it is like a string of beads, with each bead being one of twenty or so different *amino acids* that combine in various sequences, depending on whether the protein will become part of your skin, your hair, a hormone molecule, or something else.

There is plenty of protein—and all the essential amino acids you'll need—in beans, grains, vegetables, and fruits. In the past, some writers had mistakenly suggested that vegetarians needed to carefully combine various foods in order to get adequate protein. Beans and grains, for example, were a good combination. However, we have since learned that the normal combinations of plant foods that make up the diet easily provide more than enough protein. There is no need to intentionally choose special combinations of foods.[2]

However, if you're looking for extra protein for some reason, you'll find plenty in the bean group and especially in the products made from soy (e.g., tofu) or wheat (e.g., seitan) derivatives (for descriptions, see pages 195–199).

There is no reason to consume animal protein, and you're better off without it. As we've seen, diets rich in animal protein lead to significant losses of calcium through the kidneys, which is believed to be why osteoporosis is much more common in countries where meat is a dietary staple.[3] Animal protein also contributes to kidney problems, including stones.

Calcium

Green, leafy vegetables and beans are rich in calcium, without the disadvantages of dairy products. While there is somewhat less calcium in broccoli than in milk, the absorption fraction—the percentage that your body can actually use—is higher from broccoli and nearly all other greens than from milk. If you're looking for extra calcium for whatever reason, you'll find more than you need in fortified juices and soy milks.

The key in maintaining calcium balance, however, is not only to have an adequate intake, but to minimize calcium losses. That means avoiding animal protein, limiting sodium (salt) in your diet, and getting adequate exercise and sunlight for vitamin D.

Iron

Traces of iron are an essential part of the hemoglobin your red blood cells use to carry oxygen. There is plenty of healthful iron in the bean group and in green leafy vegetables—the same foods that give you calcium. When people adopt balanced plant-based diets, they easily get plenty of iron from these healthy sources. Vitamin C-rich foods, such as fruits and vegetables, increase iron absorption.

In the not-so-distant past, many people imagined they needed to eat meat to get adequate iron. It has since become clear not only that other foods can easily provide iron without meat's fat and cholesterol, but also that meat tends to tip iron balance into overload. Like other metals, iron has dangers when you overdo it, as many people unknowingly do. Iron encourages the production of unstable molecules in your body called *free radicals,* and these maladjusted molecules can damage your body tissues—leading to signs of aging—and contribute to heart disease.

Young women might occasionally run low in iron as a result of menstrual blood losses. However, before they rush to increase their iron intake they should first have their iron level checked by a doctor. Second, they should avoid dairy products, which inhibit normal iron absorption; and, third, they should make sure their diet includes plenty of green vegetables and beans. It is uncommon for anyone—even a young woman—to actually need an iron supplement, and it is never necessary to use meat for this purpose.

Zinc

Your immune system and your ability to heal wounds depend on traces of zinc, as do a great many biochemical reactions in your body. But as is the case with iron, overdoing it is risky, interfering with immune function and causing other problems. Healthy sources include legumes, nuts, and fortified breakfast cereals (e.g., Bran Flakes, granola, Grape-Nuts, Special K).

Fat

Your body needs some fat in the diet, although the amount you actually need is minuscule—just 3–4 percent of your calories. Most people in Western countries get ten times that amount. There are just two fats your body actually needs—*alpha-linolenic acid* and *linoleic acid.* While there is not a great deal of fat in beans, vegetables, and fruits, the traces of fat they do contain are relatively rich in alpha-linolenic acid. Nuts, seeds, olives, avocadoes, and soy products provide more fat. If for any reason you are looking for an especially rich source of these fats, flax oil is more than 50 percent alpha-linolenic acid. But go easy—there is no reason to have more than one tablespoon per day (and most people do not need to supplement at all.) These botanical sources provide healthy fats without the contaminants found in fish oils or other animal products. Linoleic acid is found in a great many foods, and you will not run low on it.

The bottom line is that you'll get all the fat you need from a diet of vegetables, fruits, beans, and whole grains, along with occasional nuts or other fattier plant foods.

Vitamin B$_{12}$

You need tiny traces of vitamin B$_{12}$ for healthy blood and healthy nerve function. However, this vitamin is not made by animals or plants, but by bacteria and other single-celled organisms. Animal products contain B$_{12}$ made by the bacteria in animals' intestinal tracts, so traces of it end up in meat and other animal products. However, along with it come cholesterol, fat, and animal proteins. As noted above, healthier sources include fortified cereals, such as Kellogg's Corn Flakes, Product 19, or Total, fortified soy milk, and, of course, all common multiple vitamins.

Vitamin D

Vitamin D is actually a hormone that is normally produced by sunlight on your skin. It helps you absorb calcium, among other functions. There is no need for dietary supplementation if you get regular sun exposure. If you do not, a multiple vitamin containing 400 IU of vitamin D is a good idea.

As you can see, getting good and complete nutrition is easy. So long as you're building your diet from healthful vegetables, fruits, beans, and whole grains, and adding any common source of vitamin B$_{12}$, such as a multivitamin, you've got it licked.

These guidelines provide optimal nutrition at all stages of life: childhood, adolescence, and adulthood, including pregnancy, nursing, and older age. For additional information on common nutrition questions you may wish to consult my previous books, as well as PCRM's Web site, www.pcrm.org.

And now that you know how to choose a craving-busting menu, let me take you one step further. The next chapter presents a three-week program that puts the entire program to work and makes it practically foolproof.

14

The Three-Week Kickstart Plan: Clean Your Slate for a New Beginning

B y now you have a pretty good idea of what you need to do to beat your cravings, and why. This chapter gives you a quick start with a three-week program that cleans your slate, so to speak, and lets you begin fresh, free of troublesome food habits, while giving you plenty of momentum for keeping your resolve.

We developed the techniques you'll read about in this chapter in the course of our research studies involving people who were anxious to change their eating habits in order to lose weight, lower their cholesterol levels, or beat other health problems. Some of our volunteers were highly motivated and ready to dive in, while others felt a bit more timid about changing their food habits. The Three-Week Kickstart Plan was designed to help both kinds of people.

If you are eager to start, it will channel your motivation into a practical road to success. And if you are just putting a very tentative toe in the water it will allow you to jump in for a safe and finite period. The short-term focus lets you really commit to doing it right, so your results—a healthier diet, weight loss, a decisive drop in cholesterol, or whatever dietary goal you are working toward—will come rapidly. You will see the payoff for yourself.

You will physically change as you begin this program. You will stabilize your blood sugar, increase your energy, pump up your appetite-taming leptin, and calm your hormone shifts. And your tastes will change, too. Your taste buds have a memory of about three weeks, as we have seen whenever people reduce their sugar, fat, or salt intake. It takes about three weeks for the new, lighter taste to be clearly preferred.

So the Kickstart uses a three-week time frame to allow you to shift from one set of preferences to another. It is just enough time for your taste buds to leave behind old tastes and learn new ones.

We are going to work fast. So buckle your seatbelt and let's get started!

Before You Begin

First, let's check a few things so that you can prove *to yourself* what the diet change is doing:

- You'll want to check your weight on a reliable scale. It is likely to start to drop.

- If cholesterol, blood sugar, or blood pressure are issues for you, have your doctor check them, too. They are all likely to improve, and you'll want to see your progress.

- Take stock of what you're eating now.

You can get a good snapshot of your overall diet with a three-day dietary record. This is the same diet-tracking tool we use in our research studies. It is strictly optional, but it really pays to do this at least once, because it shows *exactly* what you are eating. You might be a bit shocked at how many calories you're taking in, how much fat, or how little fiber. And it lets you see how your diet improves over time. If you're having a problem it almost always shows you what's wrong and how to improve things.

You simply take a sheet of paper and note down *everything* you eat or drink (except water) for three days, including two weekdays and one weekend day (most of us eat a bit differently on weekends, compared to weekdays.)

Using the form on page 165 (photocopy it as many times as you need to), jot down each food, condiment, or beverage on a separate line. For example, if you had toast with butter and jam, use three lines, one for each of the ingredients—toast, butter, and jam. Or if you had a baked potato topped with butter, sour cream, and black pepper, along with a cola, use five lines so you can separate out each part of the meal—potato, butter, sour cream, pepper, and your drink. Write down everything other than water.

Also note how you felt before the meal: happy, stressed, depressed, tired, or whatever. Then do the same after you've eaten, to see whether you feel the same, better, or worse. In the section marked "Why chosen?" just indicate what prompted you to pick this food at this time: hunger, taste, peer pressure (everyone else was eating it), and so on.

Jot down your foods as you go, so you don't forget. If it is more convenient, you can keep notes in a small notebook and transfer them to this form later. No one is going to see this other than you, so be thorough.

When your record is complete look it over carefully. What patterns emerge? What are the foods that you wish you hadn't eaten? Where were you when you ate them? How were you feeling beforehand? After? What is the record telling you?

If you like, you can get a detailed nutrient analysis of your diet. Just be sure to fill in quantities carefully, using a food scale (available in cookware stores) and log onto a nutrient analysis Web site, such as the University of Illinois Food Science and Human Nutrition Department site, http://www.nat.uiuc.edu/mainnat.html, or Dietsite.com.

By the way, while nutrient analyses on these sites are accurate, you'll want to disregard their nutrition guidelines that allow too much fat and cholesterol. For an adult consuming 2,000 calories per day, a good fat intake goal is about 25–45 grams each day. Cholesterol intake ideally is zero. Your protein intake should be roughly 50 grams per day. Resist the temptation to push protein intake too high (see pages 70–71).

After three weeks we'll check your eating habits again and you'll be astounded at the difference.

⊰ะ The Kickstart uses a three-week time frame to allow you to shift from one set of preferences to another. It is just enough time for your taste buds to leave behind old tastes and learn new ones.

Diet Record

Make as many copies of this page as you need. Record only one ingredient per line.

Date: _____

Time of day	Food	Amount	Cooking method	Place	Why chosen?	Feeling before	Feeling after

Diet Record—Sample

Here is a sample diet record for the morning hours. A full record would include meals and snacks throughout the entire day.

Time of day	Food	Amount	Cooking method	Place	Why chosen?	Feeling before	Feeling after
7:30 A.M.	Wheat toast	2 slices	toasted	home	hungry	hungry, tired	less hungry
7:30 A.M.	Butter	2 pats	(for toast)	home	taste	hungry, tired	less hungry
7:30 A.M.	Grape jam	2 tsp	(for toast)	home	taste	hungry, tired	less hungry
7:30 A.M.	Omelet	3 eggs	fried	home	taste	tired	overly full
7:30 A.M.	Velveeta	2 oz.	for omelet	home	taste	tired	overly full
7:30 A.M.	Coffee	1 cup	drip	home	needed a pick-up	tired	more awake
7:30 A.M.	Creamer	1 tsp	—	home	to whiten coffee	tired	more awake
10:30 A.M.	Choc. chip cookies	4	home-made	office	they were there	fine	fine
11:00 A.M.	Choc. chip cookies	3	home-made	office	they were still there	fine	a bit sick

Check your cravings. One last preliminary. Let's check the strength of your cravings with the five-minute questionnaire beginning on the next page. We'll repeat it in three weeks, so you can see how things have changed.

Cravings Questionnaire

Date: _____

Rate your desire for each of these food items during a typical day in the last week from 0 (no desire) to 7 (enormously powerful desire). Our goal is not to add them up or to try to create an overall score. Rather, these numbers allow you to compare cravings over time. When you fill out this questionnaire again, take a look at your scores for each item before and after to see how they have changed.

Rate from 0 (no desire) to 7 (enormously powerful desire)

Red meat	_____	Nonchocolate candy	_____
Poultry	_____	Fruit	_____
Fish or shellfish	_____	Green vegetables	_____
Cheese	_____	Other vegetables	_____
Cow's milk	_____	Bread	_____
Ice cream	_____	Cookies or cake	_____
Eggs	_____	Sugar	_____
Chocolate	_____	Potato chips	_____

Cleaning Your Slate

Now you have a clear picture of where you stand. You know what you're eating, what you weigh, what you crave, and perhaps additional details about your nutrient intake and health. Now it's to time get started.

- **Choose a three-week period.** Take out your calendar and pick a starting date when it will be convenient for you to make some diet changes. Because all this is a bit new, you'll want to avoid times when you are traveling, major holidays, and April 14 if you're an accountant.

  If you are a young woman, you'll get an extra benefit if you start on the first day of your period and extend the Kickstart from three to four weeks. Starting this way, at the beginning of your cycle, mellows the hormone shifts of your entire cycle much more effectively than if you were to start halfway through the month.

- **Use the New Four Food Groups.** During this time period you are going to be on as perfect a diet as possible, eating only the very best of foods. This gives your taste buds a chance to learn some new tricks and to forget some old ones. Let me first give you the basic guidelines, and then we will see how they turn into actual meals.

We will draw our menu from the New Four Food Groups that we learned about in chapter 13. To refresh your memory, this means:

- Vegetables: 4 or more servings per day.
- Legumes (beans, peas, and lentils): 3 servings per day.
- Whole grains: 8 small servings (or four normal servings) per day.
- Fruits: 3 or more servings per day.

During this three-week period avoid meat (red meat, poultry, and fish), dairy products, eggs, added oils, and high-fat foods (potato chips, olives, nuts and nut butters, seeds, and avocadoes). Steer clear of fried foods and any oily or fatty toppings, such as margarine or typical salad dressings (nonfat dressings are fine). Keep in mind that fatty foods interfere with leptin, allowing your appetite to fly out of control and encouraging hormone swings that, in turn, lead to cravings. Avoid them scrupulously for this three-week period. The other reason for avoiding fatty foods is to help your taste buds to reduce their preference for greasy tastes. This is exactly like the shift from whole milk to skim, except that you are intentionally lightening the *entire* diet.

When you select breads, cereals, or other grain products, favor those that retain their normal fiber (e.g., brown rice, rather than white rice) and also favor those with a low GI, that is, below 90 on the chart beginning on page 93. These choices will keep your blood sugar steady and hold hunger at bay.

Those are the basic guidelines: Use the New Four Food Groups, be very careful about added oils, go high-fiber, and choose low-GI foods.

So, what does all this translate into on your plate? The foods you'll now focus on are not really so different from what you already eat. At dinner your salad will be the same, except that it will have a nonfat dressing. Your soup will not be a greasy cream of chicken soup;

instead you'll have minestrone, lentil, split pea, or black bean soup. They are all hearty and satisfying, but are very low in fat and high in healthy fiber, with a stunningly low GI to block rebounding hunger.

Instead of meaty chili, have a bean chili or chunky vegetable chili, or perhaps an autumn stew of vegetables, beans, and hearty grains. Top your pasta with a marinara, primavera, or puttanesca sauce instead of with meat sauces.

The foods you will be eating will be naturally low in calories, so you should increase your portion sizes a bit so that you don't get hungry later. In a recent study we found that, when people followed these guidelines and ate until they were full, they still had a marked reduction in calorie intake, nearly 400 calories less each day. The reason is that high-fiber foods are very filling and satisfying, and by skipping meat, cheese, and oily foods there is so little fat in the diet that calorie intake plummets.

You might be saying to yourself that this is more of a change than you need. You might feel, for example, that it's just chocolate or cookies that have you enslaved, and you're not so worried about meat, cheese, or some of the other things we're leaving out. Let me encourage you to follow these guidelines anyway. Bad habits feed off each other. As we saw in chapter 9, a young woman eating meat, cheese, butter, or other fatty foods drives up the amount of estrogen in her bloodstream, leading to a severe estrogen drop at the end of the month, which then accentuates cravings for chocolate and sweets during the last week of her cycle. A similar phenomenon occurs with sugary foods. Sugary foods in the morning spark cravings later in the day. So our job is to really clean house, so to speak. It is best to break *all* your bad habits at the same time.

- **Do not intentionally limit calories.** There should be no limit on portion size or on seconds—within reason. You can eat all you want,

> ❧ Instead of meaty chili, have a bean chili or chunky vegetable chili, or perhaps an autumn stew of vegetables, beans, and hearty grains. Top your pasta with a marinara, primavera, or puttanesca sauce instead of with meat sauces.

so long as the foods you eat meet these guidelines. If you are a committed calorie counter, use the Rule of Ten that we learned about in chapter 8 to make sure you don't cut calories too severely. Simply multiply your ideal body weight by ten, which gives you the number of calories you need each day, as a minimum. An adequate food intake, along with the strong emphasis on low-fat foods, keeps your leptin system working strong, so hunger stays within bounds.

- **Take a multiple vitamin.** Any common brand is fine. It will provide vitamin B_{12}, which is important, as we saw in the last chapter. It will also ease your mind in case you're worried that you're missing something during this dietary transition.

- **Do it 100 percent.** Resist the temptation to deviate from these guidelines. Allow yourself to experience what it is like to be on as close to a perfect diet as is humanly possible.

As Mary Ann, our volunteer you met in the Introduction, said, it is easier to simply set aside tempting foods than to try to limit them to "manageable" amounts. Teasing yourself with small bits of unhealthy foods leads to "guaranteed feelings of deprivation because of having to limit so many things."

Yvonne agreed: "I find it easier to have none of the foods to which I'm addicted, rather than a little of one of them. For me, there's no such thing as two or three Twizzlers or jelly beans. Also, it helps me enormously to have good substitutes ready to eat."

Planning Your Menu

Let's pick out some breakfasts. Write down ideas on a piece of paper for healthy breakfasts that follow the guidelines above and that appeal to you. You'll find plenty of suggestions in the menu section. Old-fashioned oatmeal with cinnamon and raisins, a half cantaloupe, whole grain toast, a breakfast burrito, scrambled tofu—there are many healthy choices.

As we saw in chapter 6, I would encourage you to keep two things in mind at every breakfast: First, go high-fiber. Old-fashioned oatmeal, for example, is rich and satisfying, and its slow-release sugars will give you energy and keep your appetite at bay. Second, include a protein-rich food, such as a meat substitute (e.g. vegetarian sausage) or, as is especially common in Europe or Latin America, a bean dish. A spoonful of chickpeas, for example, might seem more normal for a lunchtime salad, but you'll find that, eaten at the beginning of your breakfast, it provides energy for later in the day, with none of the fat and cholesterol that comes from eggs, bacon, or other typical breakfast fare.

An adequate breakfast is key. So write your breakfast ideas down; they will become a shopping list.

- **Now choose the rest of your menu for the next three weeks.**
  Knowing what you're going to eat will prevent hunger and help you avoid situations where empty shelves lead to a trip to the convenience store or fast-food restaurant.

  What will you have for lunch? How about dinner? Write down the choices that appeal to you, looking through the menus and recipes in the back of this book for suggestions. How about French onion, or lentil soup, a chuckwagon stew, mushroom stroganoff, vegetable stir-fry, or a zucchini and herb calzone? Keep your list realistic, taking into account where you will be. For example, you may have more latitude at home than you would at work. Would you like to bring in some leftovers to keep in the refrigerator at the office? Perhaps a sandwich or can of soup that is healthier than what is served at the fast-food restaurant on the corner? Don't limit calories and don't skip meals.

- **Plan your snacks.** Stock up on fruit, perhaps keeping a bowl of sliced cantaloupe or melon in the refrigerator. Instant soups, carrot sticks, rice cakes, dried fruit, and many other simple snacks can be lifesavers when hunger strikes. Check out the many other healthy snack ideas in the next chapter and the recipe section.

- **Go shopping.** Stock your pantry with the foods you will need. Our goal is to be sure we never run out of healthful foods. You might find it handy to cook extra food on the weekend so it's ready during the week.

  If you haven't done so already, take a look at the health food store. Pick up some foods that may be new to you and test them out. It is worth trying the substitutes for meat, cheese, and milk that are now on the market. Try the varieties of foods from other lands, such as rice pilaf, hummus, or tabouli, now packaged for quick preparation.

Take a new look at the some of the neglected aisles at the grocery store. The produce aisles often stock meat substitutes, soy milk, and other healthy products, along with familiar as well as new and exotic fruits and vegetables. You may also find interesting products in the "health" or "dietetic" aisles. And look at the shelves with innumerable varieties of colorful dried beans.

At a library or bookstore pick up some of the cookbooks listed in the Recommended Reading list on page 316.

- **Plan your restaurants.** Think for a moment about where you will eat if you go out for lunch or for an evening dinner. As we'll see in the next chapter, ethnic restaurants offer plenty of choices, if you can convince the chef to contain his or her exuberance for oils.

- **Give away the offending foods.** If there is contraband in the refrigerator, it presents more of a temptation than you need. Throw it away or give it to a neighbor or a homeless shelter. If you're not ready to do this you're not ready to change.

  If your husband, wife, or significant other is reluctant to see unhealthy foods leave the kitchen, it is time for some encouragement and a bit of assertiveness on your part. The late Benjamin Spock, M.D., used to joke about this happening in his own life. He was in his eighties when he decided to become a vegetarian. His wife Mary helped shore up his resolve in times of weakness. She did this by throwing away anything unhealthy he might buy. He recalled how he might occasionally buy some expensive cheese, only to find it missing when he went to look for it later. "Mary," he would say, "Didn't I have a little piece of cheese in the refrigerator?" To which Mary would say, "Yes, dear, I threw it away. I love you too much to leave food like that lying around."

- **Beware of times of vulnerability.** As you're getting started, take one more look at your three-day dietary record. When did problems tend to arise, and where were you at the time? If you had a chocolate binge every afternoon as you did errands around the house, the answer may be simple: don't be hungry (adjust your mealtimes), and don't be home (plan to be somewhere where eating is impossible).

- **Plan your exercise.** In chapter 10 we saw the value of regular exercise in resetting your natural diurnal rhythm and subduing cravings. The type of exercise you do is not so important as its frequency— including it at regular intervals in your weekly routine. Using the guidelines on pages 123–124, pencil exercise into your calendar, and ask someone to join you, if you can, to help you stick to it.

- **Check your weight.** It is good to step on the scale once a week or so. If you drop about a pound per week you'll be very much like our research participants.

- **Staying on track.** Here is a simple checklist we use to help our research volunteers stay on track each day. Photocopy it and use it daily during the three-week Kickstart.

Daily Checklist

Here is your checklist of the foods you need each day. This guide will provide about 1,500 calories. At the bottom you will find ways to adjust your calorie intake to meet your own energy requirements. Photocopy this checklist and use it daily.

Food Group	Serving Recommendations
GRAINS 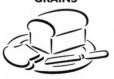 *(A serving equals about 80 calories.)* 6 of your 8 servings should be from whole grain sources like wheat bread, brown rice, whole wheat pasta, bran cereal, oatmeal, etc.	8 servings a day. A serving is ½ cup cooked grain, like oatmeal or pasta. The exception is rice. A serving of rice is ⅓ cup. One oz. of dry cereal (usually ¾ to 1 cup) is a serving. One slice of bread or half a pita bread or a tortilla is a serving. Most bagels are actually *four* servings, so watch out for that. Eight servings may sound like a lot, but, when you think about it, 1 cup of oatmeal for breakfast, a sandwich with two slices of bread for lunch, and a bowl of pasta made with 1½ cups of pasta with a slice of bread meets your 8 serving goal. Check off your servings here: ☐ ☐ ☐ ☐ ☐ ☐ ☐ ☐
LEGUMES *(A serving equals about 100 calories.)* Have at least 1 cup of beans every day.	3 servings a day. A serving is a half-cup of cooked beans, peas, or lentils, ½ cup low-fat bean spread, 1 cup low-fat soy milk, or 1 oz. of veggie meat. Check off your servings here: ☐ ☐ ☐
VEGETABLES *(A serving equals 35–50 calories.)* At least one serving should be a raw vegetable, like salad or carrot sticks.	4 servings a day. This means ½ cup cooked or 1 cup raw. As long as the vegetable isn't topped with a fatty dressing or sauce, you can go all out with vegetables. At least 1 of your vegetable servings should be calcium-containing leafy greens, such as broccoli, kale, or collards. Check off your servings here: ☐ ☐ ☐ ☐

Food Group	Serving Recommendations
FRUIT *(A serving equals 80 calories.)*	3 servings a day. A serving is ½ cup chopped, or one small piece of fruit. Many fruits are large, so a serving usually means a half an apple or a half a banana. Aim for the low-calorie, high-nutrition varieties, such as strawberries, kiwis, mangoes, blueberries, peaches, plums, oranges, grapefruit, and raspberries. Check off your servings here: ☐ ☐ ☐
SWEETS (OPTIONAL)  One sweet serving has no more than 1 gram of fat and equals 100 calories.	No more than one sweets serving per day. Your sweets should be fat-free. Try fruit if you are craving sweets. Other low-fat ideas include having a bowl of sweetened whole grain cereal with low-fat soy milk, making a soy milk/fruit smoothie, or sautéing bananas or apples (in water) with a little cinnamon or sugar. Check off no more than one serving: ☐

If you've checked off all your boxes and are still hungry, add extra servings from the vegetable or bean groups. If, on the other hand, this is too much food for you, cut out the sweets first, then subtract a grain serving or two. However, you shouldn't cut your calories too much. Most people should never go below 1,200 calories/day. Use the Rule of Ten to set your own minimum.

After Three Weeks

When you reach the three-week mark, your body is physically different. Your blood sugar and hormones are now more stable, and your body's sensitivity to leptin and to insulin has almost certainly improved. It's time to see what you've accomplished.

- **Let's do another three-day dietary record**, so you can see how much your eating habits have improved. If you analyze your record on-line, you will likely find that the amount of fat, especially saturated fat, in your diet has plummeted, as has your cholesterol intake. Protective nutrients, like vitamin C, beta-carotene, and folic acid, have probably skyrocketed, thanks to those vegetables, fruits, and beans you've been checking off each day. Over the long run the eating pattern you've just experienced improves immune strength, helps you slim down, and cuts your risk of many health problems.

- **Let's check your cravings.** This is the acid test. Fill out a fresh copy of the questionnaire on page 167 and see if, indeed, your cravings have diminished. In our studies, the vast majority of people have dramatic reductions in their desire for meat, cheese, chocolate, sugar, cookies, and potato chips, and have a new appreciation for the fruits and vegetables their mothers would have wanted them to eat.

- **Check your health.** This is a good time to stand on your scale, if you haven't already, to see if your weight is headed in the right direction. If you checked your cholesterol, blood pressure, or blood sugar before you started, plan to check them again soon. Three weeks is not enough time to see the full effect of a diet change, but it is enough for a noticeable start.

If you like, you can continue on your new, healthy menu indefinitely, and that is certainly the best course. Should you happen to sample a bit of the not-so-healthy foods you thought you loved, you will very like find they have become as uncharismatic as full-fat milk.

If you should happen to slide off the wagon, you can use the three-week program as often as you need to. It will get you back on track with the healthiest possible diet and help you leave troublesome foods behind.

In the next chapter we'll take a closer look at how healthy diets work at restaurants and fast-food outlets, and while traveling. And we'll finish up with enough recipes and food ideas to give you a great many healthy choices for any occasion.

15

On the Go: Restaurants, Fast Food, and Snacks

When we put our culinary fate in the hands of a waiter or chef it is sometimes a challenge to stick to a healthful menu. At fast-food restaurants the challenges are far greater. But our goal is not just to cope, but to make restaurant eating one of the pleasures of our newfound healthful lifestyle. And it can be.

In this chapter we'll look at how to choose restaurants and what to order when we get there. And, if we're on the road, we'll look at how to dine healthfully in the world of fast food and airline meals. And we'll finish off with a look at how to pack healthy snacks for work or travel.

On the Town

When it comes to restaurants the key is choice. For starters, it helps to think international. Ethnic restaurants often have a full range of healthful menu items:

- Italian restaurants feature minestrone, pasta and bean soup, pasta marinara or primavera, pesto dishes, and vegetables sautéed with garlic.

- Chinese restaurants have entire menu sections devoted to what will be listed as "vegetables," but are actually main dishes made from tofu, broccoli, spinach, green beans, and other ingredients, and are usually available steamed or fried. They also include plenty of soups, along with various noodle and rice dishes.

- Mexican restaurants serve bean burritos, which, if prepared without lard and not topped with cheese, are usually low in fat and free of cholesterol. Top them with salsa and have rice on the side.

You'll find Italian, Chinese, and Mexican restaurants in just about every community, no matter how small. Midsized and larger cities have many more choices:

- Japanese restaurants serve miso soup, salads, appetizers, and vegetable sushi, all of which are usually very low in fat and delicately prepared.

- Vietnamese and Thai restaurants serve dishes of soft noodles with vegetables and delicate sauces, along with tofu and endless soups and salads.

- Indian restaurants always have a great many vegetarian choices, all of which are delicious, as are their soups and appetizers, such as samosas. But make sure the waiter asks the chef to be careful about the overzealous use of oil and to skip the dairy ingredients.

- Cuban restaurants keep it simple with black beans, salsa, salad, and plantains.

- Ethiopian restaurants capitalize on the fact that some religious groups in Ethiopia follow vegan diets during certain days of the year. They have found ways of turning simple chickpeas, split peas, lentils, green beans, and peppers into delightfully spiced meals eaten with thin, soft bread, rather than cutlery.

- American restaurants—and even steak houses—now feature salad bars and vegetarian selections for those who want them.

Fast Foods

William Castelli, M.D., the former director of the famed Framingham Heart Study, used to joke that, "When you see the Golden Arches, you're probably on the road to the Pearly Gates." Indeed, fast-food restaurants have earned their reputation for fatty fare and super-sized sodas. Nonetheless, it is still possible to survive—and even flourish—in the world of fast food.

Taco Bell offers a bean burrito that if you hold the cheese is low in fat and entirely vegan. Add jalapeños to your heart's content.

In Europe, veggie burgers are nearly universal, although they've been slower to arrive in North America. Burger King has offered a meatless sandwich for years, which consisted simply of all the Whopper's vegetable toppings, minus the meat. In 2002, it introduced the BK Veggie, which is dramatically lower in fat than its other sandwiches (less than 10 grams of fat, compared to around 40 for the Whopper or Burger King's fish sandwich). Other good choices are the Veggie Delite at Subway and Wendy's Garden Pita (hold the dressing), that you can get along with a baked potato, if you'd like.

Most family-style restaurants, like Denny's or Bob Evans, offer plenty of side vegetables that combine to make a hearty meal, and Denny's offers a veggie burger.

Healthy Snacks for Air Travelers

Many airlines have eliminated in-flight meals—and even snacks—and with the long delays at airports, many travelers will find their stomachs growling long before they reach their destinations. Families traveling with children are especially prone to hunger pangs. Here are some tips for healthy travel snacks:

- **Before You Fly:** Do yourself a favor and drop by the health food store. You'll find faux-meat deli slices that resist spoiling, even when your sandwich has had a long wait in your carry-on luggage. Individual soy and rice milk cartons need no refrigeration and are better tolerated than cow's milk by people with sensitive stomachs. And pick up a pack of hummus and pita bread (it can't squash—it's already flat) for an easy in-flight snack.

- **Easy-Packin' Snacks:** A banana is healthy, but it won't do well at the bottom of your luggage. Instead, carry these easy snacks:

- Dried fruit, such as apricots or banana chips. Packaged dried assortments are in stock in every airport newsstand, as is trail mix, another good choice.
- Mandarin oranges are small, tasty, and easy to carry.
- Individual applesauce servings are convenient.
- Baby carrots are healthy and pack well.
- Rice cakes are light as a feather.
- Instant soup cups just need hot water—try lentil, split pea, and black bean soups, or veggie chili. Or pack a small pop-top can of chickpeas.

If You're Traveling with Kids

Bottled water is your best in-flight beverage. Go easy on caffeinated colas and sugary drinks that can make kids cranky.

Avoid milk. It can cause sniffles and ear troubles. Breast-feeding moms should avoid cow's milk and caffeinated beverages, too, as they can cause colic in your baby.

There's always PB & J. It's got plenty of protein, and whole-grain bread makes it a fiber-rich sandwich.

More Healthy Snacks

Even if you're not stuck at an airport you'll want to have healthy snacks on hand. My friend Eilene likes crunchy foods, so her hot-air popcorn popper is always at the ready. She tops it with various seasonings, and it is a totally healthy snack (a cup has only 30 calories and 0.3 grams of fat). Or your tastes might call for pretzels or chocolate sorbet.

You'll probably find that your preferences will drift over time. Years ago, when I first tasted rice cakes I promptly fed them to a group of ducks, who I thought might appreciate them more than I. But somehow I have come to love them, even without salt or sugar coatings. Look down this list of foods to see which ones appeal to you as quick snacks:

- Fresh fruit: bananas, apples, pears, oranges, grapes, etc.
- Precut fruit. Cantaloupe or melons can be purchased already cut into bite-sized squares, or you can prepare your own. Keep them in the refrigerator for times when cravings come on.
- Dried fruit: apricots, papaya, apples, raisins, prunes.
- Chocolate sorbet, available at all health-food stores and many regular groceries.
- Pretzels.
- Rice cakes. Go for the simple, plain varieties. You'll soon see that you don't need the sugary toppings.
- Air-popped popcorn topped with garlic salt, mixed seasonings (e.g. Spike), or nutritional yeast.
- Nonfat crackers with jam.
- Baby carrots.
- Baked sweet potatoes.
- Hot soup: minestrone, split pea, lentil.

The pace of life has changed dramatically in recent decades. We're on the go more than ever, and home cooking has been all but replaced by restaurant and fast-food dining. But, as we've seen, that does not mean we have to settle for less than a healthy meal. The choices are there, once you know where to look.

Part IV
Menus and Recipes

By now you have a pretty good handle on the whys and hows of healthy eating. It's time to dig in. This wonderful collection of recipes and cooking information was prepared by Joanne Stepaniak, M.S. Ed., an accomplished chef, author, and educator from Pittsburgh, Pennsylvania. You may have seen her previous books, *Raising Vegetarian Children, The Uncheese Cookbook,* and *Vegan Vittles,* among many others. Joanne's Web address is www.vegsource.com/joanne.

As you'll see, these recipes are fast, and most use familiar ingredients. They are also delicious and wonderfully healthful.

We'll start with a look at healthy substitutions, so when your taste buds say fatty chocolate or gooey cheese, but your good sense is not so sure, you'll be covered with healthier choices. We'll then look at a few ingredients that may be new to you, in case you've never tasted tahini or balsamic vinegar.

You'll find a week's worth of delicious craving-busting menus, followed by a generous collection of breakfasts, lunches, and dinners, complete from soups and salads to scrumptious desserts. Nutritional information is provided for each recipe.

For more recipe ideas, please take a look at Joanne's previous books or my own. And the Internet now links an enormous number of people who are taking the same steps you are. Check out www.pcrm. org, the Web site of the Physicians Committee for Responsible Medicine. Or you might visit other sites friendly to low-fat and vegetarian nutrition, such as www.VeggieChef.com, www.VRG.org, www.VegSource. com, www.vegetariantimes.com, www.vegtv.com, or www.Vegan.com.

Healthy Substitutions

Here is how to get all the taste of sweets, chocolate, cheese, and meaty dishes with little of the fat or other undesirables of less healthy choices. After you've looked at these tips, you'll also want to check the treasury of healthy choices in the recipes that follow.

Thinking Outside the Sugar Box

When it comes to replacing sugar, just one sweetener—fructose—has been proven to have a lower glycemic index than typical table sugar. Derived from fruit sugar, fructose closely resembles granulated white sugar, but it is more concentrated, so you'll need less to achieve a similar result. It has a noticeably smaller effect on blood sugar. Use it in place of sugar as an all-purpose sweetener in baking, cooking, and in hot or cold beverages.

There are other sweeteners you may wish to use in place of ordinary sugar. Their glycemic indices have not yet been established. Several, however, are considerably more flavorful than table sugar, so they allow you to use less to achieve tasty results. Even so, most of them are sugars in their own right, so I am presenting them here, not to recommend that you dig into them with gusto, but rather to show you a few options some people use temporarily as they pry themselves loose from a sugar habit. If you find it easier to not use any forms of sugar at all, you can skip this list.

Barley Malt Syrup

Dark, sticky, and boldly flavored, barley malt syrup is not as assertive as molasses, nor as sweet as honey. Barley malt syrup is a wonderful addition to winter squash and pumpkin breads, bran muffins, and hearty rye or pumpernickel breads. Use it to glaze sweet potatoes and to make winter malted "milk" shakes using frozen bananas and vanilla nondairy milk.

Brown Rice Syrup

A traditional Asian sweetener, brown rice syrup is the mildest of the liquid sweeteners. Use it to replace honey in cooking and baking, to sweeten hot or cold beverages and cereals, or as a spread for fresh breads.

Concentrated Fruit Juice Syrups

Fruit juice syrups come from juice that has had its fiber and most of its water boiled away. After opening, fruit syrups should be refrigerated.

Date Sugar

Not actually a sugar in the conventional sense, date sugar is simply ground, dehydrated dates. It is about two-thirds as sweet as white table sugar and may be ground or blended to a finer texture, if desired. Dates are high in fiber and rich in a wide variety of vitamins and minerals. Date sugar can be exchanged measure for measure for sugar in baking cakes, muffins, and quick breads. Use it in place of brown sugar to make crumb toppings for pies and fruit crisps. Don't use date sugar to sweeten beverages, however, as the tiny date pieces do not dissolve.

Evaporated Cane Juice

Evaporated cane juice refers to the boiled and extracted liquid of sugarcane stalks that is dried and crystallized naturally. This involves a chemical-free process comprising fewer steps than white cane sugar, Sucanat, or turbinado sugar (see below), allowing more of the sugarcane's natural taste, color, and nutrients to remain. Lime (calcium phosphate) is used as a catalyst to separate impurities in the freshly squeezed cane juice. Its fine, golden crystals have a faint molasses flavor, dissolve well, and very closely resemble the taste and delicate texture of white table sugar.

Frozen Fruit Juice Concentrate

Frozen juice concentrate is simply juice that has been refined to remove fiber and approximately two-thirds of the water content. It can be made into juice by blending with water. When used as a sweeteners, however, it should not be reconstituted. Fruit juice concentrates should always be stored in the freezer.

Maple Sugar

Maple sugar is dehydrated, crystallized maple syrup (see "Maple Syrup" below). It has a delectable maple flavor and can be substituted for sugar measure for measure in all types of recipes.

Maple Syrup

While this beloved sweetener is mainly sucrose, a simple sugar, it does contain several trace minerals, plus measurable amounts of calcium and iron. Maple syrup tends to be pricey, as it takes about 30 to 40 gallons of sap to produce one gallon of syrup. Store it in the refrigerator to discourage insects and retard mold.

Molasses

Molasses is the thick, dark syrup that remains after sugar crystals are removed during cane sugar refinement. It is probably the only natural sweetener that can boast any real nutritional value, being rich in iron, vitamin B$_6$, and, depending on the type, calcium and potassium. Blackstrap molasses is richest in calcium, but it is not very sweet and has a strong assertive taste and a dark brown color, making it unsuitable for many types of cooking. Use molasses in making dark rye or pumpernickel breads, in sweet potato dishes, and to make full-bodied barbecue sauces. Barbados molasses is a close relative of blackstrap, but is somewhat lighter in color and flavor. Store molasses in a tightly sealed container at room temperature.

Sorghum Syrup

Made from the stalks of a cereal grain related to millet, sweet sorghum syrup has been produced in the United States since colonial days and is especially popular in the southeastern states. Store sorghum syrup at room temperature in cooler seasons, and in the refrigerator during warm months to discourage insects and retard mold.

Stevia

Among the most concentrated natural sweeteners, stevia is derived from an herb native to Paraguay, where for centuries its leaves have been used to sweeten food and beverages and as a folk remedy for diabetes and high blood pressure. Stevia leaves are sometimes available ground into a greenish powder. The active sweetening components, called *glycosides,* are isolated and sold as a white powder or clear liquid. In these forms stevia doesn't claim to confer the benefits of the leaves, but is a potent sweetener (two hundred to three hundred times sweeter than sugar) that is calorie-free and won't raise blood sugar levels.

Stevia is intensely sweet, with a slight herbal aftertaste with a hint of black licorice flavor. Stevia is best used to sweeten hot or cold beverages. Because it has such a high sweetening quotient compared to sugar, using it to replace sugar in baked goods and desserts can be tricky and requires some trial and error. If you're up for experimenting, here are a few general guidelines:

- Start with a very small quantity. Try ¼ teaspoon of the liquid extract to replace 1 cup of white table sugar. Add just one drop at a time, tasting as you go, until you achieve the level of sweetness that tastes right to you. Be sure to measure carefully, using a measuring spoon or dropper. Too much stevia will make foods bitter.

- If the recipe you're using requires at least some sugar for body, texture, and flavor, try replacing just half the sugar with stevia, following the guidelines above.

- Stevia is a good complement to the natural sweetness of fruit, particularly citrus fruit, lemonade, fruity teas, fruit salad, smoothies, and fruit purées.

The U.S. Food and Drug Administration has approved stevia as a dietary supplement, but not as a sweetener, citing insufficient safety data. Stevia is sold in natural food stores or on the Web at www.stevia.com or www.lowcarbmall.com. While it is comparatively expensive, a little bit goes a very long way.

Sucanat

Sucanat is the trade name for a specific brand of unbleached sugarcane juice that is dehydrated and then milled into granules much like white sugar, but with a deep amber color similar to brown sugar and a moderate molasses taste. Sucanat is about 88 percent sucrose, or simple sugar, as compared to table sugar, which is 99 percent sucrose. As an all-purpose sweetener for baking, cooking, and in hot or cold drinks, use it measure for measure as a replacement for white table sugar.

Turbinado Sugar

Turbinado is granulated sugarcane that has been steam-cleaned, rather than bleached, and filtered through activated carbon. Turbinado sugar's coarse crystals retain up to 15 percent of the natural molasses, imparting a light caramel color and a gentle molasses flavor. It contains about the same amount of sucrose as refined white table sugar.

Check the shelves of your local natural food store for these and other commercial sweeteners. Experiment with them to see which ones have the flavors you prefer. You may wish to buy small quantities of several different sweeteners and try them in various recipes before purchasing larger amounts.

Here are some tips for using alternative liquid sweeteners:

- To replace white sugar with a liquid sweetener, reduce the total amount of other liquid ingredients in the recipe by about ¼ cup for each cup of liquid sweetener used.

- To liquefy liquid sweetener that has crystallized, place the jar in a pan of hot water for several minutes.

- To accurately measure liquid sweeteners and keep them from sticking to the measuring utensil, first rub a little oil in your measuring cup or spoon.

Substitute the following for the sweetening power of 1 cup of white sugar. Some experimenting may be necessary to achieve the desired results.

- barley malt: 1 to 1⅓ cups
- brown rice syrup: 1 to 1⅓ cups
- date sugar: 1 cup
- evaporated cane juice: 1 cup
- fructose: ½ cup
- maple syrup: ½ to ¾ cup
- molasses: ½ cup
- sorghum syrup: ½ cup
- Sucanat: 1 cup
- turbinado sugar: 1 cup

Getting that Chocolate Taste

One of the easiest ways to break free from chocolate is to use cocoa powder instead. Cocoa powder is made by separating most of the cocoa butter out of the chocolate liquor, making it much less fattening than chocolate.

Wondercocoa (made by Wonderslim) is real cocoa, but is even

lower in fat than other common brands. What's more, it is caffeine-free, with the caffeine extracted using a natural process. You'll find it in supermarkets and natural food stores and you can use it in any recipe that calls for cocoa.

Dutch process cocoa has been treated with alkali to reduce cocoa's natural acidity. This gives cocoa a darker appearance and milder taste. Because Dutch process cocoa is more alkaline, it may alter the chemistry in a recipe, reacting differently from natural cocoa with baking soda or baking powder. So if a recipe simply calls for cocoa, use natural cocoa. In recipes without leaveners, natural and Dutch process cocoa are interchangeable.

Sweetened cocoa drink mixes have sugar, milk solids, and other flavorings added to them, so you'll want to look for pure, unsweetened cocoa, sometimes called "baker's cocoa."

Natural unsweetened cocoa powder imparts a deep chocolate flavor to baked goods and beverages. Its intense flavor makes it well suited for use in brownies, cookies, and some chocolate cakes. The combination of natural cocoa and baking soda creates a leavening action that causes the batter to rise in the oven. Try adding cocoa powder to muffin recipes or to soy or rice milk, with a touch of sugar. For a dense, rich, chocolaty indulgence, make Instant Chocolate Pudding or Ultra-Fudge Brownies, both on page 292. You're in for a very special treat!

If your goal is to avoid migraines, try carob instead of chocolate or cocoa. Carob powder is made from the dried and ground pods of a tropical locust tree. Roasted carob powder has a rich, chocolatelike flavor and is often substituted in recipes measure for measure for cocoa powder. It is not, however, low in fat, so a switch from chocolate to carob will not trim your waistline.

Carob is somewhat sweeter than cocoa, so you may find that you need less sweetener when using it. The recipes in this book that use carob call for only unsweetened roasted carob powder, which you'll find in natural food stores and some supermarkets. Store it in a tightly sealed container at room temperature away from heat and moisture.

Natural food stores carry chocolate sorbet, low-fat Tofutti, and other chocolaty frozen desserts and ice cream alternatives that let you sidestep some of the fat and calories. Many come in rich, fudgey flavors that taste delicious without the fat of regular ice cream.

Getting that Cheese Taste

As a source of calories, fat, and cholesterol, cheese is hard to beat. Slabs of cheese weigh down grocery checkout scales everywhere. Unfortunately, bathroom scales reflect a similar trend.

Happily, breaking free of cheese is easy, and the results—on the scale, on your cholesterol level, and in how you feel every day—can be spectacular. Here are some easy kitchen tricks that will make it a breeze to get that cheese taste:

- **Dairy-free soy cheeses** now are widely available, but be sure to read the package label. While most cheese analogs take the helpful step of replacing animal fat with vegetable oils, many include milk-derived casein—one of the suspected addicting components of cheese—and some use hydrogenated oils, which are nearly as bad as animal fats in promoting cholesterol problems.

- **Avocado** can substitute for the rich "mouth feel" of cheese on sandwiches, salads, or in Mexican food. It is much lower in saturated fat than cheese, so it is not as likely to raise your cholesterol level or promote heart problems (the fat in avocados is mostly monounsaturated). Although the *type* of fat in avocadoes is far preferable to that in cheese, the overall *amount* still is high (up to 15 grams for half an avocado). So, while it won't hurt your cholesterol level, having avocados regularly might add to your waistline.

- **Nutritional yeast** is an extremely versatile topping that lends a cheesy flavor to spaghetti sauce, stews, casseroles, and even pizza. Because it is an inactive yeast it doesn't have any leavening power, as does yeast used for bread baking. Instead, it is prized for its delicious "cheesy" taste and high nutritional content. When mixed with certain seasonings, nutritional yeast also can impart a poultrylike flavor. A serving of one and one-half heaping tablespoons (16 grams) has only 47 calories, boasts 8 grams of protein, and contains only 0.8 grams of fat.

Pure nutritional yeast (Red Star Vegetarian Support Formula) is most commonly found in the bulk section of natural food stores. A serving (about 1½ to 2 tablespoons) of Vegetarian Support Formula flakes contains a full day's supply of vitamin B_{12}. Some brands of packaged nutritional yeast have been combined with whey, a byproduct of cheese processing. For packaged nutritional yeast without any additives, look for Kal domestic (not imported) nutritional yeast at your natural food store (this is Red Star Vegetarian Support Formula repackaged). Red Star Vegetarian Support Formula also may be ordered in bulk from The Mail Order Catalog, Box 180, Summertown, TN 38483. Call for current price information at 1-800-695-2241 or visit www. healthy-eating.com.

Do not confuse nutritional yeast with brewer's yeast, which is a byproduct of the brewing industry and is extremely bitter. Nutritional yeast is available in flakes or powder, but you'll probably find the flakes more versatile and delicious.

- Make the wonderful Cheesy Sauce for Macaroni (see recipe on page 265) to top any favorite pasta.
- Try your hand with Quick and Easy Alfredo Sauce (see recipe on page 264). It's unbeatable!
- Treat your family to Better-Than-Grilled Cheese sandwiches (see recipe on page 250).
- Make your own healthful cheddary cheeze spread with Chick Cheeze (see recipe on page 240) to use in sandwiches, soups, or Mexican and Italian dishes.
- Top your spaghetti or baked potatoes with scrumptious Eggplant Pecan Pesto (recipe on page 241).
- Look for vegan parmesan cheese substitute in the dairy section of your supermarket or natural food store. This soy-based cheese alternative is surprisingly similar to dairy parmesan in flavor, texture, and aroma, and can replace it measure for measure in any recipe.
- Many recipes work fine if the cheese simply is omitted. A vegetable lasagna can be delicious without cheese. For pizza, use extra sauce and veggies.
- Top casseroles and pasta with ground nuts or seeds instead of cheese.

- Stir tahini or cashew butter into soups, sauces, gravies, or spreads for added richness and a creamy texture.
- Use mashed, water-packed tofu, mixed with a little lemon juice, in place of ricotta or cottage cheese.
- Add small amounts of light miso or soy sauce to provide the saltiness of cheese in recipes and add a rich, aged flavor.

In choosing which recipes to prepare, you might find it easiest to avoid foods whose flavor depends on cheese. A quesadilla, for example, may have nothing going for it in the taste department when the cheese is omitted. Rather than trying to substitute, why not pick a veggie enchilada, bean taco, or other healthy meal instead?

Meaty Flavor Without the Meat

When people contemplate setting meat aside, their first question usually is "Where will I get my protein?" The truth is that protein is an integral part of nearly all plant foods, including vegetables and grains. Beans, seitan, tempeh, tofu, and TVP (textured vegetable protein) are high in protein and—if you use them the right way—are absolutely delicious, and they readily replace meat in many traditional recipes. They are extremely adaptable to a wide range of dishes and eating styles. Tofu, TVP, tempeh, and seitan have an uncanny way of taking on flavors and seasonings. Beans add bite and robustness to meals, and their rainbow of colors can enliven any dish. If you are unaccustomed to these amazing foods, be daring and sample them in the recipes contained in this book, or use them to replace meat in your old standards. You're in for a surprise!

In addition to these remarkable foods you'll find an ever-expanding selection of new products at your local supermarket or natural food store. In addition to veggie burgers and tofu dogs, you'll find everything imaginable, from vegetarian "chicken" nuggets to "ground round," and from meatless pepperoni and salami to turkey and even jerky. They are handy for those days you don't feel much like cooking and are convenient to add to casseroles, or keep on reserve for "emergency" lunches and dinners. No matter what you're craving, there is an appetizing choice to satisfy your urge.

Beans

Since ancient times, many varieties of beans have been a part of the growth and survival of cultures worldwide. Beans are a rich source of protein, complex carbohydrates, and soluble fiber. Whether fresh, dried, canned, frozen, or home-cooked, beans don't lose any of their usable fiber, because they remain essentially unrefined from the field to market to your table.

If beans cause you to have a little gas, here are a few tips:

1. Keep in mind that a little bit goes a long way. If you're replacing a huge steak with an equally huge serving of beans, it pays to realize that you'll still get plenty of protein and good overall nutrition with smaller servings. Complement beans with grains and vegetables.
2. Soak dried beans overnight (or for at least eight hours) and replace the soak water with fresh water before cooking. The indigestible sugars leach into the soak water and are rinsed away.
3. Cook beans for as long as possible. Heat helps break down the fiber in beans as well as the complex sugars, making them more digestible.
4. Cook beans with epazote, a pungent wild herb commonly used in Mexican and Caribbean cuisine. Epazote is a carminative—that is, it breaks down some of the complex sugars in beans, which helps reduce the production of gas.
5. Kombu, a sea vegetable, added to both the soak water and cook water tends to make beans more digestible.
6. Rinse canned beans well. This washes away excess sodium, as well as any complex sugars that have leached into the bean liquid in the can.

Tofu

Tofu, sometimes called soybean curd, is a soft, cheeselike food made by curdling fresh hot soy milk. Traditionally the curdling agent used to make tofu is *nigari,* a compound found in natural ocean water, or calcium sulfate, a naturally occurring mineral. Curds also can be produced by acidic foods, such as lemon juice or vinegar. The curds are then pressed into a solid block.

Tofu is rich in high-quality protein. It also is a good source of B-vitamins and iron. When the curdling agent used to make tofu is calcium salt, it is an excellent source of calcium. Generally, the softer the tofu, the lower the fat content. Tofu also is very low in sodium, making it a perfect food for people on sodium-restricted diets.

In recipes, tofu has the miraculous ability to take on any flavorings that are added to it. Crumble it into a pot of chili and it absorbs all the rich, spicy flavors. Blend it with cocoa and a sweetener and it turns into chocolate pudding. Cubes of firm tofu can be added to any casserole, soup, or stew for a meaty texture. Blend tofu with smoothies for a rich and creamy shake. Or mash it with seasonings and to make an eggless egg salad. The possibilities are limited only by your imagination and creativity.

Three main types of tofu are available in stores throughout North America:

- *Firm regular tofu (also called "Chinese tofu" or "water-packed tofu")* is sold in a sealed tub or box. It holds up well in stir-fry dishes, soups, or on the grill—anywhere that you want it to maintain its shape. Firm regular tofu generally is higher in protein, fat, and calcium than other types.

- *Soft regular tofu* is a good choice for recipes that call for blended tofu or for use in Asian-style dishes.

- *Silken tofu (also called "Japanese tofu")* is made by a slightly different process, that results in a creamy, custardlike product. Silken tofu works well in pureed or blended dishes, such as smoothies, puddings, and creamy soups. It comes in a variety of firmnesses, ranging from soft to extra-firm.

Tofu is sold in water-filled tubs, vacuum packs, or in aseptic brick packages. You'll find it in the produce section of grocery stores, although some stores keep it in the dairy or deli sections. Sometimes it is sold in bulk in food cooperatives or Asian markets. Unless it is aseptically packaged, it should be kept cold. As with any perishable food, check the expiration date on the package.

Once the package is open, leftover tofu should be rinsed and covered with fresh water for storage. Change the water daily to keep it fresh, and use it within a week.

Tofu can be frozen up to five months. Defrosted tofu has a pleasant caramel color and a firm texture that soaks up marinade sauces and is great for the grill.

Seitan

Seitan is a low-fat, high-protein, firm-textured food made from gluten, a protein extracted from wheat flour that is first combined with water and mixed to a bread dough consistency. The dough is then thoroughly rinsed under running water to remove most of the starch and much of the bran. What is left is firm, high-protein gluten that is simmered in a broth usually containing soy sauce and the sea vegetable *kombu*. It is then ready to be used in casseroles, stews, stir-fries, sandwiches, wraps, or just about anywhere that you might previously have used meat.

Nutritionally, seitan is a high-quality protein that provides B vitamins and iron, and contains no saturated fat or cholesterol. As a meat substitute, seitan is versatile, nutritious, and delicious. Here are a few ways you can use it in meals:

- Dice seitan and stir-fry it with your favorite vegetables. Serve over brown rice or pasta.

- Sauté thin slices of seitan in olive oil. Sandwich it between rye or pumpernickel bread, and garnish with mustard, lettuce, tomatoes, onion, and pickles.

- Make a seitan "Reuben." Thinly slice seitan and layer it on hearty, dark rye bread along with well-drained cole slaw and dairy-free Thousand Island dressing. Grill in a little oil, if desired, and serve with potato salad and a dill pickle.

- Incorporate diced bits of seitan into your favorite casserole dishes.

- Use diced seitan as a substitute for chicken or beef in hearty stews, chili, kebobs, and Mexican dishes.

Tempeh

Tempeh is a cultured cake of beans and/or grains that has been a staple food in Indonesia for centuries. It is made by cooking and dehulling grains and fermenting them for eighteen to twenty-four hours. As with other fermented foods, it is this incubation process that makes tempeh so savory and delicious.

The protein found in tempeh is every bit as high-quality as that derived from meats, and it skips all meat's disadvantages. As with all vegetable proteins, tempeh has no cholesterol, and it has a great deal less saturated fat than protein derived from animal sources. One three-ounce serving of tempeh contains seven grams of dietary fiber. In addition, the fermentation process used to make tempeh breaks down the oligosaccharides that make beans difficult for some people to digest. Another bonus is that soybeans contain significant amounts of *isoflavones,* phytoestrogens that may reduce the risk of certain kinds of cancer and may help curtail menstrual and menopausal symptoms in some women.

Fresh tempeh has a firm texture and a fragrant, mushroomlike aroma. Small black spots may occasionally appear on the surface. These spots do not necessarily indicate spoilage, but are part of the tempeh culture's life cycle. If frozen in the package, tempeh keeps well for up to a year. Once thawed, it will keep for approximately seven days in the refrigerator. Most tempeh packages are stamped with a "sell by" or "use by" date.

If the package does not state that the tempeh is "fully cooked and ready to use," you will need to steam, sauté, or bake it for twenty minutes before eating it, or make sure that the recipe in which you are using it involves cooking it for that length of time.

TVP (Texturized Vegetable Protein)

TVP is a wonderful product to substitute for ground beef. It is produced from soy flour after the soybean oil has been extracted. It then is cooked under pressure and dried. TVP has a long shelf life when stored in airtight containers in a cool dry place, and it is an excellent source of economical protein. Unlike meat, TVP contains dietary fiber and has zero cholesterol. It also contributes calcium and magnesium to the diet. Some brands are fortified with vitamins, including vitamin B_{12}.

TVP is a healthy timesaver. Whenever you are in a rush you can have tacos or Sloppy Joes in under fifteen minutes by using TVP instead of ground beef. It's also great for camping, as it is very light and just a little boiled water turns it into a meal. Once TVP is rehydrated it becomes perishable, so always store it in the refrigerator and use it within a reasonable amount of time.

TVP comes in various shapes and sizes, so how much water you need to reconstitute it will depend largely on what type you are using. The small granules or bits are easiest to rehydrate: just add them directly to soups, sauces, chili, or stew, or pour ⅞ cup boiling water or vegetable broth over 1 cup of dry TVP and let it stand for five to ten minutes. Adding a little ketchup, lemon juice, vinegar, or other acidic ingredients will help speed up the rehydration process if you are in a hurry. Using less liquid to rehydrate the TVP will create a slightly firmer and dryer texture. Alternatively, you can partially rehydrate the TVP and then add it to any moist recipe you are cooking. It will absorb some of the liquid as well as the flavor from the dish. It retains its texture well in spaghetti sauce and stews, making it an especially good choice if you anticipate saving some leftovers.

Ingredients That May Be New to You

H ere is a list of a few ingredients that may be unfamiliar to you. They are used in some of the recipes in this book, and you'll want to turn some of them into kitchen staples. You also will find descriptions of additional ingredients in the Healthy Substitutions chapter on pages 185–199.

Almond butter: Similar to peanut butter, almond butter is made from raw or roasted almonds that have been ground into a paste. It is available in natural food stores.

Arrowroot: Arrowroot is a natural thickener made from the arrowroot plant. Dissolve arrowroot in a small amount of cool liquid before adding to sauces, gravies, pie fillings, or puddings. After adding, bring to a boil stirring constantly, then lower the heat and cook until thickened.

Balsamic vinegar: Balsamic vinegar is dark brown with an exquisite flavor and subtle sweetness. It is made from sweet Trebbiano grapes and acquires its dark color and pungency from being aged in wooden barrels for a minimum of ten years. Balsamic vinegar is available in supermarkets, Italian grocery stores, and gourmet and specialty food shops.

Brown rice vinegar: This delicately flavored, amber-colored vinegar is made from either fermented brown rice or unrefined rice wine. It is available in natural food stores and some supermarkets. Beware of most grocery store "seasoned" rice vinegars, as these typically contain added sugar. Stored at room temperature, brown rice vinegar will keep indefinitely.

Miso: Miso is a salty, flavorful, fermented soybean paste that often contains rice, barley, or another grain or bean. Some specialty misos are made from chickpeas, lentils, *adzuki* beans, or other legumes instead of soybeans. Used primarily as a seasoning, miso ranges from dark and strongly flavored to light, smooth, and delicately flavored. The best kinds will be found in the refrigerated section of your natural food store, as they retain active enzymes. Store miso in a tightly covered container in the refrigerator where it will keep for several months to a year (check the "use by" date on the container).

Sesame tahini: Sesame tahini is a smooth, creamy, tan-colored paste made by finely grinding raw or roasted sesame seeds. It is an essential ingredient in many Middle Eastern recipes and adds a wonderful texture and nutty flavor to spreads, sauces, and dressings. Tahini may be very thick, like peanut butter, or thin and slightly runny, depending on the brand. As with all unrefined nut and seed butters, you'll want to store tahini in the refrigerator to keep it from becoming rancid and to keep the oil from separating. However, if the oil does separate, simply stir it back in. Sesame tahini is available in many supermarkets, Middle Eastern grocery stores, and natural food stores.

Tamari: Typical brands of "soy sauce" are little more than hydrolyzed vegetable protein, sugar, and caramel coloring. However, excellent, naturally fermented soy sauce, commonly called *tamari,* is readily available in natural food stores and some supermarkets. As you'll see on its label, it contains only soy beans, salt, water, and sometimes wheat. Good soy sauces with reduced sodium also are available. If you have a sensitivity to yeast or fermented foods, look for Bragg Liquid Aminos, a rich, savory soy product that has not been fermented. You can substitute it equally for tamari.

Toasted sesame oil: This oil is extracted from toasted sesame seeds and has a luscious, highly concentrated flavor. A few drops sprinkled over cooked grains, beans, pasta, or vegetables add outstanding flavor, especially when combined with a little tamari soy sauce. Do not use it for cooking or sautéing, as it burns easily. Refrigerate toasted sesame oil after opening. You'll find it in your natural food store.

A Week of Menus for Breaking the Food Seduction

DAY I

Breakfast
orange juice
veggie "sausage" patties
Slow-Cooker Whole Grain Porridge (page 212)
berries

Lunch
tomato soup
Better-Than-Grilled Cheese (page 250)
Banana Snack Cake with Creamy Fudge Frosting (page 296)

Dinner
Seitan and Mushroom Stroganoff (page 280)
brown rice pasta
Sesame Broccoli (page 261)
Chocolate Bonbons (page 297)

DAY 2

Breakfast
savory smoked tofu
Swiss-Style Muesli (page 212)
fresh fruit

Lunch
Sloppy Joes (page 246)
whole grain bread or bun
celery and carrot sticks
apple

Dinner
Red Bean Burritos (page 248)
tossed salad with fat-free vinaigrette
brown rice
chocolate Italian ice

DAY 3

Breakfast
orange juice
veggie "sausage" links
Maple-Walnut Granola (page 213)
sliced banana

Lunch
Yellow Split Pea Soup with "Frankfurters" (page 229)
whole grain bread or roll
tossed salad with fat-free vinaigrette
carrot and celery sticks
peach

Dinner
Cheesy Sauce for Macaroni (page 265)
Garlic Broccoli (page 251)
Ultra-Fudge Brownies (page 292)

DAY 4

Breakfast
fresh fruit
Black Bean Breakfast Burritos (page 216)
lettuce and tomato garnish

Lunch
Eggless Egg Salad Sandwich Spread (page 244)
whole grain bread or roll
sliced beets
banana

Dinner
Chuckwagon Stew (page 278)
Greens and Garlic (page 263)
Hot Carob "Cocoa" (page 303)

DAY 5

Breakfast
grapefruit half
Breakfast Scrambler (page 216)
whole grain toast with fruit-sweetened jam

Lunch
veggie burger
sautéed mushrooms
whole grain bun
condiments (ketchup, mustard, onion, No-Naise Dressing (page 239)
lettuce
tomato slices
Steak Fries (page 255)

Dinner
Mandarin Stir-Fry, with chickpeas (page 283)
brown rice
strawberries
chocolate sorbet

DAY 6

Breakfast
Slow-Cooker Whole Grain Porridge (page 212)
grapefruit half
Hot Carob "Cocoa" (page 303)

Lunch
Chickenless Chicken Salad (page 239)
mixed salad greens
tomato wedges
brown rice crackers
Apricot Confections (page 290)

Dinner
Milli's Chili (page 225)
brown rice
Garlic Broccoli (page 251)
Hot Fudge Cake (page 298)

DAY 7

Breakfast
orange juice
veggie Canadian "bacon"
Cinnamon-Raisin Oatmeal (page 209)
banana

Lunch
Fantastic Fajitas (page 249)
mixed vegetable salad
brown rice
apple

Dinner
Chili Bean Macaroni
steamed broccoli
Instant Chocolate Pudding (page 292)

Breakfasts

Morning meals should be quick and easy. As we saw in chapter 6, you'll want to be sure to include plenty of fiber for staying power through the day. That means old-fashioned oatmeal, a breakfast burrito, bran cereal, or fresh fruit. You'll also want to start off with a healthy, high-protein food, such as veggie "sausage," veggie "bacon," tofu scrambler, or even a small serving of beans or chickpeas. Some brands of breakfast meat substitutes you might try are YvesVeggie Cuisine (pepperoni, bacon, veggie dogs, bologna, deli slices, burgers) and Lightlife (lean links sausage, tofu pups, savory seitan, deli slices), among others. For high-fiber foods, there's no need to be fancy. Crack open a box of oatmeal or bran cereal, splash on some soy milk, and off you go. If you want to be both quick *and* creative, try these:

- Cinnamon-Raisin Oatmeal, page 209
- Breakfast Brown Rice, page 210
- Hot Whole Wheat with Dates, page 211
- Slow-Cooker Whole Grain Porridge, page 212
- Swiss-Style Muesli, page 212
- Breakfast Scrambler, page 216

- Fantastic Fruit Smoothie, page 220
- Banana or Mango Lassi, page 220
- Orange-Pineapple Crush, page 221
- Berry-Berry Smoothie, page 222
- Whole Grain Bagel with Banana Smoosh, page 222

Reheated leftover soups and stews can make for a speedy and nourishing breakfast. Try heartier ones with beans and whole grains to keep you energized all day. In some cultures both children and adults start every day with brown rice and vegetables, beans and rice, or tortillas and beans, as these foods have staying power and give us the stamina we need to keeping going until the next meal. A big bowl of brown rice and a portion of cooked beans truly is a powerhouse combination, particularly if you face an active or demanding day. Whenever you feel adventurous, try one of the following for a stick-to-your-ribs morning meal:

- Black Bean Breakfast Burritos, page 216
- Milli's Chili, page 225
- Red Lentil Soup, page 228
- Yellow Split Pea Soup with "Frankfurters," page 229
- Tempeh Tostadas, page 247
- Red Bean Burritos, page 248
- Fantastic Fajitas, page 249
- Cheesy Broccoli Polenta, page 282

Here are a few spur-of-the-moment standbys you can rely on:

- Bran cereal with fresh fruit and fortified vanilla soy or rice milk
- Brown rice cake with 1 tablespoon nut or seed butter and 1 teaspoon fruit-sweetened jam
- Mixed fresh fruit salad topped with chopped raw walnuts

Orange-Scented Corn Muffins

MAKES 12 MUFFINS

With just a touch of sweetness, these sugar-free muffins are a welcome treat for breakfast.

1 cup firm silken tofu, crumbled

½ cup orange juice

1 tablespoon organic canola or safflower oil

1 cup whole wheat flour

⅔ cup yellow cornmeal

1 tablespoon grated orange peel (optional)

2 teaspoons baking powder

1 teaspoon baking soda

½ teaspoon salt

Preheat oven to 350°F. Mist 12 muffin cups with nonstick cooking spray and set aside. Combine tofu, juice, and oil in blender and process into a smooth, creamy emulsion. Place remaining ingredients in a large bowl and stir with a dry wire whisk until well combined. Pour blended mixture into dry ingredients and mix just until dry ingredients are moistened. Batter will be stiff. Immediately spoon into prepared muffin cups, using an equal amount for each. Bake 20 to 25 minutes. Gently loosen muffins and turn them on their side in the muffin tin. Cover with a clean kitchen towel, and let rest for 5 minutes. This will keep them from developing a hard crust. Transfer to a cooling rack, and serve warm or at room temperature.

Per muffin: Calories: 98; Protein: 5 g; Carbohydrate: 15 g; Fat: 3 g; Sodium: 284 mg; Cholesterol: 0 mg; Fiber: 2 g.

Cinnamon-Raisin Oatmeal

MAKES 4 SERVINGS

Hearty, old-fashioned rolled oats in the morning will keep you satisfied until lunchtime. Raisins add a bit of natural sweetness with no added sugar.

4 cups water
2 cups old-fashioned rolled oats
½ cup raisins
½ teaspoon cinnamon
¼ teaspoon salt
Fortified vanilla soy or rice milk (optional)

Combine all ingredients in a heavy saucepan. Bring to a boil, lower heat, and cook, stirring occasionally, for about 10 minutes, or until cooked to your liking. Serve plain or with vanilla soy or rice milk, if desired.

VARIATIONS:

- For Cinnamon-Apricot Oatmeal, replace raisins with ½ cup chopped dried apricots. Cook as directed.
- For Cinnamon-Apple Oatmeal, reduce water to 3¼ cups and replace raisins with 1 apple, peeled and coarsely chopped. Cook as directed.
- Omit raisins, cook as directed, and top each serving with a dollop (about 1 teaspoon) of fruit-sweetened jam or jelly.

Per one-cup serving: Calories: 205; Protein: 6 g; Carbohydrate: 42 g; Fat: 3 g; Sodium: 156 mg; Cholesterol: 0 mg; Fiber: 5 g.

Breakfast Brown Rice

MAKES 4 SERVINGS

Brown rice makes a delicious warm breakfast that will jump-start your day. This recipe calls for soaking the rice overnight. Soaking the rice overnight reduces the normal cooking time considerably, making it convenient for everyday breakfasts. You can pack your lunch, take a shower, or read the paper while it's steaming.

1 cup brown rice
2 cups water
¼ teaspoon salt (optional)
1 sliced ripe banana
1 cup chopped fresh fruit or
  berries

¼ cup chopped walnuts
¼ cup raw sunflower or
  pumpkin seeds
Fortified vanilla soy or rice milk
  or soy yogurt (optional)

Place rice in a large wire mesh strainer and rinse well under running water, stirring with your fingers. Place in a large saucepan with the water. Cover and let soak 8 to 22 hours. Do not drain. In the morning, add salt, if using, and bring to a boil. Reduce heat to very low, cover, and cook until tender, about 20 to 30 minutes, or until water is absorbed. If time permits, remove from heat and let rest, covered, 5 to 10 minutes. Top each serving with some of the fruit, nuts, and seeds. Serve plain or with vanilla soy or rice milk or a dollop of soy yogurt, if desired.

Per ½-cup serving: Calories: 315; Protein: 8 g; Carbohydrate: 50 g; Fat: 11g; Sodium: 156 mg; Cholesterol: 0 mg; Fiber: 4 g.

Hot Whole Wheat with Dates

MAKES 4 SERVINGS

This satisfying porridge includes the bran and germ of the whole wheat berry. Unlike most commercial hot wheat cereals that are stripped of the grain's natural fiber and nutrition, this wholesome porridge is a beautiful earthy brown.

3½ cups water	¼ teaspoon nutmeg
1 cup bulgur	¼ teaspoon cardamom
⅔ cup chopped, pitted dates	Fortified plain or vanilla soy or
Pinch of salt	rice milk (optional)
½ teaspoon vanilla extract	

Combine water, bulgur, dates, and salt in a large saucepan and bring to a boil, stirring constantly. Reduce heat, cover, and simmer, stirring occasionally until bulgur is very tender, about 20 to 30 minutes. Remove from heat and stir in vanilla extract, nutmeg, and cardamom. Serve plain or with soy or rice milk, if desired.

Per one-cup serving: Calories: 164; Protein: 3g; Carbohydrate: 40g; Fat: less than one gram; Sodium: 83 mg; Cholesterol: 0 mg; Fiber: 5g.

Slow-Cooker Whole Grain Porridge

MAKES ABOUT 4 SERVINGS

Wake up to hot, whole grain porridge by preparing it the night before and letting it simmer in your slow-cooker while you sleep. A healthy breakfast has never been easier!

⅓ cup brown rice
⅓ cup millet
⅓ cup kamut, spelt, or wheat
  berries
3 cups hot water
½ cup raisins or chopped dried
  apricots, prunes, or apples

½ teaspoon cinnamon
¼ teaspoon salt (optional)
Fortified vanilla soy or rice milk
  (optional)

Combine grains, water, fruit, cinnamon, and salt, if using, in slow-cooker and cook on low overnight. Serve plain or with vanilla soy or rice milk, if desired.

Per ¾-cup serving: Calories: 329; Protein: 12g; Carbohydrate: 65g; Fat: 2.5g; Sodium: 155 mg; Cholesterol: 0 mg; Fiber: 8g.

Swiss-Style Muesli

MAKES 4 SERVINGS

This recipe is an adaptation of an old Swiss cereal. The texture is similar to hot porridge; however, muesli is not cooked, but is served cold. In the morning you simply stir in fresh fruit, and breakfast is ready to be served.

1½ cups old-fashioned rolled oats
¼ cup raisins
¼ cup chopped raw nuts or sunflower seeds
½ teaspoon cinnamon
2 cups fortified plain or vanilla soy or rice milk
¼ cup frozen fruit juice concentrate, thawed (undiluted)
1 small apple or pear

Combine oats, raisins, nuts, and cinnamon in a bowl. Stir together milk and juice concentrate. Pour over fruit and nut mixture and stir to mix thoroughly. Cover and refrigerate overnight. In the morning, grate or finely chop the apple or pear and add to the muesli.

TIPS:

* Sliced banana, peaches, fresh berries, or other fresh fruit may used in place of, or in addition to, the apple or pear.
* This recipe is easily halved or doubled.

Per one-cup serving: Calories: 276; Protein: 9g; Carbohydrate: 43g; Fat: 8g; Sodium: 17mg; Cholesterol: 0mg; Fiber: 6.5g.

Maple-Walnut Granola

MAKES ABOUT 10 CUPS (APPROXIMATELY 20 SERVINGS)

Serve this crunchy, satisfying cereal with lots of chopped fresh fruit or berries and plenty of plain or vanilla fortified soy or rice milk. This recipe makes a large quantity, but it will keep for a long time in airtight jars or containers in the refrigerator.

6 cups old-fashioned rolled oats
1 cup barley or brown rice flour
1 cup coarsely chopped walnuts
1 cup raw sunflower seeds
½ teaspoon salt
1 cup frozen apple juice concentrate, thawed (undiluted)
½ cup pure maple syrup
2 tablespoons organic canola oil
2 tablespoons water
2 teaspoons vanilla extract
1 cup raisins

Preheat oven to 325°F. Combine oats, flour, walnuts, sunflower seeds, and salt in a large bowl. In a separate bowl, whisk together juice concentrate, maple syrup, oil, water, and vanilla. Pour over dry ingredients and mix thoroughly until evenly moistened. Divide mixture between two large pans, spreading it out into a one-inch-thick layer. Bake until golden brown, about 50 to 60 minutes. Stir well every 15 minutes, then spread mixture back to a one-inch-thick layer before returning it to oven. When granola is finished baking, remove from oven and stir in raisins while granola is still hot. Steam from the hot cereal will help plump the raisins. Let cool completely. Store in airtight containers in the refrigerator.

TIP:

Replace or supplement the raisins with any chopped dried fruit of your choice. Good selections are dried apricots, dates, prunes, pears, apples, and figs. Try a mixture of fruit, or alternate different fruits each time you make the recipe.

Per ½-cup serving: Calories: 277; Protein: 7g; Carbohydrate: 42g; Fat: 11g; Sodium: 65mg; Cholesterol: 0mg; Fiber: 4.0g.

Zucchini Bread

MAKES 1 LOAF (ABOUT 10 TO 12 SERVINGS)

This popular quick bread can be served at breakfast, snack time, or even dessert. It's moist and satisfying without being overly sweet.

2 cups whole wheat flour
2 teaspoons baking powder
1 teaspoon baking soda
½ teaspoon cinnamon
¼ teaspoon ground cloves
1½ cups shredded zucchini
(about 2 small)
½ cup unsweetened applesauce

¼ cup apple juice concentrate, thawed (undiluted)
¼ cup pure maple syrup
1 tablespoon organic canola or safflower oil
1 teaspoon vanilla extract
½ cup chopped walnuts

Preheat oven to 350°F. Mist an 8½ × 4½-inch loaf pan with nonstick cooking spray and set aside. Place flour, baking powder, baking soda, cinnamon, and cloves in a large mixing bowl, and stir together using a dry wire whisk. Place remaining ingredients, except walnuts, in a separate bowl, stir together until well combined. Pour wet ingredients into dry ingredients. Mix just until dry ingredients are evenly moistened. Stir in walnuts, and mix until they are evenly distributed. Spoon batter into prepared loaf pan. Bake on center rack of oven for about 50 to 55 minutes, or until cake tester inserted in the center tests clean. Turn bread out onto a cooling rack and let cool completely before slicing or storing. Wrap cooled bread tightly. It will keep at room temperature up to 3 days, or refrigerate up to 7 days.

Per slice (12 per loaf): Calories: 135; Protein: 4g; Carbohydrate: 21g; Fat: 5g; Sodium: 173mg; Cholesterol: 0mg; Fiber: 3g.

Phenomenal French Toast

MAKES 6 PIECES

Serve this delectable, egg- and dairy-free French toast with fresh fruit chunks, applesauce, or fruit-sweetened preserves.

¼ cup whole wheat flour
1 teaspoon nutritional yeast flakes
¼ teaspoon salt
Pinch each: cinnamon and nutmeg
1 cup fortified plain or vanilla soy or rice milk
6 slices whole grain bread

Place flour, nutritional yeast, salt, cinnamon, and nutmeg in a medium bowl and stir with a dry whisk until well blended. Pour milk into flour mixture and whisk vigorously until well blended. Let batter sit for 10 minutes. Oil a *nonstick* skillet or griddle and place over medium-high heat. Mix batter again. Dip bread slices one at a time into batter, making sure that each is well saturated. Cook 3 to 5 minutes, or until bottom is lightly browned. Turn over and cook other side until golden. Lightly oil skillet between batches to prevent sticking.

Per slice serving: Calories: 122; Protein: 7g; Carbohydrate: 26g; Fat: 2g; Sodium: 290mg; Cholesterol: 0mg; Fiber: 4g.

Breakfast Scrambler

MAKES 4 SERVINGS

Scrambled tofu has the look and taste of scrambled eggs. It's hard to find a high-protein breakfast that is faster, easier, or more delicious.

> 2 teaspoons onion powder
> 1 teaspoon garlic powder
> ½ teaspoon turmeric
> ¼ teaspoon pepper
> ¼ teaspoon salt
> 1 teaspoon parsley flakes, lightly crumbled
>   between fingers
> 1 pound firm regular tofu, rinsed, patted dry,
>   and crumbled

Combine onion powder, garlic powder, turmeric, pepper, salt, and parsley flakes in a small bowl. Mist a regular or nonstick skillet with nonstick cooking spray. Add tofu to skillet and sprinkle seasonings over it. Cook and stir over medium heat until heated through.

TIP:

- Double, triple, or quadruple the seasonings and store in a jar. When you want a quick scramble, just add about 5 teaspoons of the seasoning mix to the tofu in your pan. For a single serving, use 4 ounces of tofu and about 1¼ teaspoons of the seasoning mix.

Per ½-cup serving: Calories: 95; Protein: 9g; Carbohydrate: 5g; Fat: 5g; Sodium: 156mg; Cholesterol: 0mg; Fiber: 1g.

Black Bean Breakfast Burritos

MAKES 12 SERVINGS

These hearty breakfast burritos freeze well and will also keep in the fridge for several days. There is a lot of room for experimentation with this recipe, so don't feel compelled to follow it exactly.

¼ cup water

1 teaspoon olive oil

1 onion, diced

½ teaspoon crushed garlic

2 bell peppers (red, orange,
yellow, or green), diced

1 tablespoon ground cumin

Pepper

3 cups drained, cooked, or
canned black beans

10 button mushrooms, sliced

2 ripe tomatoes

½ cup salsa

3 cups cooked brown rice

Salt or tamari

Tabasco sauce

Whole grain tortillas

Heat water and oil in a large saucepan or wok. When hot, add onion and sauté until limp. Add garlic, cumin, and pepper, and cook and stir 2 minutes longer. Add a little more water if necessary, to prevent sticking. Stir in black beans, mushrooms, tomatoes, and salsa, and cook and stir until mushrooms are tender, about 10 minutes. Add rice and season to taste with salt or tamari and Tabasco sauce. Serve on warm tortillas, folded or rolled up to enclose filling.

Per burrito: Calories: 193; Protein: 7g; Carbohydrate: 38g; Fat: 2g; Sodium: 235mg; Cholesterol: 0mg; Fiber: 7g.

Orange-Oat Pancakes

MAKES ABOUT 16 SMALL PANCAKES

These light and fluffy pancakes have a delicate orange flavor that is nicely complemented by Apple-Maple Fusion Topping (recipe follows).

1⅓ cups whole wheat flour

⅔ cup old-fashioned rolled oats

2 teaspoons baking powder

½ teaspoon baking soda

1 cup fortified soy or rice milk

¼ cup unsweetened applesauce

3 tablespoons frozen orange
juice concentrate, thawed
(undiluted)

Combine flour, oats, baking powder, and baking soda in a medium bowl. In a separate bowl whisk together milk, applesauce, and juice concentrate. Pour into dry ingredients and stir with a wooden spoon.

Batter will be slightly lumpy. Oil a large *nonstick* skillet and place over medium-high heat. Spoon batter into hot skillet using 2 level tablespoons for each pancake. Cook until bottoms are brown, adjusting heat as necessary. Cook second side briefly, just until golden. Lightly oil skillet between batches to prevent sticking.

Per small pancake: Calories: 58; Protein: 2g; Carbohydrate: 11g; Fat: less than one gram; Sodium: 92mg; Cholesterol: 0mg; Fiber: 2g.

Apple-Maple Fusion Topping

MAKES ABOUT 1 CUP

Pure maple syrup is unquestionably delicious, but it's also high in calories and a bit expensive. To reduce the cost to your waistline and your wallet, try this fabulous blend. It is so easy to make, adds a bit of extra nutrition, and extends the maple syrup while retaining all of its magnificent flavor. It's the perfect topping for pancakes, waffles, or French toast.

½ cup pure maple syrup
½ cup unsweetened applesauce

Stir together maple syrup and applesauce until well blended. Serve at room temperature, or warm briefly over low heat. Store leftovers in refrigerator.

Per one-cup serving: Calories: 118; Protein: less than one gram; Carbohydrate: 30g; Fat: less than one gram; Sodium: 4mg; Cholesterol: 0mg; Fiber: less than one gram.

Fresh Fruit Compote

MAKES 2 TO 4 SERVINGS

This delicious mixture of stewed, fresh, and dried fruit makes any morning sweet and special. Top each serving with a little vanilla soy or rice milk, soy yogurt, finely chopped raw nuts or seeds, or a pinch of dried, unsweetened coconut for a real treat.

1 Granny Smith apple, peeled and chunked
1 pear, peeled and chunked
1 cup water
¼ cup chopped dates, figs, or raisins
½ teaspoon cinnamon

Combine all ingredients in a medium saucepan and bring to a boil. Simmer, stirring occasionally, until fruit is tender but not mushy. Serve hot, warm, or chilled.

TIP:
• If the compote gets too sweet, add 2 to 3 teaspoons fresh lemon juice to balance the flavor.

Per ½-cup serving: Calories: 76; Protein: less than one gram; Carbohydrate: 20g; Fat: less than one gram; Sodium: 2 mg; Cholesterol: 0mg; Fiber: 3g.

Stewed Prunes

MAKES ABOUT 3 CUPS

Serve prunes hot or cold, unadorned or topped with plain or vanilla soy or rice milk or soy yogurt. Stewed prunes also make a tasty topping for plain hot oatmeal or Phenomenal French Toast, page 215.

2 cups pitted prunes
2 cups water

Combine prunes and water in a medium saucepan and bring to a boil. Reduce heat, cover, and simmer until prunes are tender, about 20 minutes. Store leftovers in refrigerator. Serve warm or chilled.

Per ½-cup serving: Calories: 135; Protein: 2g; Carbohydrate: 36g; Fat: less than one gram; Sodium: 5mg; Cholesterol: 0mg; Fiber: 4g.

Fantastic Fruit Smoothie

MAKES ABOUT 2 TO 2½ CUPS (2 SERVINGS)

Frozen fruit makes smoothies extra thick and creamy. If you don't like icy cold beverages, use fresh fruit instead. Experiment with a variety of juices and fruit, depending on what is in season.

> 1 frozen or fresh banana, broken into chunks
>   (see Tip, below)
> 1½ cups unsweetened fruit juice
>   (your choice; any kind)
> ½ cup sliced fresh or frozen unsweetened fruit or berries
> ½ cup plain, vanilla, or fruit-flavored soy yogurt
>   (optional)

Combine all ingredients in blender and process until very smooth and creamy. Serve immediately.

TIPS:

- With a few ripe bananas in your freezer you can always create a quick breakfast smoothie. Simply peel, place them in plastic bags, and store in the freezer. They will last for several weeks, depending on your freezer's temperature.
- To make your smoothie extra creamy and give it a healthy protein boost, try adding a little powdered soy milk or protein powder prior to blending.

Per one-cup serving: Calories: 211; Protein: 3g; Carbohydrate: 52g; Fat: 2g; Sodium: 18mg; Cholesterol: 0mg; Fiber: 4g.

Banana or Mango Lassi

MAKES ABOUT 2½ CUPS (2 TO 3 SERVINGS)

Lassi is a sweet and spicy beverage from India that traditionally is made with yogurt. This dairy-free version is delicious and makes a wonderful breakfast or snack.

2 cups fortified plain or vanilla soy or rice milk

1 frozen or fresh banana or 1 small ripe mango, peeled and cut into
chunks

3 pitted dates, chopped

1 teaspoon cardamom

¼ teaspoon black pepper

Combine all ingredients in blender and process until very smooth and creamy. Serve cold.

TIP:

• Lassi is best served well chilled. If the milk and fruit are cold, you can serve at once. If they are room temperature, the lassi will taste best if it is chilled in the refrigerator for at least 30 minutes before serving.

Per ¾-cup serving: Calories: 130; Protein: 5g; Carbohydrate: 23g; Fat: 3g; Sodium: 20mg; Cholesterol: 0mg; Fiber: 4g.

Orange-Pineapple Crush

MAKES 5 CUPS

Savor the tropical flavors in this quick and creamy smoothie.

1½ cups (about 12 ounces) silken tofu, crumbled

1 medium banana, broken into chunks

2 cups unsweetened orange-pineapple juice, chilled

1 (8-ounce) can unsweetened crushed pineapple, chilled

Combine all ingredients in blender and process until very smooth and creamy. Serve immediately.

Per one-cup serving: Calories: 122; Protein: 5g; Carbohydrate: 25g; Fat: 1g; Sodium: 63mg; Cholesterol: 0mg; Fiber: 1g.

Berry-Berry Smoothie

MAKES 3 CUPS

Get double the berry taste in this delicious morning beverage.

2 cups fortified vanilla soy or rice milk
1 large banana, broken into chunks
½ cup frozen unsweetened raspberries or blueberries
¼ cup frozen unsweetened raspberry juice concentrate (undiluted)

Combine all ingredients in blender and process until very smooth and creamy. Serve immediately.

Per one-cup serving: Calories: 137; Protein: 6g; Carbohydrate: 24g; Fat: 3g; Sodium: 20mg; Cholesterol: 0mg; Fiber: 5g.

Banana Smoosh

MAKES 2 SERVINGS

Here is a creamy, healthful spread to use on bagels (in place of cream cheese) or on quick breads or toast (in place of butter or margarine).

1 large ripe banana
¼ cup chopped nuts or seeds
1 tablespoon nut or seed butter (peanut, almond, cashew, sesame tahini)
1 tablespoon raisins, dried cranberries, or currants

Mash banana well with a fork or potato masher. Stir in remaining ingredients. Serve at once.

Per ¼-cup serving: Calories: 211; Protein: 4g; Carbohydrate: 21g; Fat: 14g; Sodium: 2mg; Cholesterol: 0mg; Fiber: 3g.

Soups and Stews

A great soup is soothing and satisfying, whether as a midday lunch or a light evening meal. Just add some whole grain bread or crusty rolls and a salad, and your feast is complete. Some cultures even enjoy soup for breakfast. Leftover soup can be heated and put in a thermos for meals away from home, or if your office has a microwave oven, it can be warmed up for lunch in a jiffy.

Most soups will keep in the refrigerator for seven to ten days, and if you make a big batch you can use it handily for meals throughout the week—and you'll only have to make it once. If your household is small, you can still make a large quantity and then freeze it in individual serving-size containers. Frozen soup can be defrosted in the refrigerator or microwave. When reheating leftover soup, take out only the quantity you'll be using at that particular meal. Reheating soup (or any food, for that matter) more than once makes it more receptive to foodborne pathogens. When warming leftover soup, always reheat it to the boiling point both for food safety as well as the best flavor.

Pasta, potatoes, and flour- or starch-thickened soups don't freeze well, because, when thawed they tend to lose their texture, even though the soup's flavor will remain intact. Most other soups, particularly bean soups, freeze beautifully. Bean-based soups tend to get thicker as they cool. For a thinner soup, simply add a little water or vegetable broth while reheating the soup, until you achieve the consistency you desire. Thick, leftover bean soups become very stewlike, making them ideal for topping grain, pasta, or potatoes to create a quick and filling meal.

Autumn Vegetable Bisque

MAKES ABOUT 2½ QUARTS

Simple root vegetables are elevated to the status of royalty in this elegant and creamy soup.

> 2 teaspoons olive oil
> 1 medium onion, chopped
> 1 large leek, rinsed well and sliced
> 1 teaspoon crushed garlic
> 4 cups water
> 4 cups peeled and diced root vegetables (use a mixture of turnips, parsnips, rutabaga, and carrots)
> 2 tablespoons dried parsley flakes
> 1 teaspoon salt
> ½ teaspoon pepper
> 2 cups fortified plain soy or rice milk
> 2 tablespoons white wine vinegar or fresh lemon juice
> ¼ cup thinly sliced chives or scallions for garnish

Heat oil in a large soup pot. Add onion, leek, and garlic, and sauté 8 to 10 minutes. Add water, root vegetables, parsley, salt, and pepper, and bring to a boil. Reduce heat, cover, and cook 45 to 60 minutes, stirring occasionally. Remove from heat and stir in milk. Mix well, then stir in vinegar or lemon juice. Blend in batches in blender or food processor until completely smooth. Warm gently until heated through. Do not boil. Garnish each serving with some of the chives or scallions.

Per one-cup serving: Calories: 58; Protein: 2g; Carbohydrate: 9g; Fat: 2g; Sodium: 262mg; Cholesterol: 0mg; Fiber: 3g.

Milli's Chili

MAKES 4 TO 6 SERVINGS

There's nothing like a steaming hot bowl of chili. Serve this thick, spicy stew over brown rice, quinoa, polenta, or whole grain pasta, or with Orange Scented Corn Muffins, page 209, on the side. Cooked greens or a tossed green salad will round out the meal.

2 teaspoons olive oil	1½ cups whole corn kernels
1 large onion, chopped	(fresh, frozen, or canned)
1 green bell pepper, diced	1½ tablespoons chili powder
1 red bell pepper, diced	1 tablespoon oregano
1 cup diced celery	2½ teaspoons ground cumin
1 teaspoon crushed garlic	1 to 2 teaspoons Tabasco sauce
1 (28-ounce) can crushed	1 teaspoon paprika (sweet or
tomatoes	hot)
2 cups drained cooked or	1 teaspoon salt
canned pinto or red kidney	½ teaspoon pepper
beans (one 15-ounce can)	Chopped cilantro and/or red
1 (14.5 ounce) can diced	onion for garnish (optional)
tomatoes, with juice	

Heat oil in a large soup pot. Add onion, peppers, and celery, and sauté until vegetables are tender—about 8 minutes. Add garlic and sauté 1 minute longer. Stir in remaining ingredients, except garnishes, and bring to a boil. Reduce heat and simmer, stirring occasionally, 25 to 30 minutes. Serve hot, garnished with cilantro and/or red onion, if desired.

Per one-cup serving: Calories: 202; Protein: 9g; Carbohydrate: 40g; Fat: 3g; Sodium: 960mg; Cholesterol: 0mg; Fiber: 12g.

Bean and Barley Chowder

MAKES ABOUT 2 QUARTS

Barley is delicious, not to mention an excellent source of soluble fiber, which reduces blood cholesterol levels. The longer you cook this thick and hearty soup, the creamier and richer tasting it becomes.

8 cups water or vegetable stock
1 cup dry baby lima beans, soaked overnight and drained
1 cup chopped onions
1 cup chopped carrots
1 stalk celery, finely chopped
½ cup pearl barley
1 tablespoon crushed garlic
1 teaspoon thyme
Salt and pepper

Place water and beans in a large soup pot and bring to a boil. Add remaining ingredients, except salt and pepper. Return to a boil, reduce heat to medium, cover, and simmer until barley and beans are tender and broth is creamy, about 1½ to 2 hours. Season with salt and pepper to taste. Serve hot.

Per one-cup serving: Calories: 116; Protein: 6g; Carbohydrate: 24g; Fat: less than one gram; Sodium: 134mg; Cholesterol: 0mg; Fiber: 6.5g.

Cream of Cauliflower and Lima Bean Soup

MAKES ABOUT 2 QUARTS

This is a creamy blended soup with a few whole lima beans added for extra texture. Be sure to use fordhook lima beans, which are large, sweet, and meaty.

16 ounces frozen Fordhook lima beans
1 teaspoon olive oil
1½ cups chopped onions
2 teaspoons whole caraway seeds, or 1½ teaspoons
    ground caraway
1 teaspoon crushed garlic
1 medium cauliflower cut into small florets
5 cups water
Salt and pepper
Minced fresh parsley (optional)

Cook lima beans according to package directions. Drain and divide in half. Heat oil in a large soup pot over medium-high heat. When hot, add onions, caraway seeds, and garlic, and sauté until onions are soft, about 10 to 15 minutes. Add cauliflower and water and bring to a boil. Reduce heat, cover, and simmer until cauliflower is very tender, about 10 to 12 minutes. In a blender, purée soup in batches along with half the reserved lima beans. Return blended soup to pot and stir in remaining whole lima beans. Season with salt and pepper. Warm over medium-low heat until beans are heated through and soup is hot. Garnish with chopped parsley if desired.

Per one-cup serving: Calories: 57; Protein: 3g; Carbohydrate: 10g; Fat: less than one gram; Sodium: 149mg; Cholesterol: 0mg; Fiber: 3g.

French Onion Soup

MAKES ABOUT 1½ QUARTS

A "beefy" tasting classic!

1 tablespoon olive oil
2 large or 3 medium onions,
  sliced or chopped
1 teaspoon crushed garlic
¼ cup flour (any kind—your
  choice)
4 cups vegetable broth or water

¼ cup low-sodium tamari
French bread (1 slice per
  serving), or ¼ cup baked
  croutons per serving
Nondairy parmesan substitute,
  such as Soymage or
  Parmazano (optional)

Place oil in a large soup pot, and heat over medium-high heat. When hot, add onions and garlic and sauté 5 minutes. Stir in flour, mixing well. Stir in water and tamari and bring to a boil. Reduce heat to low, cover, and simmer until onions are tender, about 20 minutes. Just before serving, place a slice of French bread or some croutons in the bottom of each soup bowl. Ladle soup on top, sprinkle with nondairy parmesan substitute, if desired, and serve at once.

Per one-cup serving: Calories: 177; Protein: 6g; Carbohydrate: 30g; Fat: 4g; Sodium: 893mg; Cholesterol: 0mg; Fiber: 3.5g.

Cheddary Soup

MAKES ABOUT 5 CUPS

Surprisingly, there is no cheese in this thick, rich, cheddary-tasting soup. You'll be amazed how satisfying it tastes.

1 medium potato, peeled and
   coarsely chopped
1 medium carrot, peeled and
   coarsely chopped
1 medium onion, coarsely
   chopped
1 cup water
1½ cups (about 12 ounces) firm
   silken tofu, crumbled

½ cup nutritional yeast flakes
2 tablespoons fresh lemon juice
1¼ teaspoons salt
1 teaspoon onion powder
¼ teaspoon garlic powder
1 cup fortified plain soy or rice
   milk

Place potato, carrot, onion, and water in a large soup pot and bring to a boil. Reduce heat to medium, cover, and simmer, stirring once or twice until vegetables are tender, about 10 minutes. Remove from heat and stir in remaining ingredients. In a blender, purée soup in batches until completely smooth. Transfer to a clean soup pot, and heat over medium-low to warm through, stirring often until hot. Do not boil.

Per one-cup serving: Calories: 145; Protein: 14g; Carbohydrate: 17g; Fat: 3.5g; Sodium: 625mg; Cholesterol: 0mg; Fiber: 5g.

Red Lentil Soup

MAKES 6 SERVINGS

This soup is so nutritious and so simple to prepare, you'll want to make it often. Its flavor is exquisite.

7 cups water
2½ cups dried red lentils
1 large onion, minced
1 teaspoon turmeric
Large pinch of cayenne pepper

2 to 4 tablespoons fresh lemon
   juice
1 teaspoon ground cumin
Salt and pepper

Combine water, lentils, onion, turmeric, and cayenne pepper in a large soup pot and bring to a boil. Reduce heat, partially cover, and simmer until lentils have disintegrated, about 30 to 60 minutes. Stir in lemon juice, cumin, salt, and pepper to taste.

Per one-cup serving: Calories: 288; Protein: 23g; Carbohydrate: 50g; Fat: 1g; Sodium: 212mg; Cholesterol: 0mg; Fiber: 25g.

Yellow Split Pea Soup with "Frankfurters"

MAKES 8 TO 10 SERVINGS

A creamy, appetizing, substantial soup that will really stick to your ribs.

2 tablespoons olive oil
1 large onion, chopped
2 medium carrots, sliced
2 cups yellow split peas, soaked overnight
8 cups water
2 bay leaves
Salt and pepper
8 meatless "hot dogs," sliced
2 to 4 tablespoons fresh lemon juice

Heat oil in a large soup pot. When hot add onion and carrots and sauté until soft. Drain peas, rinse well, and add to the pot along with the water. Bring to a boil. Reduce heat, cover, and simmer, stirring occasionally, until peas have practically disintegrated, about 1½ to 2 hours. Purée soup in batches in a blender and return to the pot. Add bay leaves, salt, and pepper. Thin with additional water if soup is too thick. Simmer 30 minutes longer. Remove bay leaves. Add sliced "hot dogs" and lemon juice and cook a few minutes more. Serve hot.

Per ¾-cup serving: Calories: 146; Protein: 12g; Carbohydrate: 16g; Fat: 3g; Sodium: 590mg; Cholesterol: 0mg; Fiber: 5g.

Spicy Noodle Soup

MAKES 6 SERVINGS

This enchanting, unusual soup abounds with exotic spices and vivid flavor.

2 teaspoons olive oil

1 large onion, finely chopped

2 teaspoons crushed garlic

1 teaspoon caraway seed, whole or ground

5½ cups water

¼ cup minced celery

3 tablespoons tomato paste

1 tablespoon sweet paprika

1 teaspoon ground cumin

½ teaspoon turmeric

¼ teaspoon cayenne pepper

4 bay leaves

Salt and pepper

1½ cups fine noodles (vermicelli) broken into small pieces

2 tablespoons minced fresh cilantro or parsley

Heat oil in a large soup pot. When hot, add onion and sauté over medium heat until soft and golden, about 15 minutes. Add garlic and caraway seeds and sauté a few minutes more. Stir in remaining ingredients, except noodles and cilantro, and bring to a boil. Reduce heat and simmer 5 minutes. Stir in noodles, cover, and cook 15 minutes longer. Stir in cilantro, and serve at once.

Per one-cup serving: Calories: 90; Protein: 3g; Carbohydrate: 16g; Fat: 2g; Sodium: 78mg; Cholesterol: 0mg; Fiber: 2g.

Green Pea and Spinach Soup

MAKES 6 SERVINGS

This brilliant green soup is as nutritious as it is delicious and satisfying.

5½ cups water

1 medium onion, sliced

4 medium carrots, peeled and sliced

1 large leek, cleaned well and sliced

½ teaspoon basil

1 large bunch spinach, stems removed
1 cup thawed frozen peas
Salt and pepper
2 to 3 teaspoons fresh lemon juice

In a large soup pot, combine water, onion, carrots, leek, and basil and bring to a boil. Reduce heat, cover, and simmer until vegetables are tender, about 25 to 30 minutes. Stir in spinach and peas and cook a few minutes until spinach wilts. Remove from heat. Purée soup in batches in a blender until smooth and return to the pot. Season with salt and pepper to taste. Add enough lemon juice to heighten flavor. Serve hot.

Per one-cup serving: Calories: 61; Protein: 3g; Carbohydrate: 13g; Fat: less than one gram; Sodium: 255mg; Cholesterol: 0mg; Fiber: 4g.

Salads, Spreads, and Sandwiches

Whether used as starters or main dishes, salads, dips, and sandwiches can make for hearty fare. In many homes they are the focal point of the meal and often are served any hour of the day or evening. Salads featuring beans or grains can be especially substantial and satisfying. Those that consist mostly of vegetables and a light dressing work well as side salads or snacks. Salads are fun, quick and easy to prepare, and are a great way to serve healthy vegetables. They typically are low in fat, readily lend themselves to creativity, and always accept little bits of leftovers from last night's feast.

Almost anything can be the basis for a salad: cold or warm pasta, grains, potatoes, sweet potatoes, or winter squash; cooked or raw vegetables; peas, beans, or lentils; and even fruit. Fresh herbs as well as nuts, seeds, and sprouts complement salads perfectly. Keep an open mind about salads and let the recipes in this book be a springboard for your own imagination.

Spreads make wonderful snacks. They're perfect for stuffing into celery sticks, smearing on crackers, or using as a dip for raw veggies, pretzels, or baked chips. A large dollop of a high-protein spread on a baked potato makes for a very filling meal. Spreads really come into their own when they are used as sandwich fillings. Add whole grain bread or a whole grain bun, a few of the trimmings (lettuce, tomatoes, onions, pickles, sprouts, peppers, or whatever strikes your fancy), and you've got a simple, nourishing meal in minutes. Try layering a corn or flour tortilla, chapati, or lavish with your favorite spread and fixings. Then just roll it up for a handy supper. Spreads are incredibly versatile, so let your creativity run wild.

Sandwiches run the gamut from basic peanut butter and jelly to veggie burgers with the works. In between are international favorites such as burritos, tostadas, and fajitas. Sandwiches can be much more wholesome than greasy cheese on standard-issue white bread, and far healthier than fatty meats on a bun. Have fun with sandwiches—they aren't just for lunch. Try a bean burrito for breakfast or tostadas served family-style for dinner. Don't forget that hot soup and a sandwich are always a perfect match.

Rice, Zucchini and Corn Salad

MAKES 6 SERVINGS

Here is a nourishing whole grain salad that will quash the hungriest of appetites.

3 cups cooked brown rice, or a mixture of brown and wild rice
1 pound small zucchini, cut in half lengthwise and sliced into half moons
2 cups cooked whole corn kernels (fresh, frozen, or canned)

¼ cup thinly sliced scallions
3 tablespoons fresh lemon juice
2 tablespoons extra-virgin olive oil
2 teaspoons Dijon mustard
2 teaspoons dillweed
½ teaspoon salt

Combine rice, zucchini, corn, and scallions in a large bowl. Whisk together remaining ingredients. Pour over rice and vegetables and toss well. Serve warm or thoroughly chilled.

Per one-cup serving: Calories: 212; Protein: 5g; Carbohydrate: 37g; Fat: 6g; Sodium: 242mg. Cholesterol: 0mg; Fiber: 4g.

Citrus Fruit and Grain Salad

MAKES 6 SERVINGS

Tart and juicy, this scrumptious salad uses fresh fruit and pantry staples to create the centerpiece of a meal.

4 cups cooked whole grain
(brown rice, wild rice, bulgur, or barley, or a combination)
2 navel oranges, peeled and chopped
½ cup minced fresh parsley
⅓ cup raisins

3 tablespoons fresh lemon juice
2 tablespoons extra-virgin olive oil
1 tablespoon wine vinegar (red, white, or balsamic)
2 teaspoons Dijon mustard
Salt and pepper

Combine grain, oranges, parsley, and raisins in a large bowl. In a small bowl whisk together oil, lemon juice, vinegar, and mustard. Pour over rice and fruit and toss well. Season with salt and pepper and toss again. Serve chilled.

Per one-cup serving: Calories: 240; Protein: 4g; Carbohydrate: 44g; Fat: 6g; Sodium: 243mg; Cholesterol: 0mg; Fiber: 4g.

Tunisian Potato Salad

MAKES 6 SERVINGS

Using just a few commonplace ingredients, this unique and tangy vinaigrette potato salad is sure to be a hit with your family and friends.

1 pound new potatoes
¼ cup fresh lemon juice
2 tablespoons extra-virgin olive oil
2 tablespoons water
1 teaspoon ground cumin
½ teaspoon paprika
Good pinch of cayenne pepper
Salt

Boil potatoes in salted water until tender. Cut in half if small, or quarters if large. Dress with lemon juice, olive oil, water, cumin, paprika, cayenne, and salt. Toss gently. Serve warm or thoroughly chilled.

Per ¾-cup serving: Calories: 82; Protein: 1g; Carbohydrate: 10g; Fat: 5g; Sodium: 354mg; Cholesterol: 0mg; Fiber: 1g.

Noodles in Nut Sauce

MAKES 8 SERVINGS

Enticing, enchanting, and irresistible!

⅓ cup natural peanut butter or other nut or seed butter
2 tablespoons low-sodium tamari
1½ tablespoons brown rice vinegar
1 tablespoon toasted sesame oil
1 teaspoon pure maple syrup or brown rice syrup
½ teaspoon ground ginger
½ teaspoon crushed garlic
Cayenne pepper
Water
12 ounces thin whole wheat or brown rice spaghetti
Thinly sliced scallions for garnish (optional)
Toasted sesame seeds for garnish (optional)

Combine nut butter, tamari, vinegar, oil, syrup, ginger, garlic, and cayenne pepper to taste in a large bowl. Stir vigorously until smooth and well combined. Gradually whisk in enough water, about 1 cup, to make a pourable sauce. Boil noodles in lightly salted water. Drain well. Rinse under cold water to cool, then drain again. Add to the bowl with the sauce and toss until evenly coated. Chill thoroughly before serving. The noodles will absorb any excess sauce as they chill. Garnish with scallions and/or toasted sesame seeds, if desired.

Per ½-cup serving: Calories: 248; Protein: 8g; Carbohydrate: 36g; Fat: 8g; Sodium: 195mg; Cholesterol: 0mg; Fiber: 2g.

Fresh Spring Salad

MAKES 8 SERVINGS

What a pleasing lunch or side salad! It's superb in spring and summer when there is an abundance of fresh vegetables and herbs, but it's equally delightful year round.

>   1 head romaine lettuce or 2 heads bibb lettuce
>   2 ripe tomatoes
>   1 cucumber, peeled
>   1 green bell pepper
>   8 red radishes
>   Minced mild red onions or thinly sliced scallions
>   Minced fresh cilantro, parsley, basil, or dillweed
>   3 to 4 tablespoons fresh lemon juice
>   1½ tablespoons extra-virgin olive oil
>   Salt and pepper

Finely chop or dice lettuce, tomatoes, cucumber, pepper, and radishes, if using. Place in a bowl along with the onion and fresh herbs. Dress with lemon juice, oil, salt, and pepper, to taste, just before serving.

Per one-cup serving: Calories: 54; Protein: 2g; carbohydrate: 7g; Fat: 3g; Sodium: 157mg; Cholesterol: 0mg; Fiber: 2g.

Tang Tsel

MAKES 4 SERVINGS

The humble cabbage rises to prominence in this simple but incredibly delicious salad that is based on an old Himalayan recipe.

>   1 cup thinly sliced or shredded green cabbage
>   1 cup thinly sliced or shredded red cabbage
>   1 small tomato, seeded and sliced into thin slivers
>   ¼ cup brown rice vinegar
>   2 teaspoons toasted sesame oil

Combine cabbage and tomato in a medium bowl and toss gently. Sprinkle vinegar and sesame oil over vegetables and toss again to mix thoroughly. Serve at once or chill.

Per one-cup serving: Calories: 38; Protein: 1g; Carbohydrate: 4g; Fat: 2.5g; Sodium: 8mg; Cholesterol: 0mg; Fiber: 1g.

Spicy Cucumber Salad

MAKES 4 SERVINGS

This light, refreshing salad is aromatic and tantalizing with just a bit of a pungent bite.

> 2 cups thinly sliced English cucumbers
> Salt
> 2 tablespoons brown rice vinegar
> 2 teaspoons toasted sesame oil
> Pinch of cayenne pepper

Sprinkle cucumbers with plenty of salt and leave to drain in a colander for at least 30 minutes until they soften and lose their juices. Rinse under cold water and drain well. Transfer to a medium bowl and sprinkle with vinegar and oil. Season with cayenne pepper. Toss to mix thoroughly. Serve at once or chill.

Per ½-cup serving: Calories: 29; Protein: less than one gram; Carbohydrate: 2g; Fat: 2.5g; Sodium: 292mg; Cholesterol: 0mg; Fiber: less than one gram.

Salad of Chickpeas, Tomato and Walnuts

MAKES 4 SERVINGS

This delightful salad is a fine example of how simple ingredients often create the most memorable dishes. Serve it with a hearty whole grain bread to dip into the flavorful dressing.

2 cups drained cooked or canned chickpeas (one 15-ounce can)

1 medium tomato, chopped

¼ cup walnuts broken into pieces

¼ cup raisins

¼ cup minced fresh parsley

2 tablespoons fresh lemon juice

1½ teaspoons extra-virgin olive oil

Salt and pepper

Combine all the ingredients in a large bowl. Toss to mix well.

Per ¾-cup serving: Calories: 236; Protein: 9g; Carbohydrate: 33g; Fat: 9g; Sodium: 302mg; Cholesterol: 0mg; Fiber: 8g.

Chicka-Dee Pea Salad

MAKES 2 TO 4 SERVINGS

For an attractive luncheon, scoop this salad onto lettuce-lined plates, garnish it with a little paprika, and surround it with fresh tomato wedges. Alternatively, spread it on whole grain bread or stuff it into whole wheat pitas with lettuce and fresh tomato slices.

2 cups drained cooked or canned chickpeas (one 15-ounce can)

½ cup finely diced celery

2 tablespoons fresh lemon juice

1½ teaspoons extra-virgin olive oil

1 thinly sliced scallion, or grated onion to taste

2 tablespoons minced fresh parsley (optional)

2 teaspoons well-drained pickle relish or chopped pickles

2 teaspoons brown mustard

¼ teaspoon paprika

Salt and pepper

Chop beans in a food processor or mash them well with a potato masher or fork. Stir in remaining ingredients and mix thoroughly. Chill before serving.

Per ¾-cup serving: Calories: 197; Protein: 7g; Carbohydrate: 29g; Fat: 7g; Sodium: 699mg; Cholesterol: 0mg; Fiber: 6g.

Chickenless Chicken Salad

MAKES 4 CUPS (ABOUT 6 SERVINGS)

This salad is a wonderful pretender—it has all the ingredients that make a great "chicken" salad, but without the bird! Serve it on a bed of fresh, crisp greens or as a hearty sandwich filling.

1 pound extra-firm regular tofu, rinsed and patted dry
1 cup water
¼ cup low-sodium tamari
½ cup finely diced celery
½ cup finely diced red bell pepper
Thinly sliced scallions or grated onion (optional)
1 cup No-Naise Dressing (recipe follows)

Preheat oven to 400°F. Mist a baking sheet with nonstick cooking spray or line with parchment paper and set aside. Cut tofu into ¼-inch-thick slices. Place in two shallow dishes, large enough to fit the tofu in a single layer. Combine water and tamari and pour over tofu. Let marinate 15 to 30 minutes. Remove tofu from marinade and place in a single layer on prepared baking sheet. Bake until it is deep, golden brown and the surface is dry, about 30 minutes. Allow tofu to cool until it can be easily handled, then slice into very thin strips or shreds. Transfer to a bowl with the vegetables and add thinly sliced scallions or grated onion, if desired. Add just enough No-Naise Dressing to the salad to moisten it to your liking. Toss gently until everything is evenly coated. Chill before serving.

Per ⅔-cup serving: Calories: 323; Protein: 21g; Carbohydrate: 8g; Fat: 26g; Sodium: 690mg; Cholesterol: 0mg; Fiber: less than one gram.

No-Naise Dressing

MAKES ABOUT 1½ CUPS

This is the perfect low-fat substitute for traditional egg-laden mayonnaise. Be sure to include the Dijon mustard when making the Chickenless Chicken Salad, as it will give the salad a little extra bite.

1½ cups (about 12 ounces) firm silken tofu, crumbled

3 tablespoons fresh lemon juice

2 teaspoons Dijon mustard (optional)

½ teaspoon salt

¼ teaspoon dry mustard

2 tablespoons organic canola oil or extra-virgin olive oil

Place all ingredients, except oil, in blender or food processor and process until smooth and creamy. With appliance running, drizzle in the oil in a slow, steady stream through the opening in the lid. Store in refrigerator. Will keep for 7 to 10 days.

Per 2-tablespoon serving: Calories: 18; Protein: 1g; Carbohydrate: less than one gram; Fat: 1g; Sodium: 103mg; Cholesterol: 0mg; Fiber: 0g.

Chick Cheeze

MAKES ABOUT 2 CUPS

This cheddar-style spread is sharp, tangy, and rich. Use it as a spread for bread or crackers, a dip for veggies, or a topping for grains, pizza, or potatoes. Stir it into sauces, gravies, soups, or casseroles whenever you want to add a spark of cheesy flavor.

2 cups drained cooked or canned chickpeas (one 15-ounce can)

3 tablespoons nutritional yeast flakes

2 tablespoons sesame tahini

2 tablespoons white wine vinegar

1½ tablespoons light miso

1 tablespoon extra-virgin olive oil

1 teaspoon onion powder

¾ teaspoon salt

½ teaspoon paprika

¼ teaspoon garlic powder

¼ teaspoon dry mustard

Combine all ingredients in food processor fitted with a metal blade. Process into a smooth paste, stopping to scrape down sides of work bowl as necessary. Chill several hours or overnight before serving, to allow flavors to blend. Keeps about 7 days in the refrigerator.

Per one-quarter-cup serving: Calories: 115; Protein: 5g; Carbohydrate: 14g; Fat: 5g; Sodium: 437mg; Cholesterol: 0mg; Fiber: 4g.

Eggplant Pecan Pesto

MAKES ABOUT 3 CUPS

Here's a superb dairy-free pesto that is very simple to prepare. It is equally delicious as a dip or topping served at room temperature, or as a warm sauce over pasta or grains.

½ cup water, more or less as needed
1 medium onion, diced
½ teaspoon crushed garlic
1 large eggplant, peeled
1 cup pecans
½ cup fresh basil, firmly packed
2 to 3 tablespoons fresh lemon juice
2 to 4 tablespoons light miso

Heat water in a large nonstick skillet. Add onion and garlic and cook over medium-high heat for 5 minutes. Meanwhile, cut eggplant into ½-inch cubes. Add to onion, cover, and reduce heat to medium. Cook, stirring often, until eggplant is very soft, about 25 to 30 minutes. If necessary, add a little more water to keep eggplant from sticking to pan. When tender, transfer eggplant mixture to blender. Add remaining ingredients and process until completely smooth. Mixture will be thick. Serve immediately while warm or at room temperature. Store leftovers in refrigerator and reheat to serve.

Per one-half-cup serving: Calories: 150g; Protein: 3g; Carbohydrate: 8g; Fat: 13g; Sodium: 84mg; Cholesterol: 0mg; Fiber: 3g.

Green Bean and Walnut Paté

MAKES ABOUT 2 CUPS

Serve this classic "meaty" spread on a bed of lettuce garnished with tomatoes, or as a spread for whole grain crackers, matzo, or bread.

2 teaspoons olive oil
1 large onion, diced
2 cups steamed green beans, cooled and coarsely chopped
½ pound firm regular tofu, rinsed
1 cup chopped walnuts
Pinch of ground allspice
Salt and pepper

Heat oil in a skillet over medium-high heat. Add onion and sauté until dark brown and caramelized, about 30 to 60 minutes. If onion sticks to the pan, add a little water. Slice tofu into thick slabs and simmer in enough water to cover for 10 minutes. Drain well and transfer to a bowl. Cool then mash. Combine tofu, onion, green beans, and walnuts in food processor, and process into a smooth paste. Season with allspice, salt, and pepper to taste. Chill thoroughly before serving.

Per tablespoon: Calories: 36; Protein: 1g; Carbohydrate: 2g; Fat: 3g; Sodium: 40mg; Cholesterol: 0mg; Fiber: 1g.

Savory Spinach Spread

MAKES ABOUT 2 CUPS

Serve this delightfully creamy spread on crackers, pita triangles, or thinly sliced French bread.

1½ cups (about 12 ounces) firm silken tofu, crumbled
1 tablespoon fresh lemon juice
¾ teaspoon onion powder
½ teaspoon tarragon
¼ teaspoon garlic powder
¼ teaspoon salt

1 (10-ounce) box frozen chopped spinach, thawed
1 cup shredded carrots
¼ cup thinly sliced scallions

Combine tofu, lemon juice, onion powder, tarragon, garlic powder, and salt in blender or food processor and blend until smooth and creamy. Transfer to a medium bowl. Squeeze spinach as dry as possible. Stir into tofu along with carrots and scallions. Mix well. Chill thoroughly before serving.

Per one-half-cup serving: Calories: 90; Protein: 9g; Carbohydrate: 10g; Fat: 2.5g; Sodium: 249mg; Cholesterol: 0mg; Fiber: 3g.

Colorful Chili Dip

MAKES 2 CUPS

Serve this zesty dip with baked corn chips or whole grain crackers or as a sandwich spread.

2 cups drained cooked or canned pinto beans (one 15-ounce can)
1 medium scallion, sliced
2 tablespoons balsamic vinegar
1 teaspoon chili powder
½ teaspoon ground cumin
½ teaspoon oregano
Several shakes Tabasco sauce, to taste
¼ cup minced red bell pepper
¼ cup minced green bell pepper

Combine all ingredients except bell peppers in food processor fitted with a metal blade. Blend until smooth and creamy. Transfer to a bowl and stir in bell peppers. Mix well. Chill thoroughly before serving.

Per one-half-cup serving: Calories: 134; Protein: 8g; Carbohydrate: 25g; Fat: less than one gram; Sodium: 14mg; Cholesterol: 0mg; Fiber: 8g.

Spicy Peanut Spread

MAKES ABOUT 2½ CUPS

This sassy spread is full of surprises. Although it contains rich peanut butter, the fat is reduced a bit by using tofu for a creamy texture and salsa to pump up the flavor. It makes a hearty, "meaty" sandwich filling or dip.

    1 pound firm regular tofu, rinsed
    ½ cup natural peanut butter
    ½ cup prepared salsa
    2 tablespoons balsamic vinegar
    4 scallions, thinly sliced
    2 stalks celery, minced
    ¼ cup minced fresh cilantro

Slice tofu into thick slabs and simmer in enough water to cover for 10 minutes. Drain well and let cool. Combine tofu, peanut butter, salsa, and vinegar in food processor and process into a smooth paste. Transfer to a bowl and stir in scallions, celery, and cilantro. Chill thoroughly before serving.

Per one-quarter cup serving: Calories: 133; Protein: 7g; Carbohydrate: 8g; Fat: 8g; Sodium: 156mg; Cholesterol: 0mg; Fiber: 2g.

Eggless Egg Salad Sandwich Spread

MAKES ABOUT 2½ CUPS

This well seasoned, high-protein spread proves that tofu can be delicious.

    1 pound firm regular tofu
    ¼ cup No-Naise Dressing (page 239)
    ¼ cup nutritional yeast flakes
    2 tablespoons sesame tahini
    2 tablespoons balsamic vinegar
    2 tablespoons sweet pickle relish

2 tablespoons minced onion
1 tablespoon Dijon mustard
½ teaspoon crushed garlic
Salt, black pepper, and cayenne pepper

Slice tofu into thick slabs and simmer in enough water to cover for 10 minutes. Drain well and transfer to a bowl. Cool, then mash. Stir in remaining ingredients and mix well. Season with salt, black pepper, and cayenne pepper to taste.

Per one-cup serving: Calories: 279; Protein: 27g; Carbohydrate: 23g; Fat: 12g; Sodium: 583mg; Cholesterol: 0mg; Fiber: 9g.

Italian Chickpea Spread

MAKES ABOUT 1½ CUPS

Enjoy this delicious, low-fat spread in sandwiches or on crackers. It's satisfying and light.

2 cups drained cooked or canned chickpeas (one 15-ounce can)
2 tablespoons water
2 teaspoons extra-virgin olive oil
1 tablespoon balsamic vinegar or fresh lemon juice
½ teaspoon basil
½ teaspoon oregano
¼ to ½ teaspoon crushed garlic
Salt and pepper

Combine all ingredients in food processor and process into a smooth paste, stopping to scrape down sides of work bowl as necessary. Chill several hours or overnight before serving to allow flavors to blend. Keeps 5 to 7 days in the refrigerator.

Per one-half-cup serving: Calories: 212; Protein: 10g; Carbohydrate: 31g; Fat: 6g; Sodium: 654mg; Cholesterol: 0mg; Fiber: 9g.

Sloppy Joes

MAKES 4 SERVINGS

This quick sandwich staple is the vegetarian version of beef-based Sloppy Joes that both kids and grownups adore.

2 teaspoons olive oil

1 medium onion, diced

8 ounces tempeh, well crumbled

2 tablespoons low-sodium tamari

½ cup ketchup

1 teaspoon prepared yellow mustard

1 teaspoon apple cider vinegar

1 teaspoon sweetener of your choice

4 whole grain burger buns, split

Heat oil in a medium saucepan. When hot, add onion, tempeh, and tamari and sauté until onion is tender and lightly browned, about 10 minutes. Add remaining ingredients except the buns and mix well. Reduce heat to medium and simmer uncovered for 10 minutes, stirring often. Spoon hot mixture over split buns. Serve at once.

VARIATION:

If preferred, replace tempeh with 1 cup TVP (texturized vegetable protein) that has been rehydrated in ⅞ cup of boiling water. Let rest for 5 minutes, then proceed with recipe as directed.

Per one-quarter-cup serving: Calories: 253; Protein: 15g; Carbohydrate: 31g; Fat: 8g; Sodium: 696mg; Cholesterol: 0mg; Fiber: 3g.

Tempeh Tostadas

MAKES 4 TO 8 SERVINGS (1 OR 2 TACOS PER PERSON)

For a Tex-Mex treat, serve these south-of-the-border specialties with plenty of your favorite toppings.

8 ounces tempeh, steamed 20 minutes, cooled, and crumbled

2 tablespoons low-sodium tamari

2 teaspoons chili powder

1 teaspoon garlic powder

½ teaspoon ground cumin

½ teaspoon dried oregano

Tabasco sauce, to taste

8 corn tortillas

2 teaspoons olive oil

½ cup finely chopped onion

Topping Options (select one or more)

1 to 2 cups shredded lettuce

2 ripe tomatoes, chopped

1 small avocado, cut into chunks

½ cup shredded carrot

½ cup prepared salsa

½ cup minced fresh cilantro

½ cup sliced black olives

2 to 4 scallions, sliced

4 to 6 tablespoons No-Naise Dressing, (page 239)

¼ cup finely chopped red onion

Combine crumbled tempeh, tamari, chili powder, garlic powder, cumin, oregano, and Tabasco sauce, and toss until thoroughly combined. Warm tortillas one by one in a dry skillet, then stack in a clean towel to keep warm. Heat oil in the skillet. When hot, add onion, and sauté until tender, about 10 to 15 minutes. Add reserved tempeh to skillet and sauté until lightly browned, about 4 to 6 minutes. Spoon an equal portion of the tempeh mixture onto each of the reserved tortillas. Add your favorite toppings, or place bowls of several different toppings on the table. To eat, gently fold the tortillas, and pick them up with your hands.

Per tostada: Calories: 134; Protein: 7.5g; Carbohydrate: 17g; Fat: 5g; Sodium: 205mg; Cholesterol: 0mg; Fiber: 2g.

Red Bean Burritos

MAKES 2 TO 4 SERVINGS (1 OR 2 BURRITOS PER PERSON)

Burritos are always fun, and they make a satisfying lunch or dinner.

4 whole wheat flour tortillas (lard-free)

2 cups drained cooked or canned pinto beans (one 15-ounce can)

½ cup prepared salsa

2 tablespoons finely chopped red or green bell pepper

1 teaspoon chili powder

¼ teaspoon garlic powder

¼ teaspoon ground cumin

¼ teaspoon oregano

Tabasco sauce, to taste

Topping Options (select one or more):

½ to 1 cup shredded lettuce

1 ripe tomato, chopped

½ of a small avocado, cut into chunks

¼ cup shredded carrot

¼ cup chopped, fresh cilantro leaves

¼ cup sliced black olives

1 to 2 scallions, sliced

2 to 3 tablespoons No-Naise Dressing (page 239)

2 tablespoons finely chopped red onion

Warm the tortillas one by one in a dry skillet. Stack them in a clean towel to keep warm. Combine the beans, salsa, bell pepper, and seasonings in a medium saucepan. Bring to a boil, reduce heat, and simmer uncovered 5 minutes, stirring occasionally. Remove from heat. Mash beans slightly with the back of a wooden spoon, fork, or potato masher. Spoon an equal portion of the bean mixture onto each of the tortillas, placing it in a strip along one side, slightly off center. Add your favorite toppings, and roll tortillas around the filling. To eat, carefully pick up a burrito with your hands, or use a knife and fork.

Per burrito: Calories: 184; Protein: 9g; Carbohydrate: 36g; Fat: 1g; Sodium: 122mg; Cholesterol: 0mg; Fiber: 9g.

Fantastic Fajitas

MAKES 4 SERVINGS

These vegetarian fajitas contain marinated tempeh that is browned and coupled with sautéed vegetables and fresh salad greens. Then everything is rolled burrito-style in warm flour tortillas. A spoonful of spicy salsa makes a delicious garnish.

8 ounces tempeh, steamed 20 minutes, cooled, and cut into ¼-inch- × 2½-inch strips

¼ cup red wine vinegar

¼ cup orange juice

2 tablespoons low-sodium tamari

2 teaspoons oregano

½ teaspoon ground cumin

Tabasco sauce, to taste

2 teaspoons olive oil

1 medium onion, cut into 8 wedges and separated

1 red or green bell pepper, cut into ½-inch- × 2-inch strips

4 whole wheat flour tortillas (lard-free)

Diced tomatoes, sliced scallions, shredded lettuce (optional)

Place tempeh strips in a large ceramic or glass bowl. In a separate bowl combine vinegar, orange juice, tamari, oregano, cumin, and Tabasco sauce. Mix well and pour over tempeh. Toss *very gently* so tempeh strips do not get broken, making sure each piece is well coated. Cover bowl and set aside. Allow tempeh to marinate 10 to 15 minutes. Meanwhile, warm tortillas in a dry skillet, and stack in a clean towel to keep warm. Heat 1 teaspoon of the oil in skillet. Drain tempeh strips and, when oil is hot, add to skillet in a single layer. Cook in two batches if necessary. Cook tempeh until bottom side is golden brown, about 5 minutes. Carefully turn strips over and brown other side about 3 minutes longer. Remove from skillet and transfer to a plate. Heat remaining teaspoon of oil in skillet. When oil is hot, add onion and pepper and sauté until tender, about 5 to 8 minutes. To assemble fajitas, spoon equal amounts of the tempeh and onion-pepper mixture onto each tortilla, placing them in a strip slightly off center. Top with tomatoes, scallion, and lettuce, if desired. Roll up each tortilla to enclose filling.

Per ¾-cup serving: Calories: 221; Protein: 14g; Carbohydrate: 24g; Fat: 9g; Sodium: 356mg; Cholesterol: 0mg; Fiber: 3g.

Better-Than-Grilled Cheese

MAKES 4 SANDWICHES

These longtime sandwich favorites have all the goo and glory we love, but now they are low-fat and dairy-free! If you like, serve them with a dab of grainy mustard spread on top.

⅔ cup water
¼ cup nutritional yeast flakes
2 tablespoons flour (any kind—your choice)
2 tablespoons fresh lemon juice
2 tablespoons sesame tahini
1½ tablespoons ketchup
2 teaspoons cornstarch
1 teaspoon onion powder
¼ teaspoon each: garlic powder, turmeric, dry mustard, and salt
8 slices whole grain bread

Combine all ingredients except bread in a medium saucepan and whisk until mixture is smooth. Bring to a boil, stirring constantly with the wire whisk. Reduce heat to low and cook, stirring constantly, until mixture is very thick and smooth. Remove from heat. Place 4 of the bread slices on a flat surface. Cover one side of each slice evenly with the cooked mixture. Top with remaining bread slices. Grill sandwiches in a large nonstick skillet or a heavy skillet misted with nonstick cooking spray or coated with a small amount of vegetable oil. Brown each side well, carefully turning over once. Slice sandwiches in half diagonally and serve at once.

Per sandwich: Calories: 354; Protein: 27g; Carbohydrate: 59g; Fat: 8g; Sodium: 712mg; Cholesterol: 0mg; Fiber: 15g.

Vegetables, Sides, and Sauces

Vegetables have lept from being mere afterthoughts to a position front and center on a healthy plate. They are rich in varied and subtle flavors and give you the benefits of vitamins, minerals, and other essential nutrients. Don't be shy with vegetables. If you like, you can turn them into a complete meal.

Garlic Broccoli

MAKES 4 SERVINGS

What a tasty way to serve greens!

1 large bunch broccoli	Salt
1 teaspoon olive oil	½ teaspoon crushed garlic
1 small onion, cut in half and thinly sliced	2 tablespoons capers

Cut broccoli into bite-size florets. Peel stems and cut in half lengthwise, then slice into 1-inch-long pieces. Heat oil in a large skillet. When hot, add onions and sprinkle lightly with salt. Cover and cook, stirring occasionally, just until onions are soft. Stir in garlic and cook 1 minute, then add capers and prepared broccoli and sprinkle with a little more salt to taste. Cover and cook, stirring occasionally, until broccoli is bright green and tender-crisp.

Per one-cup serving: Calories: 44; Protein: 3g; Carbohydrate: 7g; Fat: 2g; Sodium: 442mg; Cholesterol: 0mg; Fiber: 3g.

Barbecued Eggplant Steaks

MAKES 4 SERVINGS

These delicious, easy-to-prepare eggplant slices make an appealing side dish. Leftovers are great as a quick and tasty sandwich filling or as a burger alternative. Be sure to use a barbecue sauce with a flavor you adore, as the sauce is the heart of the recipe.

    1 medium eggplant
    Bottled barbecue sauce, as needed
    Salt

Cut eggplant into ½-inch-thick slices and sprinkle generously with salt. Place on a rack or in a colander in the sink and let rest for 30 minutes. Rinse off salt and pat dry with a clean kitchen towel. Preheat oven to 375°F. Mist a baking sheet with nonstick cooking spray and arrange eggplant slices in a single layer. Brush or spoon barbecue sauce over each slice and bake for 15 minutes. Turn slices over and brush or spoon barbecue sauce on other side. Bake 10 to 20 minutes longer, or until fork tender.

Per "steak": Calories: 50; Protein: 1g; Carbohydrate: 12g; Fat: less than one gram; Sodium: 484mg; Cholesterol: 0mg; Fiber: 3g.

Wilted Spinach

MAKES 4 SERVINGS

Wilted fresh spinach makes a vivid, almost-instant addition to any meal.

    2 bunches fresh spinach, stems removed
    1 teaspoon olive oil
    1 small onion, minced
    ½ teaspoon crushed garlic
    Pinch each: salt, pepper, nutmeg

Wash spinach well to remove any dirt, grit, or sand. Heat oil in a large skillet. When hot, add onion. Reduce heat, cover, and cook, stirring occasionally until limp. Stir in garlic and cook 1 minute longer. Add spinach and sprinkle lightly with salt, pepper, and nutmeg. Cover and cook just until wilted. Remove cover and cook a few minutes longer until all the liquid cooks off. Do not overcook!

Per one-half-cup serving: Calories: 12; Protein: less than one gram; Carbohydrate: 2g; Fat: less than one gram; Sodium: 310mg; Cholesterol: 0mg; Fiber: 2g.

Squash Pudding

MAKES 4 SERVINGS

Mashed winter squash is a sweet and colorful alternative to ordinary mashed potatoes. It's also the perfect holiday side dish in place of yams, and it even makes a tasty dessert, especially if you add a few toasted, chopped pecans.

    4 cups peeled butternut squash cut into cubes
    3 tablespoons pure maple syrup
    2 tablespoons sesame tahini, peanut butter, or almond butter
    ½ teaspoon vanilla extract
    Salt

Steam squash cubes until very soft. Transfer to a food processor along with the remaining ingredients and process until very smooth. Season with salt to taste. Serve hot.

Per one-half-cup serving: Calories: 148; Protein: 3g; Carbohydrate: 28g; Fat: 4g; Sodium: 300mg; Cholesterol: 0mg; Fiber: less than one gram.

Broccoli or Asparagus with Quick Hollandaise Sauce

MAKES 4 TO 6 SERVINGS

Hollandaise sauce makes all vegetables take notice. This version, however, is egg-and butter-free and very simple to prepare. Try it on asparagus for a classic dish, or on carrots or cauliflower, too. Your taste buds will applaud you!

> 4 to 6 cups bite-size broccoli florets, or 2 pounds trimmed asparagus spears
> 1 cup Quick Hollandaise Sauce (recipe follows)

Steam the broccoli or asparagus until bright green and tender-crisp. Serve with sauce on the side.

Per one-half-cup serving: Calories: 108; Protein: 9g; Carbohydrate: 11g; Fat: 5g; Sodium: 21mg; Cholesterol: 0mg; Fiber: 5g.

Quick Hollandaise Sauce

MAKES ABOUT 1 CUP

> 1 cup firm silken tofu, crumbled
> 2 tablespoons water
> 1 tablespoon fresh lemon juice
> 1 tablespoon nutritional yeast flakes
>
> 1 tablespoon sesame tahini
> 2 teaspoons extra-virgin olive oil
> 1 teaspoon prepared yellow mustard
> ½ teaspoon tarragon

Combine all ingredients in blender or food processor and process until smooth and very creamy. Chill. Stir before serving.

Per 2-tablespoon serving: Calories: 63; Protein: 4g; Carbohydrate: 4g; Fat: 4g; Sodium: 12mg; Cholesterol: 0mg; Fiber: 2g.

Steak Fries

MAKES 2 TO 4 SERVINGS

Thick, oven-baked french fries are low in fat but resonate with fabulous flavor.

2 large russet potatoes
1½ teaspoons olive oil
1 teaspoon paprika, or ½ teaspoon curry or chili powder
¼ teaspoon salt
Dash each: pepper, garlic powder, and turmeric

Preheat oven to 450°F. Line a large baking sheet with parchment paper (for easy cleanup) and set aside. Scrub potatoes well and remove any eyes and discolored areas. Peel, if desired, and cut into wedges or french fry shapes. Place in a large bowl, sprinkle with oil, and toss to coat evenly. Sprinkle with seasonings and toss again so all pieces are evenly coated. Arrange in a single layer on prepared baking sheet. Bake until golden brown and fork tender, about 30 minutes. For more even browning, turn over once midway through the cooking cycle.

Per one-half-cup serving: Calories: 80; Protein: 2g; Carbohydrate: 14g; Fat: 2g; Sodium: 148mg; Cholesterol: 0mg; Fiber: 2g.

Crusty Carrot Sticks

MAKES 2 TO 4 SERVINGS

One of the easiest and most delicious ways to serve nutritious, naturally sweet carrots.

> 1 pound carrots
> 1½ teaspoons extra-virgin olive oil
> 3 tablespoons nutritional yeast flakes
> Seasoned salt or salt-herb blend

Peel and trim carrots and cut into sticks about ½-inch thick by 3 inches long. Steam until tender. Transfer to a large bowl. Sprinkle with oil and toss gently. Sprinkle with nutritional yeast and season with salt blend to taste. Toss again until yeast and seasoning are evenly distributed.

Per one-half-cup serving: Calories: 154; Protein: 14g; Carbohydrate: 22g; Fat: 4g; Sodium: 140mg; Cholesterol: 0mg; Fiber: 9g.

Italian-Style Zucchini

MAKES 4 SERVINGS

Seasoned zucchini harmonizes with almost every meal.

> 1 teaspoon olive oil
> ½ teaspoon crushed garlic
> 2 medium zucchini, sliced on diagonal
> 1 to 2 teaspoons dried basil
> Salt and pepper

Heat oil in a large skillet. When hot add garlic and cook for 1 minute. Stir in zucchini, basil, salt, and pepper. Cover and cook, stirring once or twice, for 5 minutes. Uncover and cook until zucchini is fork-tender.

Per one-half-cup serving: Calories: 19; Protein: less than one gram; Carbohydrate: 2g; Fat: 1g; Sodium: 147mg; Cholesterol: 0mg; Fiber: less than one gram.

Stewed Green Beans and Tomatoes

MAKES 4 SERVINGS

This tasty combination of green beans, tomatoes, and onions is a classic Middle Eastern dish. Serve it with hearty, whole grain bread or pita bread.

2 teaspoons olive oil
1 large onion, quartered and thinly sliced
1 teaspoon crushed garlic
1½ pounds fresh green beans, trimmed and cut into 2-inch pieces
1 (28-ounce) can chopped tomatoes, undrained
Salt and pepper

Heat oil in a large skillet. When hot add onion, reduce heat, cover, and cook slowly until onion is limp. Add garlic and cook 1 minute more. Add green beans and sauté a few minutes. Cover and let beans steam in their own juices for 15 minutes. Add tomatoes and their juice, cover, and cook over low heat, stirring occasionally, for 30 to 35 minutes, or until beans are very tender. If mixture cooks dry add a little water. Season with salt and pepper to taste.

Per one-cup serving: Calories: 65; Protein: 3g; Carbohydrate: 11g; Fat: 2g; Sodium: 379mg; Cholesterol: 0mg; Fiber: 5g.

Green Peppers and Tomatoes

MAKES 4 TO 6 SERVINGS

This sumptuous, quick-cooked vegetable salad may be served either warm or cold. Be sure to pass plenty of pita bread to dip into the incredible sauce.

4 medium green bell peppers, seeded and diced
1 tablespoon olive oil
2 teaspoons crushed garlic

3 cups chopped fresh or canned tomatoes, undrained
2 tablespoons ground coriander
½ teaspoon salt

Heat oil in a large skillet. When hot add green peppers and cook until tender. Stir in garlic and sauté for 1 minute. Stir in tomatoes, coriander, and salt. Cover and cook 5 minutes longer. Serve warm or chilled.

Per one-cup serving: Calories: 71; Protein: 3g; Carbohydrate: 10g; Fat: 3g; Sodium: 450mg; Cholesterol: 0mg; Fiber: 3g.

Easy Baked Beans

MAKES 6 SERVINGS

Here is a time-honored classic made simple.

> 2 teaspoons olive oil
> 2 large onions, minced
> 2 teaspoons crushed garlic
> 1 (6-ounce) can unsalted tomato paste
> ¼ cup low-sodium tamari
> 2 to 4 tablespoons light molasses or pure maple syrup
> 2 teaspoons prepared yellow mustard
> 4 cups drained cooked or canned navy or pinto beans
>   (two 15-ounce cans)

Preheat oven to 350°F. Mist a medium casserole dish with nonstick cooking spray and set aside. Heat oil in a large skillet. When hot add onion and garlic and sauté until onion is well browned and very tender. Meanwhile, combine tomato paste, tamari, molasses or maple syrup, and mustard in a large bowl. Mix well to form a smooth, thick sauce. Add beans and mix gently. Stir cooked onion into beans and spoon mixture into prepared casserole dish. Cover tightly and bake for 30 minutes.

Per one-half-cup serving: Calories: 182; Protein: 9g; Carbohydrate: 34g; Fat: 2g; Sodium: 436mg; Cholesterol: 0mg; Fiber: 7g.

Sautéed Mushrooms and Scallions

MAKES 4 SERVINGS

Simple but delicious, this perky side dish is bound to become a family favorite.

1 pound button mushrooms, thinly sliced
2 teaspoons olive oil
1 teaspoon whole cumin seeds
8 scallions, thinly sliced
1¼ teaspoons salt
1 tablespoon fresh lemon juice
Good pinch each: black pepper and cayenne pepper

Heat oil in a large skillet. When hot add cumin seeds and let sizzle for several seconds. Add scallions and stir-fry a minute or two. Add mushrooms and salt and sauté just until tender. Season with lemon juice, black pepper, and cayenne.

Per one-half-cup serving: Calories: 65; Protein: 4g; Carbohydrate: 6g; Fat: 5g; Sodium: 737mg; Cholesterol: 0mg; Fiber: 2g.

Sweet and Salty Southern Braised Turnips

MAKES 4 TO 6 SERVINGS

Gently braised turnips are surprisingly delicious. Be sure to peel them deeply, as their skin can be fairly thick. You can braise the turnip's greens right along with them, if you are lucky enough to find them attached.

1 tablespoon organic canola or safflower oil
2 pounds turnips, peeled and cut into 1-inch dice
1 cup water
2 tablespoons low-sodium tamari
1 tablespoon sugar or other sweetener of your choice
1 teaspoon toasted sesame oil

Heat oil in a large skillet. When hot add turnips and stir-fry until light browned all over, about 5 to 8 minutes. Add water, tamari, and sugar, and bring to a boil. Cover, reduce heat, and simmer, stirring occasionally, until turnips are tender, about 15 minutes. Sprinkle with toasted sesame oil, toss gently, and serve.

Per one-half-cup serving: Calories: 80; Protein: 2g; Carbohydrate: 12g; Fat: 3g; Sodium: 305mg; Cholesterol: 0mg; Fiber: 3g.

Fried Pepper and Tomato Salad

MAKES 8 SERVINGS

This unusual dish is more like a vegetable jam or spread than a conventional salad. It is traditionally served on bread accompanied with fresh lemon wedges.

4 red bell peppers, cut into ¾-inch pieces
1 tablespoon olive oil
2 ripe tomatoes, chopped
½ teaspoon crushed garlic
1 to 2 teaspoons sugar or other sweetener of your choice
Salt and pepper

Heat oil in a large skillet. Add peppers and fry over low heat until soft and lightly browned. Add tomatoes, garlic, sugar, salt, and pepper and simmer uncovered until the mixture is very thick, about 30 minutes. Serve warm or cold.

Per one-half-cup serving: Calories: 46; Protein: 1g; Carbohydrate: 7g; Fat: 2g; Sodium: 77mg; Cholesterol: 0mg; Fiber: 2g.

Pilaki (cooked vegetable salad)

MAKES 6 TO 8 SERVINGS

When you serve this cooked and chilled salad everyone will beg for second helpings!

1 tablespoon olive oil	1 teaspoon ground cumin
2 large onions, cut in half and sliced	Good pinch of cayenne pepper
½ teaspoon crushed garlic	¾ cup water
4 green bell peppers, sliced into narrow strips	Salt and pepper
	3 tablespoons fresh lemon juice
2 large tomatoes, chopped	Minced fresh parsley (optional)

Heat oil in a large skillet. Add onions and garlic and sauté until onions are soft. Add green peppers, tomatoes, cumin, and cayenne. Sauté 5 minutes. Add water and bring to a simmer. Simmer uncovered, stirring occasionally, until liquid has cooked off and peppers are tender, about 40 to 45 minutes. Season with lemon juice, salt, and pepper. Chill thoroughly. Garnish with parsley just before serving, if desired.

Per one-half-cup serving: Calories: 80; Protein: 2g; Carbohydrate: 12g; Fat: 4g; Sodium: 737mg; Cholesterol: 0mg; Fiber: 2g.

Sesame Broccoli

MAKES 6 SERVINGS

A feast for the eyes as well as the palate, this attractive combination complements almost any main dish. Served chilled, Sesame Broccoli makes an unusual and appetizing salad.

6 cups broccoli florets	2 tablespoons lightly toasted sesame seeds
1 tablespoon olive oil	
1 red bell pepper, sliced into matchsticks	1 tablespoon dark sesame oil
	Salt or natural soy sauce
½ teaspoon crushed garlic	

Steam broccoli until tender-crisp. Transfer to a bowl. Heat olive oil in a medium skillet. Add pepper and sauté until tender. Stir in garlic and cook 30 seconds. Remove from heat and pour over broccoli. Add remaining ingredients and toss gently. Serve warm or thoroughly chilled.

Per one-cup serving: Calories: 89; Protein: 3g; Carbohydrate: 7g; Fat: 6g; Sodium: 122mg; Cholesterol: 0mg; Fiber: 4g.

Caponata (Italian cold eggplant salad)

MAKES 6 TO 8 SERVINGS

This tantalizing, sweet-and-sour vegetable mixture is irresistible. Try it as a side dish, as a spread for whole grain bread or rolls, or as a topping for baked potatoes, pasta, or rice.

2 pounds eggplant, peeled and cubed
1 large onion, chopped
1 tablespoon olive oil
½ teaspoon crushed garlic
4 ripe tomatoes, peeled and chopped
3 stalks celery, sliced or chopped

½ cup pitted green olives, cut lengthwise into quarters
4 to 6 tablespoons wine vinegar
1½ to 3 tablespoons sugar or other sweetener of your choice
2 tablespoons capers
Salt and pepper

Place eggplant in a colander and sprinkle generously with salt. Put a plate on top of the eggplant and a weight (such as a pan of water) on the plate. Let sit for 1 hour. Then rinse eggplant, and pat dry with a clean kitchen towel. Heat oil in a large skillet or saucepan. When hot add onion and sauté until soft. Add garlic and sauté for 1 minute. Add eggplant, tomatoes, celery, olives, vinegar, sugar (start with the smaller amounts of vinegar and sugar and add more to taste at the end, if necessary), capers, salt, and pepper. Bring to a boil. Reduce heat slightly and simmer, stirring often, until tomatoes have cooked down to a thick sauce, about 25 to 30 minutes. Chill thoroughly before serving.

Per one-cup serving: Calories: 97; Protein: 2g; Carbohydrate: 16g; Fat: 3g; Sodium: 377mg; Cholesterol: 0mg; Fiber: 4g.

Greens and Garlic

MAKES 4 SERVINGS

This is an absolutely spectacular way to serve greens! Don't be intimidated by the large quantity of garlic. Thinly sliced garlic is surprisingly mild, because very little of its pungent oil is released.

Vegetable mix
8 cups greens, thinly sliced, torn, or chopped into small pieces
   (see Tip below)
1 tablespoon olive oil
6 to 8 cloves garlic, very thinly sliced
¼ to ½ cup water, as needed

Seasoning options
Tabasco sauce
Fresh lemon juice
Salt, black pepper, cayenne pepper

Heat oil in a very large saucepan. When hot add garlic and stir-fry 30 seconds. Add greens, toss to coat with the oil, and stir-fry until slightly wilted, about 2 to 5 minutes. Pour in just enough water to cover bottom of the pan and bring to a boil. Reduce heat slightly, cover, and steam, stirring occasionally for 12 to 18 minutes, or until greens are tender. There should be very little liquid left in the saucepan. If there is liquid, simmer uncovered briefly until it cooks off. If greens are cooking dry, add a little more water so they do not burn. Stir in seasoning options of your choice. Serve hot or warm.

TIP:
• For the greens, use collards, kale, mustard greens, turnip greens, beet greens, or a mixture of two or more.

Per one-half-cup serving: Calories: 68; Protein: 2g; Carbohydrate: 8g; Fat: 4g; Sodium: 46mg; Cholesterol: 0mg; Fiber: 4g.

Savory Brown Gravy

MAKES ABOUT 3 CUPS

This versatile gravy is great on everything from beans to mashed potatoes.

¼ cup arrowroot or cornstarch
⅓ cup low-sodium tamari
3 cups vegetable broth or water
1 teaspoon garlic powder
¼ cup sesame tahini

Combine arrowroot or cornstarch and tamari in a medium saucepan. Mix well to make a smooth, thin paste. Gradually whisk in broth or water and garlic powder. Cook over medium-high heat, stirring constantly with a wire whisk until gravy thickens and comes to a boil. Remove from heat and beat in tahini using the wire whisk. Serve at once.

TIP:
• This makes a very thick gravy. If you prefer a thinner consistency gradually beat in a little more water, about 1 or 2 teaspoons at a time, until it is the consistency you desire.

Per one-half-cup serving: Calories: 26; Protein: 1g; Carbohydrate: 3g; Fat: 2g; Sodium: 261mg; Cholesterol: 0mg; Fiber: less than one gram.

Quick and Easy Alfredo Sauce

MAKES ABOUT 4 CUPS

Use this amazing sauce to top pasta, vegetables, potatoes, or grains.

1½ cups (about 12 ounces) firm
silken tofu
2 cups plain soy or rice milk
1 teaspoon onion powder
½ teaspoon garlic powder

½ teaspoon salt
Pinch of ground nutmeg
1 cup parmesan cheese
alternative, such as Soymage
or Parmazano

Combine all ingredients except parmesan cheese alternative in a blender or food processor and process until very smooth and creamy. Transfer mixture to a medium saucepan and cook over low heat, stirring constantly until warmed through. Do not boil. Remove from heat and stir in parmesan cheese alternative. Adjust seasonings, if necessary. Serve at once.

Per one-half-cup serving: Calories: 93; Protein: 11g; Carbohydrate: 6g; Fat: 4g; Sodium: 423mg; Cholesterol: 0mg; Fiber: less than one gram.

Cheesy Sauce for Macaroni

MAKES ABOUT 2½ CUPS

This recipe is very adaptable, so feel to experiment with whatever herbs, spices, and seasonings you prefer. This is the quintessential sauce for healthier versions of macaroni and cheese.

½ cup flour (any kind—your choice)
½ cup nutritional yeast flakes
1 teaspoon salt
¼ teaspoon onion powder
¼ teaspoon garlic powder
¼ teaspoon hot or sweet paprika
2 cups water or plain soy milk
2 tablespoons olive oil
½ teaspoon prepared mustard (any kind—your choice)

Combine flour, yeast flakes, salt, onion powder, garlic powder, and paprika in a medium saucepan. Gradually whisk in water, olive oil, and mustard. Cook over medium heat, stirring almost constantly with a wire whisk until bubbly, thick, and smooth.

TIP:
• Leftover sauce should be stored in the refrigerator. It will become very thick and firm when chilled, but will turn "melty" again when gently reheated. A double boiler works well for reheating. Thin with a little water or plain soy milk if desired.

Per one-cup serving: Calories: 160; Protein: 9g; Carbohydrate: 15g; Fat: 8g; Sodium: 485g; Cholesterol: 0mg; Fiber: 5g.

Main Dishes

For many people, setting aside meaty, cheesy dishes leaves them uncertain what to put in their place. Never fear—today there is an incredible array of meatless options that are absolutely delicious, simple to prepare, satisfying, hearty, and—dare we say—"meaty." Just add a salad or a few side dishes, and perhaps a whole grain bread, and you're all set.

You'll be delighted with the rich, new flavors you find here, and your body will thank you for their health value. A few recipes will use ingredients that may be new to you. Give yourself a chance to try them—you'll be very glad you did.

Before we get to the recipes themselves let's take a look at whole grains, a staple food for much of the world, often neglected in the West.

Storing and Cooking Whole Grains

Whole grains are a staple part of nearly all cuisines around the world, and for thousands of years they have been valued for their simplicity of preparation and nutritional value. If you like, whole grains work very well as the center of a meal, as they are filling and abundantly nutritious. They can function as the foundation for a chunky tomato sauce, vegetable stew, leftover soup, or saucy bean dish, and they will add substance and balance to lighter fare. You even could build effortless, impromptu meals around whole grains just by adding some beans, seasoned tofu, or tempeh, and whatever fresh vegetables you have on hand.

Planning meals around whole grains is fun and exciting because there is such a wide variety available to us. One visit to any well-stocked natural food store quickly reveals a multitude of options. Each grain has its own unique flavor and characteristics, so it can be a bit overwhelming trying to learn about all of them at once. Focus on one or two, adding more to your repertoire as you are ready.

At each kernel's core, called the "germ," is a tiny nutrient-packed seed that provides fat, protein, carbohydrates, and vitamins, and is capable of sprouting into a new plant. The surrounding endosperm layer is comprised of complex carbohydrates encased in protein that provides energy for the grain embryo. The bran is a hard protective coat that is rich in fiber, vitamins, and minerals. Whole grains are an excellent source of long-lasting energy and a rich source of B vitamins, vitamin E, and several minerals, including calcium, phosphorous, and iron.

Whole grains require different treatment than refined foods and must be handled with care. Grains with the germ intact contain oils that will go rancid rapidly if kept at room temperature, especially in hot weather. Store whole grains in the freezer or refrigerator in zippered plastic bags or airtight containers, labeled with the date of purchase. They will remain fresh for about 4 to 5 months.

Rinsing

Whole grains should be thoroughly rinsed before cooking, to remove dust or natural coatings that may impart a bitter taste. Clean the grain just before you are ready to use it, rinsing only the quantity you are planning to cook.

Toasting

Toasting grains refers to browning them in the cooking pot before they are simmered. Browning makes grains taste nuttier. It also allows them to absorb liquid more readily and cook more evenly. Depending on the grain, toasting can take from a few minutes to 10 or even 15 minutes, so it is a step that most people omit, with one exception—millet. The flavor of millet is really enhanced by toasting. It also cooks more completely and develops a fluffier, more pilaf-like texture. To toast grains:

1. Place the rinsed grain in a large, heavy-bottomed pot over medium heat. Stir with a wooden spoon until any remaining water has evaporated and the grain looks dry.
2. At this time some cooks add a teaspoon or so of oil for each cup of grain used. Although purely optional, a small amount of oil enhances the toasting process and helps to keep the grains separate and fluffy.
3. Reduce the heat slightly and continue stirring. Once the grains emit a roasted, nutty aroma and turn a shade or two darker, the toasting process is complete.
4. Pour the liquid into the pot and proceed with simmering the grain. Stand back a bit when you add the liquid, as it will sputter.

How to Cook Whole Grains

- Always cook grain in a heavy-bottomed pot with a tight-fitting lid. A loose-fitting lid is inefficient and may extend the cooking time or cause uneven results.

- The best liquids to use for cooking grains are water, bean broth (the water from cooked beans), or vegetable broth. Do not add salt to the grain if the liquid you are using contains salt.

- Bring the simmer liquid to a rolling boil before stirring in the grain.

- Cooking times for grains can vary greatly, depending on their age and storage conditions. If the grain is not completely cooked after the cooking time has elapsed and the water has been absorbed, stir in a few tablespoons of boiling water.

Cover the pot tightly and continue to cook the grain over very low heat until it is sufficiently done.

- If liquid remains after the grain is tender, drain it in a strainer. Then return it to the cooking pot and reheat it over very low heat to dry it out.

- If you have trouble with grains scorching or sticking to the bottom of your pot, use a heat diffuser.

- Fluff the grain with a fork before serving.

- Refrigerating leftover grain is the best way to store it, but cold grains tend to dry out and harden. To rehydrate place the grain on a vegetable steamer and put in a pot filled with an inch or two of water. Bring the water to a simmer, cover, and steam the grain, stirring once or twice with a fork until it is soft and hot, about 2 to 3 minutes.

Grain Cooking Times

Grain (1 cup)	Liquid (cups)	Optional Salt (teaspoons)	Minutes	Yield (cups)	Characteristics
Barley (hulled)	3	½–¾	1½ hrs. + 10 min. st*	3½–4	Has a pleasant, hearty texture; can be substituted for brown rice in any recipe.
Barley (pearl)	3	½–¾	50 + 10 min. st*	3½	See above.
Buckwheat (kasha)	2	½–¾	10–12 + 5 min. st*	2	Toasted buckwheat has a robust flavor; perfect for cold-weather fare.
Bulgur	2	½–¾	20 + 5 min. st*	3	Made by soaking and cooking the whole wheat kernel, then removing 5 percent of the bran and cracking the remaining kernel into small pieces. Bulgur can be used in salads, soups, breads, and desserts.
Couscous	2	½–¾	1 hr. + + 5 min. st*	3	Not a whole grain, couscous is a tiny beaded pasta made from durum wheat. Often served as a pilaf, couscous is a good source of protein.
Millet†	2½	½–¾	20–25 + 5 min. st*	3½	A handy alternative to rice; light toasting gives it a pleasing aroma and almost nutty flavor. It adds texture and flavor to breads, or can be ground and used interchangeably with cornmeal.
Quinoa	2	½–¾	15 + 5 min. st*	3–3½	This prize of the Incas is a superior source of protein as well as calcium, iron,

Grain (1 cup)	Liquid (cups)	Optional Salt (teaspoons)	Minutes	Yield (cups)	Characteristics
Quinoa (cont.)					vitamins, and potassium. Tasty and quick cooking, it's a welcome addition to almost any dish, from salads to desserts.
Rice, Basmati White	2	½	15–20 + 5 min. st*	3	Originally from Thailand and India, now also grown in California. A long-grain rice with a nutty, popcornlike fragrance.
Rice, Long Grain Brown	2¼	½	40 + 10 min. st*	3	Cooks to a firm, fluffy texture, with a mild, slightly nutty flavor. A good all-purpose rice.
Rice, Short Grain Brown	2¼	½	45–50 + 10 min. st*	3	Cooks to a nuttier texture than long grain brown rice with a slightly sweeter taste. If cooked beyond the "done" stage and with a little extra water it becomes sticky and is very suitable for vegetable sushi or rice pudding.
Wild Rice	2¾	¼†	50–55 + 10 min. st*	2½–3	Not really a rice, but a wild grass. Originally harvested by hand in boats by the native peoples of what is now Minnesota and the surrounding Great Lakes region, wild rice is a wonderful, nutty-flavored addition to any rice dish. Nutritionally, wild rice is superior to most grains, being high in protein, B vitamins, iron, and phosphorous.

*Standing time (covered)
†Toast before boiling for enhanced flavor and/or even cooking

272 Breaking the Food Seduction

Oven-Roasted Tom Tofu

MAKES 8 SLICES (ABOUT 4 SERVINGS)

Marinated tofu is coated with a seasoned flour and baked, creating succulent slices that can be used as an entrée or in sandwiches. Serve it with mashed potatoes and gravy (see Tip that follows recipe), bread stuffing, green beans, cranberry sauce, and a salad—you'll have a veritable holiday feast!

1 pound firm regular tofu, rinsed and patted dry

Marinade:
¾ cup water
3 tablespoons low-sodium tamari
3 tablespoons nutritional yeast flakes
½ teaspoon poultry seasoning
½ teaspoon ground coriander
½ teaspoon onion powder
½ teaspoon garlic powder

Coating Mix:
½ cup whole wheat flour
¼ cup yellow cornmeal
¼ cup nutritional yeast flakes
½ teaspoon onion powder
½ teaspoon salt
⅛ teaspoon pepper

Cut tofu into eight ½-inch-thick slices and place in a wide, shallow mixing bowl. Whisk together marinade ingredients and pour over tofu. Turn slices over so all sides are well coated. Cover bowl and place in refrigerator. Let marinate several hours or overnight, turning slices over occasionally, or spooning the marinade over them from time to time.

When ready to cook, preheat oven to 400°F. Mist a baking sheet with nonstick cooking spray, or line with parchment paper, and set aside. Combine ingredients for coating mix in a shallow bowl. Remove each slice of tofu from marinade one at a time and dredge in coating mix, covering it well all over. Place on prepared baking sheet as soon as it is coated. Mist the tops lightly with olive oil or nonstick cooking spray.

Bake until the bottoms are golden brown, about 15 minutes. Turn over slices and bake until other side is golden brown, about 15 minutes longer.

TIP:

• Save leftover marinade and thicken with a small amount of flour, arrowroot, or cornstarch to make a delicious gravy.

Per two-slice serving: Calories: 298; Protein: 27g; Carbohydrate: 28g; Fat: 11g; Sodium: 770mg; Cholesterol: 0mg; Fiber: 8g.

Oven-Barbecued Tofu Steaks

MAKES 4 SERVINGS

You can prepare these tender tofu steaks as mild or spicy as you like by adjusting the quantities of cayenne and black pepper. They make a great entrée or sandwich filling.

1 pound firm regular tofu
2 tablespoons salt-free tomato paste
2 tablespoons light molasses
2 tablespoons low-sodium tamari
2 tablespoons water
2 tablespoons balsamic vinegar
1 teaspoon olive oil
½ teaspoon dry mustard
½ teaspoon onion powder
½ teaspoon ground cinnamon
Black and cayenne pepper
Finely chopped scallions, for garnish (optional)

Preheat oven to 375°F. Mist a baking sheet with nonstick cooking spray, or line with parchment paper, and set aside. Rinse tofu and pat dry, then wrap it in a clean kitchen towel and press it gently all over with your hands to extract as much moisture as possible. Slice horizontally into four equal slabs and place on prepared baking sheet. Whisk together remaining ingredients except scallions until well combined.

Season with pepper and cayenne to taste. Spread some of the sauce mixture evenly over the top of the tofu slabs. Carefully turn slabs over and spread other side with some of the remaining sauce. If time permits, let the steaks rest at room temperature for 10 minutes to allow the flavor of the sauce to penetrate the tofu. Bake steaks for 20 minutes, basting occasionally with any remaining sauce. Serve hot, warm, or cold, garnished with scallions, if desired.

TIP:
- To infuse the tofu with a deeper barbecued flavor, marinate steaks in the refrigerator 4 to 6 hours, or even overnight, before baking.

Per slice: Calories: 226; Protein: 19g; Carbohydrate: 16g; Fat: 11g; Sodium: 325mg; Cholesterol: 0mg; Fiber: 4g.

Roadhouse Hash

MAKES 4 TO 6 SERVINGS

You'll never miss eggs or hash again, once you taste this hearty, cholesterol-free dish. Turmeric imparts a beautiful golden color and nutritional yeast flakes add a delicious egg-like flavor. Roadhouse Hash is wonderful for leisurely breakfasts, brunches, lunches, and dinners.

1½ teaspoons olive oil or organic canola or safflower oil
½ cup grated carrots
½ cup diced red or green bell peppers
½ cup thinly sliced scallions
¼ teaspoon turmeric
1 pound firm regular tofu, rinsed, patted dry and crumbled
1 cup drained cooked or canned red kidney beans
2 tablespoons nutritional yeast flakes
Seasoned salt (such as Spike, Herbamare, or garlic salt) and pepper
2 tablespoons minced fresh parsley (optional)

Heat oil in a large skillet over medium-high heat. When hot, add carrots, peppers, scallions, and turmeric, and sauté 3 to 4 minutes. Add tofu, beans, nutritional yeast flakes, seasoned salt, and pepper. Mix well and continue to cook, stirring almost constantly, for 5 to 7 minutes, or until hot. Stir in parsley, if using, and mix well. Serve at once.

Per one-half-cup serving: Calories: 125; Protein: 10g; Carbohydrate: 13g; Fat: 5g; Sodium: 255mg; Cholesterol: 0mg; Fiber: 5g.

Sweet and Sour Tempeh

MAKES 4 SERVINGS

This savory entrée always receives rave reviews. Serve it with a salad and a cooked grain of your choice.

2 teaspoons olive oil	¼ cup apple cider vinegar
8 ounces tempeh, cut into cubes	¼ cup water
1 cup grated carrots	1 tablespoon sweetener of your
1 red bell pepper sliced into	choice
strips	2 tablespoons low-sodium
1 green bell pepper sliced into	tamari
strips	1 tablespoon cornstarch
½ teaspoon crushed garlic	1 teaspoon ground ginger
2 cups canned pineapple	2 scallions thinly sliced
chunks packed in juice	(optional)

Heat oil in a large skillet. When hot add tempeh and cook 15 to 20 minutes, stirring almost constantly until browned all over. Add carrots, peppers, and garlic, and sauté with the tempeh until peppers are tender. Drain pineapple, but reserve ½ cup of the juice. Combine reserved juice and remaining ingredients except the pineapple chunks and scallion in a small bowl or measuring cup. Whisk together until well combined. Pour over tempeh and vegetables, then add pineapple chunks. Cook, stirring constantly, until sauce is just thickened, about 2 minutes. Serve hot, garnished with scallions if desired.

Per one-cup serving: Calories: 251; Protein: 12g; Carbohydrate: 34g; Fat: 9g; Sodium: 331mg; Cholesterol: 0mg; Fiber: 3g.

Quick Barbecued Tempeh

MAKES 4 SERVINGS

This incredibly simple dish is a fabulous choice for the outdoor grill. In cool weather cook it on an indoor grill or in the oven. Leftovers make a great sandwich filling.

    16 ounces tempeh
    1 large onion, halved and thinly sliced
    2 cups bottled barbecue sauce

Cut tempeh into 1-inch chunks. Steam over boiling water for 15 minutes. Place tempeh and sliced onion in a deep glass or ceramic dish and pour barbecue sauce over all. Toss gently and marinate in refrigerator for at least 1 hour. Cook on outdoor or indoor grill until browned and heated through. Baste frequently with barbecue sauce. Alternatively, bake in a covered casserole dish in a 350°F. oven for 30 minutes.

Per one-half-cup serving: Calories: 328; Protein: 24g; Carbohydrate: 30g; Fat: 9g; Sodium: 680mg; Cholesterol: 0mg; Fiber: 2g.

Southern Beans and Greens

MAKES 4 SERVINGS

This traditional Southern combination creates a beautiful dish with a heavenly blend of flavors and a surprisingly meaty texture. Serve it with rice or another grain on the side. It also makes an excellent topping for warm corn bread, or a delicious filling for pita pockets, tortillas, or chapatis.

    3 cups drained canned or cooked beans (your choice—any kind)
    1 cup vegetable broth or water
    ½ teaspoon crushed garlic
    4 cups chopped kale, stems and center ribs removed, lightly packed
    1 teaspoon olive oil
    Salt and pepper
    Tabasco sauce

Combine beans, broth or water, and garlic in a large saucepan. Place chopped kale on top of beans and bring to a boil. Cover, reduce heat to low, and simmer until kale is tender, about 15 to 20 minutes. Remove from heat and stir in oil, salt, pepper, and Tabasco sauce to taste.

Per one-cup serving: Calories: 250; Protein: 15g; Carbohydrate: 45g; Fat: 3g; Sodium: 309mg; Cholesterol: 0mg; Fiber: 10g.

Seitan Cassoulet

MAKES 4 SERVINGS

What was a classic lamb stew is now healthful, meatless, and chock-full of unbeatable flavor. Serve it with crusty rolls to dip in the fabulous gravy.

4 large carrots, peeled and sliced into 1-inch chunks
2 cups vegetable broth, water, or flat beer
2 stalks celery sliced diagonally into ½-inch pieces
1 teaspoon dried rosemary finely crushed
2 bay leaves
2 teaspoons olive oil
2 cups chopped onions
Heaping ¼ cup whole wheat flour
1 cup water
3 cups drained cooked or canned white beans
2 cups seitan chunks
2 tablespoons low-sodium tamari
Salt and pepper

Combine carrots, broth (or water, or beer), celery, rosemary, and bay leaves in a large saucepan and bring to a boil. Reduce heat to medium, cover, and simmer until vegetables are tender, about 20 minutes. Meanwhile, heat oil in a large skillet. When hot add onion and sauté until tender, about 10 minutes. Stir in flour and mix well. Then *gradually* stir in 1 cup water and mix vigorously until sauce is smooth. Remove from heat. When vegetables are tender stir in onion mixture and mix well. Stir in beans, seitan, and tamari. Bring to a boil stirring constantly, then reduce heat to medium. Simmer stew about 5 minutes until sauce thickens and the beans and seitan are hot. Remove bay leaves. Season with salt and pepper to taste. Ladle into soup bowls. Serve hot.

Per one-cup serving: Calories: 558; Protein: 50g; Carbohydrate: 80g; Fat: 5g; Sodium: 797mg; Cholesterol: 0mg; Fiber: 17g.

Chuckwagon Stew

MAKES 4 SERVINGS

Plenty of herbs and seasonings make a sensational broth for this stew. Bread for dipping into the gravy is absolutely essential. Come and get it!

3 cups vegetable broth or water	½ cup ketchup
8 ounces tempeh cut into ½-inch cubes	¼ cup low-sodium tamari
	1 teaspoon garlic powder
4 medium carrots, peeled and sliced	1 teaspoon dried tarragon
	¼ teaspoon pepper
2 medium potatoes, peeled and cut into bite-size chunks	¼ cup whole wheat flour
	⅓ cup cold water
2 medium onions cut into wedges	1 to 2 tablespoons minced fresh parsley for garnish (optional)

Combine broth or water, tempeh, vegetables, ketchup, tamari, garlic powder, tarragon, and pepper in a large saucepan and bring to a boil. Reduce heat to medium-low, cover, and simmer, stirring occasionally, until vegetables are tender, about 30 minutes. Place flour in a small bowl or measuring cup. Gradually stir in cold water, beating vigorously with a fork until mixture is smooth. Stir into the simmering stew. Cook, stirring constantly, until gravy is thickened and bubbly. Ladle into soup bowls. Garnish each serving with parsley, if desired.

TIP:
Choose reduced-sodium ingredient brands to trim sodium substantially.

Per one-cup serving: Calories: 405; Protein: 21g; Carbohydrate: 66g; Fat: 6g; Sodium: 1389mg; Cholesterol: 0mg; Fiber: 9g.

Broccoli Strudel

MAKES 4 TO 6 SERVINGS

This strudel consists of a phyllo dough crust filled with broccoli, onions, and seasoned tofu "cheese." It's elegant enough for company, yet simple enough for everyday fare.

6 sheets phyllo dough, thawed if frozen
1 teaspoon olive oil
1½ cups chopped onions
1 teaspoon crushed garlic
2 cups bite-size broccoli florets
1 pound firm regular tofu, rinsed, patted dry, and finely crumbled or
    mashed
2 tablespoons low-sodium tamari
2 teaspoons oregano
½ teaspoon nutmeg

Preheat oven to 350°F. Mist an 8-inch-square glass baking pan with nonstick cooking spray and set aside. Cover phyllo dough with a clean, damp kitchen towel and plastic wrap to prevent it from drying out. Heat oil in a large skillet. When hot add onions and garlic and sauté until onion is translucent, about 5 minutes. Add broccoli and continue to sauté until broccoli is bright green and tender-crisp, about 8 to 10 minutes longer. Transfer mixture to a large bowl. Add tofu, tamari, oregano, and nutmeg, and mix well. Arrange half of the phyllo sheets in the prepared baking dish, easing them in gently. Let edges of the dough hang over the sides of the dish. Spoon broccoli-tofu mixture into the phyllo dough, pressing it in gently to make a smooth, even layer. Separate remaining sheets of phyllo dough. Place them, one at a time, on top of the broccoli-tofu mixture. Lightly mist each one with olive oil or nonstick cooking spray. Fold in edges of phyllo dough 6 and mist top with a little more oil or cooking spray. Bake until crust is golden brown, about 25 to 30 minutes.

Per one-half-cup serving: Calories: 168; Protein: 7g; Carbohydrate: 18g; Fat: 7g; Sodium: 311mg; Cholesterol: 0mg; Fiber: 3g.

Seitan and Mushroom Stroganoff

MAKES 4 SERVINGS

This creamy stroganoff is perfect over rice, toast, or wide noodles. Just add a crunchy tossed salad on the side to complete your meal.

2 tablespoons cornstarch or arrowroot
3 tablespoons low-sodium tamari
1⅓ cups vegetable broth or water
½ teaspoon garlic powder
2 tablespoons sesame tahini
1 teaspoon olive oil
2 cups thinly sliced onions
1 teaspoon crushed garlic
4 cups sliced mushrooms
2 cups thinly sliced seitan strips
Pepper

For the gravy, combine cornstarch or arrowroot and tamari in a 2-quart saucepan. Mix well to make a thin, smooth paste. Gradually whisk in vegetable broth, or water, and garlic powder. Cook over medium-high heat, stirring constantly with a wire whisk until gravy thickens and comes to a boil. Remove from heat and vigorously whisk in tahini. Cover and set aside. Heat oil in a large skillet. When hot add onion and garlic and sauté 10 minutes. Add mushrooms and cook, stirring often, 5 to 7 minutes longer. Stir in seitan strips and reserved gravy. Reduce heat to low and cook, stirring often, just until the seitan is heated through, about 5 to 10 minutes. Season with pepper to taste. Serve at once.

Per one-cup serving: Calories: 373; Protein: 39g; Carbohydrate: 38g; Fat: 9g; Sodium: 657mg; Cholesterol: 0mg; Fiber: 6g.

Portobello Mushroom Steaks

MAKES 4 SERVINGS

These large, meaty mushrooms make an exquisite entrée, especially when surrounded by brightly colored vegetables such as green and yellow squash and red bell peppers or cherry tomatoes. The beefy-tasting sauce mingles with the mushroom juices to create a rich, flavorful gravy. You won't believe how scrumptious, chewy, simple, and satisfying plant-based "steaks" can be!

¼ cup ketchup
2 tablespoons balsamic vinegar
½ teaspoon crushed garlic
4 medium portobello mushrooms
Olive oil, as needed
Salt and pepper
Minced fresh parsley, chives, or scallions for garnish (optional)

Combine ketchup, vinegar, and garlic and set aside. Carefully remove mushroom stems, but leave caps whole. Rinse caps under water, gently rubbing with the surface of your thumb to remove any dirt. Place a thin layer of olive oil in a large skillet and heat over medium-high heat. If you do not have a skillet large enough to comfortably hold all four mushrooms at once, cook them in two batches or use two skillets. Place mushrooms in skillet, stem-side up. Cover and cook about 5 minutes. Turn over, reduce heat to medium, cover and continue to cook until fork-tender in the center, about 5 minutes longer. Season with salt and pepper. Spoon reserved sauce equally over each mushroom. Garnish with fresh herbs, if desired. Serve whole, or slice mushrooms on the bias (with the knife held at an angle).

Per "steak": Calories: 72; Protein: 4g; Carbohydrate: 11g; Fat: 1g; Sodium: 482mg; Cholesterol: 0mg; Fiber: 4g.

Cheesy Broccoli Polenta

MAKES 4 SERVINGS

Hot polenta is simply great for breakfast. It also makes an interesting main dish or side. Nutritional yeast flakes add a cheeselike touch, while broccoli adds flavor, nutrition, and beautiful flecks of green. Do not be tempted to substitute cornmeal for the corn grits, because you will not have good results. Use only the more coarsely ground, whole grain grits (polenta), which can be found in natural food stores and many super-markets. To round out your dinner, serve with steamed carrots or sliced tomatoes topped with fresh basil. Add a tossed salad with baby greens dressed with a splash of balsamic vinegar.

5 cups water

1⅓ cups yellow corn grits (polenta)

1 to 2 cups finely chopped broccoli

¼ cup nutritional yeast flakes

2 teaspoons olive oil (optional)

1 teaspoon salt

Bring water to a boil in a heavy-bottomed saucepan. Add broccoli and simmer until tender, about 5 minutes. Remove from heat and slowly stir in grits, stirring briskly with a long-handled wooden spoon. Return to a boil stirring constantly. Reduce heat to very low, cover, and cook, stirring occasionally, until very thick, about 20 to 40 minutes. Stir in nutritional yeast flakes, olive oil, if using, and salt, and mix until well combined.

TIPS:

• If the polenta sticks to the bottom of your saucepan slip a heat diffuser underneath.

• For less stirring and sticking, after the grits and broccoli come to a boil transfer the mixture to a double boiler to finish cooking.

Per one-cup serving: Calories: 111; Protein: 7g; Carbohydrate: 16g; Fat: 3g; Sodium: 782mg; Cholesterol: 0mg; Fiber: 3g.

Mandarin Stir-Fry

MAKES ABOUT 4 SERVINGS

The marinade used here adds a sweet and pungent flavor to this hearty, protein-rich dish. Serve it over brown rice, quinoa, or noodles.

3 tablespoons low-sodium tamari
1 tablespoon minced fresh ginger or ginger paste
1½ tablespoons pure maple syrup
1½ cups drained cooked or canned chickpeas (one 15-ounce can),
    or cubed firm regular tofu or tempeh, or seitan strips
2 teaspoons olive oil
1 large onion halved and thinly sliced
2 medium carrots thinly sliced on diagonal
4 cups bite-size broccoli florets
1 small zucchini or 1 cup snow pea pods, sliced on the diagonal

In a large bowl, whisk together tamari, ginger, and syrup. Add chickpeas, cubed tofu, tempeh, or seitan strips. Toss gently so all pieces are coated with marinade. Let marinate in refrigerator for 30 to 60 minutes or longer, stirring occasionally. Heat oil in a large wok or skillet over high heat. Add onion and sauté until golden brown, about 2 to 5 minutes. Add carrots and cook until just tender-crisp, about 2 to 5 minutes. Add marinated mixture and broccoli and cook until broccoli turns bright green, about 2 minutes. Add zucchini or snow pea pods and cook until tender-crisp and everything is warmed through, about 2 minutes more.

Per one-cup serving: Calories: 214; Protein: 10g; Carbohydrate: 36g; Fat: 4g; Sodium: 649mg; Cholesterol: 0mg; Fiber: 9g.

Stuffed Vegetable Rolls

MAKES ABOUT 4 SERVINGS

This is a variation of stuffed cabbage rolls using vibrant greens in place of the cabbage. Kale and collard greens are exceptionally high in calcium and other important vitamins and minerals. This recipe is a delicious way to incorporate these amazing greens into your repertoire, and it's actually quite simple to pull together. Serve the rolls with well-seasoned mashed potatoes for a hearty and delectable meal.

12 very large kale or collard
    leaves
1 cup vegetable broth or water
1 cup finely diced zucchini
1 small red bell pepper, finely
    chopped
⅔ cup medium-grind bulgur
¼ cup raisins or currants
1 teaspoon basil

½ teaspoon marjoram
½ teaspoon garlic powder
½ teaspoon salt
¼ teaspoon pepper
½ cup chopped walnuts
1 tablespoon fresh lemon juice
2 cups tomato sauce
Several drops Tabasco sauce

Thoroughly clean the kale or collard greens and carefully cut off the stems. Bring a large pot of water to the boil. Add the whole leaves to the pot, reduce heat, and simmer until leaves are bright green, wilted, and tender, about 12 to 15 minutes. Carefully drain leaves and let cool until they can be handled easily.

Meanwhile, combine water, zucchini, bell pepper, bulgur, raisins or currants, herbs, garlic powder, salt, and pepper in a large saucepan and bring to a boil. Reduce heat to medium, cover, and simmer 8 minutes. Remove from heat and let rest, covered, 5 to 10 minutes. Stir in walnuts and lemon juice.

Lay cooked leaves on a flat surface. Place about ⅓ cup of bulgur mixture on each leaf in a strip near the stem end. Fold in the two lengthwise sides. Then, starting at the unfolded edge of the stem end, carefully roll up each leaf to enclose filling, forming a neat packet. Save any extra filling to serve on the side.

Stir Tabasco sauce to taste into tomato sauce. Then spoon ⅔ cup of the sauce into a shallow, 4-quart baking dish. Place vegetable rolls, seam side down, in a single layer over the sauce. Spoon remaining sauce over the rolls. Cover with foil and bake for 20 minutes. Serve hot.

Per roll: Calories: 251; Protein: 9g; Carbohydrate: 36g; Fat: 11g; Sodium: 1171mg; Cholesterol: 0mg; Fiber: 9g.

Zucchini and Herb Calzones

MAKES 4 CALZONES

Stuff bread, not birds! That's exactly what you'll do with this tantalizing recipe. The cheesy tofu filling tastes like a rich, well-seasoned ricotta. Serve these scrumptious calzones plain or, if you prefer, topped with a spoonful or two of tomato sauce. Although the directions may appear lengthy, this is a very simple recipe to prepare.

Dough:
1 teaspoon active dry yeast
¾ cup warm water (between 105°F. to 115°F.)
2 teaspoons sweetener of your choice
½ teaspoon salt
2 to 3 cups whole wheat flour—more or less (as needed)

Ricotta-Style Filling:
1 teaspoon olive oil
1 cup zucchini cut into ¼-inch cubes
½ teaspoon crushed garlic
½ pound firm regular tofu, rinsed and patted dry
2 tablespoons minced fresh parsley
1 teaspoon basil
½ teaspoon oregano
½ teaspoon salt
⅛ teaspoon ground nutmeg
⅛ teaspoon pepper

To make the dough, place yeast in a large bowl and pour the warm water over it. Let rest 5 minutes. Add sweetener and salt, then, using a wooden spoon, beat in enough flour to make a soft but kneadable dough. Turn dough out onto a floured board and knead 5 minutes. Lightly oil a clean, large bowl, and place dough in it. Turn dough over so it is lightly oiled on all sides. Cover bowl with a clean, damp kitchen towel and let rise in a warm place for 1 hour.

Meanwhile, heat oil in a 9- or 10-inch skillet. When hot add zucchini and garlic and sauté until zucchini is just tender, about 3 to 5 minutes.

Place tofu in a medium bowl and mash well. Add parsley, basil, oregano, salt, nutmeg, and pepper and mix well. Fold in cooked zucchini and set aside.

Preheat oven to 400°F. Mist a baking sheet with nonstick cooking spray or line with parchment paper, and set aside. Punch down dough and divide it into 4 equal balls. Keep dough covered with the same towel that covered the bowl and work with 1 ball of dough at a time. Place the ball on a lightly floured board and roll into a 6-inch round. Place ¼ of the filling (about ½ cup for each calzone) slightly off the center of the round, and fold the dough over. Seal edges of the calzone by crimping them with your fingers or with the tines of a fork dipped in flour. Prick them in a few places on top with the tines of the fork. Place calzones on prepared baking sheet as soon as they are formed. Mist tops lightly with nonstick cooking spray or olive oil. Bake on center rack of oven until lightly browned, about 20 minutes.

Per calzone: Calories: 373; Protein: 18g; Carbohydrate: 70g; Fat: 6g; Sodium: 594mg; Cholesterol: 0mg; Fiber: 12g.

Chili Bean Macaroni

MAKES 4 SERVINGS

Spicy beans and pasta make a hearty meal the whole family will enjoy. Serve it with a tossed green salad for a quick and easy supper.

    2 cups dry elbow macaroni
    1 teaspoon olive oil
    1½ cups chopped onions
    1 medium green bell pepper, chopped

½ cup finely chopped celery

1 teaspoon chili powder

1 teaspoon ground cumin

1 teaspoon basil

1 (14- or 16-ounce) can diced tomatoes, with juice

2 cups drained cooked or canned red kidney beans
  (one 15-ounce can)

¼ cup low-sodium tamari, or 2 tablespoons balsamic vinegar

Cook macaroni according to package directions. Drain well and place in a covered saucepan or bowl to keep the pasta warm. Set aside. Meanwhile, heat oil in a large skillet. When hot, add onion, bell pepper, and celery. Sauté until tender, about 10 to 12 minutes. Stir in chili powder, cumin, and basil. Mix well, and cook and stir 1 minute longer. Remove from heat and set aside. Add tomatoes and their juice to the reserved pasta. Stir in beans, cooked vegetables, and tamari or vinegar. Mix well. Cook over medium-low heat, stirring often, until warmed through.

Per one-cup serving: Calories: 406; Protein: 18g; Carbohydrate: 77g; Fat: 3g; Sodium: 1116mg; Cholesterol: 0mg; Fiber: 14g.

Satisfying Desserts

When the chocolate urge strikes we've got you covered. In this section you'll find amazing recipes for chocolate pudding and sauce, fudge brownies, frosting, cake, cookies, bars, and confections. They're so good, the whole family will gobble them up, and you'll be proud to serve them to company. Don't let on that they're healthful, because no one would ever guess! You'll also find a full range of other dessert delights.

For some people, desserts are like special occasions that only come around once in awhile. For others, a meal isn't complete without something sweet at the finish. Whatever your dessert desire, there are bound to be recipes in this section that will fit the bill.

Of course, the most wholesome sweet ending to a well-balanced meal is some fresh fruit, one or two pieces of dried fruit, or a small handful of raisins. These provide nutrition along with their sweetness, so you aren't simply consuming empty calories. A spoonful of unsweetened applesauce or apple butter is another pleasing way to end a meal, as is an ice-cold glass of chocolate or vanilla soy milk, rice milk, almond milk, or oat milk, or chilled *amazake,* a naturally sweet beverage made from sweet brown rice. Frozen Italian ice or dairy-free chocolate or fruit sorbet also make quick and refreshing sweet treats.

You'll want to savor these simple, fruit-based recipes for delightful desserts that won't fill you out or weigh you down:

- Date and Walnut Balls, page 290
- Apricot Confections, page 290
- Stuffed Dates, page 291
- Fresh Fruit Compote, page 218
- Stewed Prunes, page 219
- Fantastic Fruit Smoothie, page 220
- Banana or Mango Lassi, page 220
- Orange-Pineapple Crush, page 221
- Berry-Berry Smoothie, page 222
- Squash Pudding, page 253

Crispy Rice Bars

MAKES 16 SQUARES

These crunchy, nutty squares make a delicious dessert or sweet snack.

⅔ cup brown rice syrup
¼ cup natural almond butter or peanut butter
½ teaspoon vanilla extract
2 cups crisped rice cereal

Additions (choose one):
½ cup lightly roasted chopped almonds or walnuts
½ cup currants, raisins, or finely chopped apricots
½ cup nondairy carob chips

Mist an 8-inch-square pan with nonstick cooking spray and set aside. Place brown rice syrup and nut butter in a small saucepan and warm until mixture is softened and smooth. Remove from heat and stir in vanilla extract. Combine cereal and the addition of your choice in a large bowl. Pour warm mixture over cereal mix and combine carefully, using a wooden spoon. Work as quickly as possible (this is especially important if using carob chips so they do not melt). Pack mixture evenly into prepared pan, pressing gently with your fingers. Cover pan with plastic wrap and chill until firm. Slice into squares and store in an airtight container in the refrigerator.

Per bar: Calories: 75; Protein: less than one gram; Carbohydrate: 14g; Fat: 2g; Sodium: 49mg; Cholesterol: 0mg; Fiber: less than one gram.

Date and Walnut Balls

MAKES ABOUT 30 BALLS

Moist, sweet dates are nature's candy. Their gentle sweetness is highlighted in these delectable fruit and nut balls.

> 1¼ cups walnuts
> ½ pound soft and moist pitted dates
> 4 to 5 tablespoons hot water, as needed

Coarsely chop half the walnuts and very finely grind the rest. Process dates into a soft paste in a food processor, adding just enough hot water, one tablespoon at a time, to make a stiff but pliable mixture. Transfer to a bowl and work in the coarsely chopped walnuts with your hands. Lightly oil your hands so the paste does not stick. Take small lumps of paste and roll into 1-inch balls. Roll each ball in the finely ground walnuts. Store leftovers in the refrigerator.

Per ball: Calories: 43; Protein: 1g; Carbohydrate: 4g; Fat: 3g; Sodium: less than one mg; Cholesterol: 0mg; Fiber: 1g.

Apricot Confections

MAKES 25 TO 30 PIECES

Apricots are an excellent source of vitamin A and potassium. These impressive confections are simply wonderful!

> ½ pound dried, unsulfured apricots
> Hot water as needed

½ cup coarsely chopped pistachios
Confectioners sugar
About 30 pistachio halves, to decorate

Pulse apricots in food processor, then grind to a smooth paste, adding a very small amount of hot water, one teaspoon at a time, only if necessary. Transfer to a bowl and work in the pistachios with your hands. Wet or oil your hands so the paste does not stick. Take small lumps of the paste and roll into marble-size balls. Roll in confectioners sugar and press a pistachio half on top of each. Store leftovers in the refrigerator.

Per confection: Calories: 35; Protein: less than one gram; Carbohydrate: 7g; Fat: 1g; Sodium: 17mg; Cholesterol: 0mg; Fiber: less than one gram.

Stuffed Dates

MAKES AS MANY AS YOU LIKE

This incredibly simple, naturally sweet recipe is satisfying and delicious. It's even elegant enough to serve to dinner guests.

Dates (preferably Medjool)
Nut butter (natural peanut, almond, or cashew)
Whole blanched almonds

Carefully slit dates with a sharp knife and remove pit. Fill slit with about ½ teaspoon nut butter. Then gently press in 1 whole blanched almond.

Per date: Calories: 61; Protein: 1.5g; Carbohydrate: 7g; Fat: 3g; Sodium: less than one mg; Cholesterol: 0mg; Fiber: 1g.

Instant Chocolate Pudding

MAKES ABOUT 1¾ CUPS

Great homemade chocolate pudding in under five minutes? You bet! You'll be an instant believer with this remarkable recipe.

> 1½ cups (about 12 ounces) firm silken tofu, crumbled
> ¼ to ½ cup dark brown sugar, unbleached cane sugar, or
>   pure maple syrup
> ⅓ cup unsweetened cocoa or carob powder
> 2 teaspoons vanilla extract
> Pinch of salt (optional)

Place all ingredients in food processor and blend several minutes until smooth and creamy. Chill in the refrigerator until serving time.

TIP:

- Start with the smaller amount of sugar and add a little more, as needed to suit your taste.

Per ¾-cup serving: Calories: 143; Protein: 10g; Carbohydrate: 20g; Fat: 4g; Sodium: 144mg; Cholesterol: 0mg; Fiber: 3g.

Ultra-Fudge Brownies

MAKES 12 TO 16 BROWNIES

The ultimate fudge brownie experience.

> 1¼ cups whole wheat flour
> 1 cup sugar
> ½ cup unsweetened cocoa or
>   carob powder
> ¼ teaspoon baking powder
> ¼ teaspoon salt
> 2 tablespoons organic canola or
>   safflower oil
>
> 1 tablespoon vanilla extract
> ¾ cup firm silken tofu,
>   crumbled
> ½ cup water
> ½ cup pure maple syrup
> ½ to 1 cup chopped walnuts

Preheat oven to 350°F. Mist an 8-inch-square glass baking pan with nonstick cooking spray and set aside. Combine flour, sugar, carob or cocoa powder, baking powder, and salt in a medium bowl and stir together until well combined. Combine tofu, water, maple syrup, carob or cocoa powder, oil, and vanilla in blender and process until completely smooth. Pour into the dry ingredients and stir until well combined. Fold in walnuts. Pour batter evenly into prepared pan. Bake on center rack of oven for 40 minutes, or until a cake tester inserted in the center comes out clean. Cool brownies in the pan. Cut and serve.

Per brownie: Calories: 183; Protein: 4g; Carbohydrate: 28g; Fat: 7g; Sodium: 49mg; Cholesterol: 0mg; Fiber: 3g.

Blonde Brownies

MAKES 12 TO 16 BROWNIES

Not too sweet, not too moist, these scrumptious blonde brownies are just right.

1¾ cups whole-wheat flour	½ cup firm silken tofu,
⅔ cup sugar	crumbled
½ cup nondairy chocolate or	½ cup pure maple syrup
carob chips	2 tablespoons organic canola or
½ cup chopped walnuts	safflower oil
½ teaspoon salt	1 tablespoon vanilla extract

Preheat oven to 350°F. Mist an 8-inch-square baking pan with nonstick cooking spray and set aside. In a large bowl combine flour, sugar, chocolate or carob chips, walnuts, and salt. Mix with a dry wire whisk. Blend tofu, maple syrup, oil, and vanilla extract in a food processor or blender. Pour into flour mixture and stir until everything is evenly moistened. Batter will be stiff. Spoon into prepared baking pan. Bake 35 minutes, or until a toothpick inserted in the center comes out clean. Cool thoroughly before cutting and serving.

Per brownie: Calories: 156; Protein: 4g; Carbohydrate: 21g; Fat: 7g; Sodium: 75mg; Cholesterol: 0mg; Fiber: 2g.

Strawberry Shortcake

MAKES 4 SERVINGS

Fresh strawberries are a sign of summer. For fun, cut the shortcakes into different shapes using cookie cutters.

2½ cups sliced fresh strawberries
4 teaspoons sugar
1 cup whole wheat flour
1½ teaspoons baking powder
¼ teaspoon baking soda
¼ teaspoon salt
1½ tablespoons organic canola or safflower oil
1 tablespoon frozen apple juice concentrate, thawed (undiluted)
About ⅓ cup fortified plain or vanilla soy or rice milk, as needed
½ cup Tofu Whipped Topping (page 295), or other nondairy
    whipped topping

Combine strawberries and sugar, and toss gently. Let stand 30 minutes. Preheat oven to 450°F. To make the shortcakes, combine flour, baking powder, baking soda, and salt in a large bowl and stir with a dry wire whisk. Combine oil and juice concentrate in a small measuring cup and beat with a fork until well blended. Pour into flour mixture, and cut in with a pastry blender or fork until the mixture resembles fine crumbs. Using a fork, stir in just enough milk so dough leaves the sides of the bowl and rounds up into a ball. (Too much milk will make the dough sticky, not enough milk will make the shortcakes dry.) Turn dough out onto a lightly floured surface and knead lightly 20 to 25 times, about 30 seconds, then gently smooth into a ball. Roll or pat dough into a ½-inch-thick circle and cut with a floured 3-inch biscuit cutter into 4 rounds. Place shortcakes on a dry baking sheet as soon as they are cut, spacing them about 1-inch apart. Bake on center rack of oven until golden brown, about 10 to 12 minutes. Immediately transfer to a cooling rack.

Carefully split shortcakes crosswise while they are warm, and spread with a small amount of the whipped topping. Place bottom halves of shortcakes on four dessert plates, and spoon half of the strawberries over them. Cover with the top halves of the shortcakes.

Spoon on remaining strawberries, and top with the remaining whipped topping.

TIP:

• If desired, any other fresh, seasonal berries of your choice may be substituted for the strawberries.

Per shortcake: Calories: 230; Protein: 5g; Carbohydrate: 37g; Fat: 8g; Sodium: 385mg; Cholesterol: 0mg; Fiber: 6g.

Tofu Whipped Topping

MAKES ABOUT 1½ CUPS

This incredibly easy whipped topping has a mesmerizing flavor. It's a wonderful touch to homemade confections.

1½ cups (about 12 ounces) firm silken tofu, crumbled
¼ cup pure maple syrup
1 tablespoon organic canola or safflower oil
2 teaspoons vanilla extract
Pinch of ground nutmeg

Combine all ingredients in food processor and process until completely smooth and very creamy. Store in an airtight container in the refrigerator.

TIP:

• The secret to the ultra-creamy consistency of this topping is processing it for several minutes, which eliminates any graininess. After the long processing time the texture will be miraculously transformed. A food processor should be used, because the mixture is too thick to process effectively in a blender.

Per one-half-cup serving: Calories: 160; Protein: 7g; Carbohydrate: 20g; Fat: 6g; Sodium: 98mg; Cholesterol: 0mg; Fiber: 0g.

Banana Snack Cake with Creamy Fudge Frosting

MAKES 12 TO 16 SERVINGS

A popular cake for snacking or for dessert.

1½ cups mashed ripe banana (about 3 to 4 medium bananas)
½ cup pure maple syrup
2 tablespoons organic canola or safflower oil
2 teaspoons vanilla extract

2¼ cups whole wheat flour
1 tablespoon baking powder
1 teaspoon baking soda
1 cup coarsely chopped or broken walnuts
1½ cups Creamy Fudge Frosting (recipe follows)

Preheat oven to 350°F. Mist an 8-inch square glass baking pan with nonstick cooking spray and set aside. Combine banana, syrup, oil, and vanilla extract in a large bowl and mix well. Place remaining ingredients, except walnuts and frosting, in a separate large bowl and stir together. Gradually stir dry ingredients into wet ingredients, sprinkling in about ⅓ at a time. Mix until well combined. Batter will be very thick. Stir in walnuts. Spoon batter into prepared baking pan. Bake on center rack of oven for 30 to 35 minutes, or until a cake tester inserted in the center comes out clean. Cool in the pan on a cooling rack. Frost with Creamy Fudge Frosting. Cool completely before cutting.

Per slice: Calories: 241; Protein: 5g; Carbohydrate: 35g; Fat: 11g; Sodium: 160mg; Cholesterol: 0mg; Fiber: 4g.

Creamy Fudge Frosting

MAKES 3 CUPS

Spread this extraordinary fudge frosting on your favorite cake, muffins, or cookies.

1½ cups (about 12 ounces) firm silken tofu
¾ cup pure maple syrup

⅔ cup natural almond or cashew butter
½ cup unsweetened cocoa or carob powder
1 tablespoon vanilla extract

Combine all ingredients in a food processor and process until smooth and creamy. Store any unused frosting in the refrigerator.

Per one-quarter-cup serving: Calories: 171; Protein: 4g; Carbohydrate: 21g; Fat: 9g; Sodium: 15mg; Cholesterol: 0mg; Fiber: 2g.

Chocolate Bonbons

MAKES ABOUT 40 BONBONS

These rich, fudgey balls will satisfy your chocolate cravings instantly!

¼ cup brown rice syrup
¼ cup natural almond or peanut butter
1½ tablespoons unsweetened cocoa or carob powder
1 tablespoon organic canola or safflower oil
½ teaspoon vanilla extract
2 brown rice cakes, finely crushed, or 1¼ cups puffed or crisped
   brown rice cereal

Place syrup, nut butter, cocoa or carob powder, and oil in a medium saucepan. Warm over low heat until melted and well combined. Remove from heat and stir in vanilla. Using a sturdy wooden spoon, stir in crushed rice cakes or rice cereal until thoroughly incorporated. Let cool until mixture can be handled easily. Roll between your hands into marble-size balls. Place each ball as it is formed on a sheet of waxed paper or parchment paper. Store in an airtight container at room temperature.

Per bonbon: Calories: 21; Protein: less than one gram; Carbohydrate: 3g; Fat: 1g; Sodium: 10mg; Cholesterol: 0mg; Fiber: less than one gram.

Tootsie Roll Heaven

MAKES ABOUT 24 ROLLS (ABOUT 1½ INCHES IN LENGTH)

It takes two strong hands to blend this recipe, but the results are worth the effort.

>   1 cup unsweetened cocoa or carob powder
>   ⅓ cup natural peanut, almond, or cashew butter
>   ¼ cup pure maple syrup
>   2 tablespoons brown rice syrup
>   ½ cup oat flour (see Tip) or wheat germ

Combine all ingredients in a large bowl and stir with a large, sturdy spoon. Finish mixing with your hands until mixture is very well combined. Mold into 24 small "tootsie rolls," about 1½ inches in length. Line a baking sheet with waxed paper or parchment paper and arrange rolls in a single layer. Freeze until very firm (about 1 to 2 hours). Store in freezer or refrigerator.

TIP
*   To make oat flour, whirl rolled oats in a dry blender until finely ground and powdery.

Per roll: Calories: 51; Protein: 1g; Carbohydrate: 9g; Fat: 2g; Sodium: 4mg; Cholesterol: 0mg; Fiber: 2g.

Hot Fudge Cake

MAKES ABOUT 8 SERVINGS

This cake tastes so rich it's hard to believe there's virtually no fat and no eggs in it. For the best flavor, serve it chilled, if you can wait that long. It's also delicious warm or at room temperature.

>   1 cup whole wheat flour
>   ½ cup unsweetened cocoa powder
>   2 teaspoons baking powder

¼ teaspoon salt
½ cup fortified vanilla soy or rice milk
¼ cup unsweetened applesauce
1 teaspoon vanilla extract
1 cup dark brown sugar
1¾ cups hot water

Preheat oven to 350°F. Mist an 8-inch-square baking pan with nonstick cooking spray. Combine flour, baking powder, salt, and ¼ cup of the cocoa powder in a large bowl. In a separate bowl combine milk and apple sauce. Pour into flour mixture and mix well. Spoon batter into prepared pan. In a clean bowl combine brown sugar and remaining ¼ cup cocoa. Gradually beat in hot water using a wire whisk and blend thoroughly. Pour evenly over batter in pan. Bake on center rack of oven for 40 to 45 minutes. Remove and cool in pan on a cooling rack. There will be a layer of moist, brownie-style cake on top and a layer of fudge sauce underneath. To serve, spoon fudge sauce on top of each serving of cake.

Per slice: Calories: 143; Protein: 3g; Carbohydrate: 33g; Fat: 1g; Sodium: 188mg; Cholesterol: 0mg; Fiber: 4g.

Incredible Hot Fudge Sauce

MAKES 1½ CUPS

Serve warm as a topping for cake, desserts, non-dairy ice cream or sorbet, or as a dipping sauce for fruit.

½ cup unsweetened cocoa or carob powder
2 tablespoons cornstarch or arrowroot
1¼ cups fortified vanilla soy or rice milk
½ cup pure maple syrup

Combine cocoa or carob powder and cornstarch or arrowroot in a small bowl and stir with a dry wire whisk. Transfer to a small saucepan and gradually whisk in ½ cup of the milk. Slowly whisk in remaining milk and maple syrup, and mix well. Cook over medium heat whisking constantly for 2 to 3 minutes or until thickened. Store in an airtight container in the refrigerator. Reheat as needed.

Per one-half-cup serving: Calories: 232; Protein: 5g; Carbohydrate: 52g; Fat: 3g; Sodium: 48mg; Cholesterol: 0mg; Fiber: 5g.

Oatmeal Carob Chippers

MAKES ABOUT 4 DOZEN COOKIES

These old-fashioned carob chip cookies will really satisfy your sweet tooth.

3 cups rolled oats
1¼ cups whole wheat flour
¼ cup shredded coconut
½ teaspoon baking soda
1 cup water
1 cup unsweetened apple juice
¼ cup brown rice syrup
3 tablespoons organic canola or safflower oil
⅔ cup nondairy carob chips
½ cup chopped walnuts or pecans

Preheat oven to 350°F. Mist baking sheets with nonstick cooking spray or line with parchment paper. Combine oats, flour, coconut, and baking soda in a large bowl. In a separate bowl whisk together water, juice, syrup, and oil until well combined. Pour into flour mixture and mix well. Stir in carob chips and nuts. Drop rounded spoonfuls onto prepared baking sheets and press flat with palm of hand. Bake 20 to 25 minutes. Cool on a rack.

Per cookie: Calories: 74; Protein: 2g; Carbohydrate: 10g; Fat: 3g; Sodium: 16mg; Cholesterol: 0mg; Fiber: less than one gram.

Carob Fondue

MAKES 8 SERVINGS

Dip your favorite fresh fruit—strawberries, bananas, pineapple, melon balls, orange sections, or whatever—into this rich dark sauce for a very special delight.

> 1 (10-ounce) package carob chips
> ⅔ cup fortified vanilla soy or rice milk
> ½ cup brown rice syrup
> ¼ teaspoon ground nutmeg
> ¼ teaspoon ground cardamom

Combine all ingredients in a heavy-bottomed medium saucepan and warm over very low heat, stirring often, until chips have melted and mixture is smooth and creamy. Transfer to a fondue pot and keep warm over a low flame.

Per ¼-cup serving: Calories: 251; Protein: 5g; Carbohydrate: 34g; Fat: 12g; Sodium: 32mg; Cholesterol: 0mg; Fiber: 2g.

Carob Walnut Fudge

MAKES 16 SQUARES

When the chocolate cravings hit hard, indulge in a piece of this luscious fudge for instant relief.

> 1 cup nut butter (almond, peanut, cashew, or sunflower)
> 1 cup brown rice syrup (see Tip below)
> 1 cup unsweetened carob or cocoa powder
> ½ cup chopped walnuts

Mist an 8-inch-square pan with nonstick cooking spray and set aside. Combine nut butter and syrup in a saucepan and heat over low heat, stirring almost constantly until mixture is soft and blended. Remove from heat and beat in carob powder with a sturdy wooden spoon. When well blended, stir in walnuts. Spread evenly into prepared pan, pushing mixture into corners. Chill in refrigerator. Cut into squares when cool and firm.

TIP:

- To easily release brown rice syrup from measuring cup, lightly oil the cup before measuring, or mist it with nonstick cooking spray.

Per square of fudge: Calories: 194; Protein: 4g; Carbohydrate: 22g; Fat: 13g; Sodium: 27mg; Cholesterol: 0mg; Fiber: 3g.

Puffy Bars

MAKES 8 LARGE BARS

Decadently delicious!

> 4 cups unsweetened puffed rice cereal
> ¾ cup brown rice syrup
> ¼ cup natural almond butter
> 1 teaspoon almond extract
> ¼ cup nondairy carob chips

Mist an 8-inch-square baking pan with nonstick cooking spray and set aside. Place cereal in a large bowl. Combine rice syrup and almond butter in a small saucepan and heat over low heat, stirring often, until soft and blended. Pour over cereal and mix until evenly coated. Stir in carob chips and mix again. Press into prepared pan, cover with plastic wrap, and chill for 30 to 60 minutes before serving.

Per bar: Calories: 242; Protein: 3g; Carbohydrate: 38g; Fat: 9g; Sodium: 37mg; Cholesterol: 0mg; Fiber: 1g.

Almond Fudge Cookies

MAKES 2 DOZEN COOKIES

Festive and rich, these cookies are extra delicious when served with a glass of ice-cold nondairy almond milk.

1 cup whole wheat flour
½ cup oat flour (see Tip on page 298)
½ cup unsweetened carob powder, sifted
½ teaspoon baking powder
¼ teaspoon salt
½ cup pure maple syrup
¼ cup organic canola or safflower oil
1 teaspoon vanilla extract
24 whole blanched almonds

Preheat oven to 350°F. Mist baking sheets with nonstick cooking spray or line with parchment paper and set aside. Combine flour, carob powder, baking, powder, and salt in a large bowl and stir together with a dry wire whisk. In a separate bowl combine syrup, oil, and vanilla extract. Pour into dry ingredients and mix thoroughly. Dough will be stiff. Form into 24 walnut-size balls using water-moistened hands and place on prepared baking sheets. Place one whole almond in the center of each ball, pressing it down lightly. Bake 12 minutes. Transfer to a cooling rack. Cool completely before storing.

Per cookie: Calories: 75; Protein: 1g; Carbohydrate: 12g; Fat: 3g; Sodium: 34mg; Cholesterol: 0mg; Fiber: 2g.

Hot Carob "Cocoa"

MAKES 1 SERVING

A cup of Hot Carob "Cocoa" is a nice treat or simple dessert. It is surprisingly thick and creamy tasting, even when made with water, and its flavor is reminiscent of bittersweet chocolate. Because carob is somewhat sweeter than cocoa powder, you may not need to add much, if any, sweetener.

2 tablespoons unsweetened carob powder

¼ teaspoon cornstarch or arrowroot

6 to 8 ounces water or fortified vanilla soy or rice milk

¼ teaspoon vanilla extract (omit if using vanilla soy or rice milk)

Sweetener of your choice (optional)

In a small saucepan whisk together carob and arrowroot or cornstarch. Gradually whisk in water or milk, keeping the mixture as smooth as possible. Heat, stirring often, until steaming hot. Stir in vanilla extract, if using, and sweetener to taste.

TIPS:

- If you prefer, you can substitute unsweetened cocoa powder for the carob powder, or try a combination of the two as you wean yourself off chocolate.
- This recipe is easily doubled, tripled, or quadrupled.

Per one-cup serving: Calories: 129; Protein: 7g; Carbohydrate: 22g; Fat: 4g; Sodium: 100mg; Cholesterol: 0mg; Fiber: 5g.

Notes

(A key to the abbreviated journal titles can be found on pages 312–313.)

Introduction

1. Ludwig DS, Majzoub JA, Al-Zahrani A, Dallal GE, Blanco I, Roberts SB. High glycemic index foods, overeating, and obesity. *Pediatrics* 1999;103:656.
2. Drewnowski A., Krahn DD, Demitrack MA, Nairn K, Gosnell BA. Taste responses and preferences for sweet high-fat foods: evidence for opioid involvement. *Physiol Behav* 1992;51:371–9.
3. Shah NP. Effects of milk-derived bioactives: an overview. *Br J Nutr* 2000;84(suppl1): S3–S10.

1. The Seduction Begins: How Foods Addict You

1. Drewnowski A., Krahn DD, Demitrack MA, Nairn K, Gosnell BA. Taste responses and preferences for sweet high-fat foods: evidence for opioid involvement. *Physiol Behav* 1992;51:371–9.
2. Kim SW, Grant JE, Adson DE, Shin YC. Double-blind naltrexone and placebo comparison study in the treatment of pathological gambling. *Biol Psychiatr* 2001;49:914–21.
3. Wang GJ, Volkow ND, Logan J, et al. Brain dopamine and obesity. *Lancet* 2001;357:354–7.
4. Thompson J, Thomas N, Singleton A, Piggott M, Lloyd S, Perry EK, Morris CM, Perry RH, Ferrier IN, Court JA. D2 dopamine receptor gene (DRD2) Taq1 A polymorphism: reduced dopamine D2 receptor binding in the human striatum associated with the A1 allele. *Pharmacogenetics* 1997;7:479–84.

5. Noble EP. Addiction and its reward process through polymorphisms of the D2 dopamine receptor gene: a review. *Eur Psychiatry* 2000;15:79–89.
6. Noble EP, St. Jeor ST, Ritchie T, Syndulko K, St. Jeor SC, Fitch RJ, Brunner RL, Sparkes RS. D2 dopamine receptor gene and cigarette smoking: a reward gene? *Med Hypotheses* 1994a;42:257–60.
7. Noble EP, Noble RE, Ritchie T, Syndulko K, Bohlman MC, Noble LA, Zhang Y, Sparkes RS, Grandy DK. D2 dopamine receptor gene and obesity. *Int J Eating Disord* 1994b;15:205–17.
8. Stahl SM. The psychopharmacology of sex, part 1: neurotransmitters and the 3 phases of the human sexual response. *J Clin Psychiatry* 2001;62:80–1.
9. Spitz MR, Shi H, Yang F, Hudmon KS, Jiang H, Chamberlain RM, et al. Case-control study of the D2 dopamine receptor gene and smoking status in lung cancer patients. *J Natl Cancer Inst* 1998;90:358–63.
10. Knowler WC, Barrett-Conner E, Fowler SE, Hamman RF, Lachin JM, Walker EA, Nathan DM. Reduction in the incidence of type 2 diabetes with lifestyle intervention or metformin. *N Engl J Med* 2002;346:393–403.

2. Sweet Nothings: The Sugar Seduction

1. Blass EM, Camp CA. The ontogeny of face recognition: eye contact and sweet taste induce face preference in 9- and 12-week-old human infants. *Devel Psychol* 2001;37:762–74.
2. Brink PJ. Addiction to sugar. *West J Nurs Res* 1993;15:280–1.
3. Smith BA, Fillion TJ, Blass EM. Orally mediated sources of calming in 1-to 3-day-old infants. *Devel Psychol* 1990;26:731–7.
4. Blass EM, Ciaramitaro V. Oral determinants of state, affect, and action in newborn humans. *Monogr Soc Res Child Dev* 1994;59:1–96.
5. Morley JE, Levine AS, Yamada T, et al. Effect of exorphins on gastrointestinal function, hormonal release, and appetite. *Gastroenterology* 1983;84:1517–23.
6. Fukudome S, Yoshikawa M. Gluten exorphin C:A novel opioid peptide derived from wheat gluten. *FEBS Lett* 1993 Jan 18;316(1):17–9.
7. Dohan FC. Genetic hypothesis of idiopathic schizophrenia: its exorphin connection. *Schizophr Bull* 1988;14:489–94.

3. Give Me Chocolate or Give Me Death: The Chocolate Seduction

1. Drewnowski A, Krahn DD, Demitrack MA, Nairn K, and Gosnell BA. Taste responses and preferences for sweet high-fat foods: evidence for opioid involvement. *Physiol Behav* 1992;51:371–379.
2. Pennington JAT. *Bowes and Church's Food Values of Portions Commonly Used, Seventeenth Edition* (Philadelphia: Lippincott-Raven, 1998), p. 383.
3. Koehler PE, Eitenmiller RR. High pressure liquid chromatographic analysis of tyramine, phenylethylamine and tryptamine in sausage, cheese, and chocolate. *J of Food Sci* 1978;43:1245–7.

4. Hurst WJ, Martin RA, Zoumas, BL. Biogenic amines in chocolate: a review. *Nutr Rep Intl* 1982;26:1081–6.
5. di Tomaso E, Beltramo M, Piomelli D. Brain cannabinoids in chocolate. *Nature* 1996;382:677–8.
6. Tuomisto T, Hetherington MM, Morris MF, Tuomisto MT, Turjanmaa V, Lappalainen R. Psychological and physiological characteristics of sweet food "addiction." *Int J Eat Disord* 1999;25:169–75.
7. Michener W, Rozin P. Pharmacological versus sensory factors in the satiation of chocolate craving. *Physiol Behav* 1994;56:419–22.
8. Macdiarmid JI, Hetherington MM. Mood modulation by food: an exploration of affect and cravings in "chocolate addicts." *Br J Clin Psychol* 1995;34:129–38.
9. Drewnowski A. Taste preferences and food intake. *Annu Rev Nutr* 1997;17:237–53.
10. Michell GF, Mebane AH, Billings CK. Effect of bupropion on chocolate craving. *Am J Psychiatry* 1989;146:119–20.
11. Shapira NA, Goldsmith TD, McElroy SL. Treatment of binge-eating disorder with topiramate: a clinical case series. *J Clin Psychiatry* 2000 May;61(5):368–72.

4. Opiates on a Cracker: The Cheese Seduction

1. Hazum E, Sabatka JJ, Chang KJ, Brent DA, Findlay JWA, Cuatrecasas P. Morphine in cow and human milk: Could dietary morphine constitute a ligand for specific morphine (μ) receptors? *Science* 1981;213:1010–2.
2. Benyhe S. Morphine: new aspects in the study of an ancient compound. *Life Sci* 1994;55:969–79.
3. Meisel H, FitzGerald RJ. Opioid peptides encrypted in intact milk protein sequences. *Br J Nutr* 2000;84(suppl 1):S27–S31.
4. Panksepp J, Normansell L, Siviy S, Rossi J, Zolovick AJ. Casomorphins reduce separation distress in chicks. *Peptides* 1984;5:829–31.
5. Shah NP. Effects of milk-derived bioactives: an overview. *Br J Nutr* 2000;84 (suppl 1):S3–S10.
6. Meisel H. Chemical characterization of opioid activity of an exorphin isolated from in vivo digests of casein. *FEBS Letters* 1986;196:223–7.
7. Teschemacher H, Umbach M, Hamel U, et al. No evidence for the presence of β-casomorphin in human plasma after ingestion of cows' milk or milk products. *J Dairy Res* 1986; 53:135–8.
8. Umbach M, Teschemacher H, Praetorius K, Hirschhäuser R, Bostedt H. Demonstration of a β-casomorphin immunoreactive material in the plasma of newborn calves after milk intake. *Regulatory Peptides* 1985;12:223–30.
9. Chabance B, Marteau P, Rambaud JC, Migliore-Samour D, Boynard M, Perrotin P, Guillet R, Jollès P, Fiat AM. Casein peptide release and passage to the blood in humans during digestion of milk or yogurt. *Biochimie* 1998;80:155–65.
10. Clyne PS, Kulczycki A. Human breast milk contains bovine IgG. Relationship to infant colic? *Pediatrics* 1991;87:439–44.

11. Lindström LH, Nyberg F, Terenius L, et al. CSF and plasma β-casomorphin-like opioid peptides in postpartum psychosis. *Am J Psychiatry* 1984;141:1059–66.
12. Nyberg F, Lindström LH, Terenius L. Reduced beta-casein levels in milk samples from patients with postpartum psychosis. *Biol Psychiatry* 1988;23:115–22.
13. Nyberg F, Lieberman H, Lindström LH, Lyrenäs S, Koch G, Terenius L. Immuno-reactive β-casomorphin-8 in cerebrospinal fluid from pregnant and lactating women: correlation with plasma levels. *J Clin Endocrinol Metab* 1989;68:283–9.
14. Chaytor JP, Crathorne B, Saxby MJ. The identification and significance of 2-phenylethylamine in foods. *J Sci Fd Agric* 1975;26:593–8.
15. Teschemacher H, Koch G, Brantl V. Milk protein-derived opioid receptor ligands. *Biopolymers* 1997;43:99–117.
16. Ratner D, Eshel E, Vigder K. Juvenile rheumatoid arthritis and milk allergy. *J Royal Soc Med* 1985;78:410–13.
17. Giovannucci E, Rimm EB, Wolk A, Ascherio A, Stampfer MJ, Colditz GA, Willett WC. Calcium and fructose intake in relation to risk of prostate cancer. *Cancer Res* 1998;58:442–7.
18. Chan JM, Stampfer MJ, Ma J, Gann PH, Gaziano JM, Giovannucci E. Dairy products, calcium, and prostate cancer risk in the Physicians' Health Study. *Am J Clin Nutr* 2001;74:549–54.
19. Heaney RP, McCarron DA, Dawson-Hughes B, et al. Dietary changes favorably affect bone remodeling in older adults. *J Am Dietetic Asso* 1999;99:1228–33.
20. Cohen P. Serum insulin-like growth factor-I levels and prostate cancer risk— interpreting the evidence. *J Natl Cancer Inst* 1998;90:876–9.
21. Peyrat JP, Bonneterre J, Hecquet B, et al. Plasma insulin-like growth factor-1 (IGF-1) concentrations in human breast cancer. *Eur J Cancer* 1993;29A:492–7.
22. Hankinson SE, Willett WC, Colditz GA, et al. Circulating concentrations of insulin-like growth factor-1 and risk of breast cancer. *Lancet* 1998;351:1393–6.
23. Ross RK, Henderson BE. Do diet and androgens alter prostate cancer risk via a common aetiologic pathway? *J Natl Cancer Inst* 1994;86:252–254.
24. Lloyd T, Chinchilli VM, Johnson-Rollings N, Kieselhorst K, Eggli DF, Marcus R. Adult female hip bone density reflects teenage sports-exercise patterns but not teenage calcium intake. *Pediatrics* 2000;106:40–4.
25. Feskanich D, Willett WC, Stampfer MJ, Colditz GA. Milk, dietary calcium, and bone fractures in women: a 12-year prospective study. *Am J Publ Health* 1997; 87:992–7.

5. The Sizzle: The Meat Seduction

1. Barnard ND, Nicholson A, Howard JL. The medical costs attributable to meat consumption. *Prev Med* 1995;24:646–55.
2. Yeomans MR, Wright P, Macleod HA, Critchley JAJH. Effects of nalmefene on feeding in humans. *Psychopharmacology* 1990;100:426–32.
3. Holt SHA, Brand Miller JC, Petocz P. An insulin index of foods; the insulin demand generated by 1000-kJ portions of common foods. *Am J Clin Nutr* 1997; 66:1264–76.

4. Ornish D, Brown SE, Scherwitz LW, Billings JH, Armstrong WT, Ports TA. Can lifestyle changes reverse coronary heart disease? *Lancet* 1990;336:129–33.

5. Hunninghake DB, Stein EA, Dujovne CA. The efficacy of intensive dietary therapy alone or combined with lovastatin in outpatients with hypercholesterolemia. *N Engl J Med* 1993;328:1213–9.

6. Nicholson AS, Sklar M, Barnard ND, Gore S, Sullivan R, Browning S. Toward improved management of NIDDM: a randomized, controlled, pilot intervention using a low-fat, vegetarian diet. *Prev Med* 1999;29:87–91.

7. Yaffe K, Barrett-Connor E, Lin F, Grady D. Serum lipoprotein levels, statin use, and cognitive function in older women. *Arch Neurol* 2002;59:378–84.

8. Seshadri S, Beiser A, Selhub J, et al. Plasma homocysteine as a risk factor for dementia and Alzheimer's disease. *N Engl J Med* 2002;346:476–83.

9. Thorogood M, Mann J, Appleby P, McPherson K. Risk of death from cancer and ischaemic heart disease in meat and non-meat eaters. *Brit Med J* 1994;308:1667–70.

10. Willett WC, Stampfer MJ, Colditz GA, Rosner BA, Speizer FE. Relation of meat, fat, and fiber intake to the risk of colon cancer in a prospective study among women. *N Engl J Med* 1990;323:1664–72.

11. Giovannucci E, Rimm EB, Stampfer MJ, Colditz GA, Ascherio A, Willett WC. Intake of fat, meat, and fiber in relation to risk of colon cancer in men. *Cancer Res* 1994;54:2390–7.

12. Sinha R, Rothman N, Brown ED, et al. High concentrations of the carcinogen 2-amino-1-methyl-6-phenylimidazo-[4,5] pyridine [PhIP] occur in chicken but are dependent on the cooking method. *Cancer Res* 1995;55:4516–19.

13. Breslau NA, Brinkley L, Hill KD, Pak CYC. Relationship of animal-protein-rich diet to kidney stone formation and calcium metabolism. *J Clin Endocrinol* 1988;66:140–6.

14. Abelow, BJ, Holford, TR, Insogna KL. Cross-cultural association between dietary animal protein and hip fracture: a hypothesis. *Calcif Tissue Int* 1992;50:14–18.

15. Feskanich D, Willett WC, Stampfer MJ, Colditz GA. Protein consumption and bone fractures in women. *Am J Epidemiol* 1996;143:472–9.

16. Westman EC, Yancy WS, Edman JS, Tomlin KF, Perkins CE. Effect of 6-month adherence to a very low carbohydrate diet program. *Am J Med* 2002;113:30–6.

17. Ornish D, Scherwitz LW, Billings JH, Brown SE, Gould KL, Merritt TA, Sparler S, Armstrong WT, Ports TA, Kirkeeide RL, Hogeboom C, Brand RJ. Intensive lifestyle changes for reversal of coronary heart disease. *JAMA* 1998;280:2001–7.

18. Reddy ST, Wang CY, Sakhaee K, Brinkley L, Pak CY. Effect of low-carbohydrate, high-protein diets on acid-base balance, stone-forming propensity, and calcium metabolism. *Am J Kidney Dis* 2002;40:265–74.

6. Step 1: Start With a Healthy Breakfast

1. Boutelle K, Neumark-Sztainer D, Story M, Resnick M. Weight control behaviors among obese, overweight, and nonoverweight adolescents. *J Pediatr Psychol* 2002 Sep;27(6):531–40.

2. Smith AP. Stress, breakfast cereal consumption and cortisol. *Nutr Neurosci* 2002 Apr;5(2):141–4.
3. Chen MY, Liao JC. Relationship between attendance at breakfast and school achievement among nursing students. *J Nurs Res* 2002 Mar;10(1):15–21.
4. Holt SH, Delargy HJ, Lawton CL, Blundell JE. The effects of high-carbohydrate vs high-fat breakfasts on feelings of fullness and alertness, and subsequent food intake. *Int J Food Sci Nutr* 1999;50:13–28.
5. Ludwig DS, Majzoub JA, Al-Zahrani A, Dallal GE, Blanco I, Roberts SB. High glycemic index foods, overeating, and obesity. *Pediatrics* 1999;103:656.

7. Step 2: Choose Foods That Hold Your Blood Sugar Steady

1. Howarth NC, Saltzman E, Roberts SB. Dietary fiber and weight regulation. *Nutr Rev* 2001;59:129–39.
2. Ludwig DS, Pereira MA, Kroenke CH, et al. Dietary fiber, weight gain, and cardiovascular disease risk factors in young adults. *JAMA* 1999;282:1539–46.
3. Kabir M, Oppert JM, Vidal H, Bruzzo F, Fiquet C, Wursch P, Slama G, Rizkalla SW. Four-week low-glycemic-index breakfast with a modest amount of soluble fibers in type 2 diabetic men. *Metab* 2002 Jul;51(7):819–26.
4. Jenkins DJ, Kendall CW, Augustin LS, Martini MC, Axelsen M, Faulkner D, Vidgen E, Parker T, Lau H, Connelly PW, Teitel J, Singer W, Vandenbroucke AC, Leiter LA, Josse RG. Effect of wheat bran on glycemic control and risk factors for cardiovascular disease in type 2 diabetes. *Diabetes Care* 2002 Sep;25(9):1522–8.
5. Lovejoy JC, Windhauser MM, Rood JC, de la Bretonne JA. Effect of a controlled high-fat versus low-fat diet on insulin sensitivity and leptin levels in African American and caucasian women. *Metab* 1998;47:1520–4.

8. Step 3: Boost Appetite-Taming Leptin

1. Montague CT, Farooqi IS, Whitehead JP, et al. Congenital leptin deficiency is associated with severe early-onset obesity in humans. *Nature* 1997;387:903–8.
2. Farooqi IS, Jebb SA, Langmack G, et al. Effects of recombinant leptin therapy in a child with congenital leptin deficiency. *N Engl J Med* 1999;341:879–84.
3. Cella F, Adami GF, Giordano G, Cordera R. Effects of dietary restriction on serum leptin concentration in obese women. *Int J Obes* 1999;23:494–7.
4. Fox C, Esparza J, Nicolson M, Bennett PH, Schulz LO, Valencia ME, Ravussin E. Plasma leptin concentrations in Pima Indians living in drastically different environments. *Diabetes Care* 1999 Mar;22(3):413–7.
5. Heshka JT, Jones PJ. A role for dietary fat in leptin receptor, OB-Rb, function. *Life Sci* 2001;69:987–1003.
6. Reseland JE, Haugen F, Hollung K, et al. Reduction of leptin gene expression by dietary polyunsaturated fatty acids. *J Lipid Res* 2001;42:743–50.
7. Weyer C, Walford RL, Harper IT, Milner M, MacCallum T, Tataranni PA, Ravussin E. Energy metabolism after 2 y of energy restriction: the biosphere 2 experiment. *Am J Clin Nutr* 2000;72:946–53.

8. Chu NF, Stampfer MJ, Spiegelman D, Rifai N, Hotamisligil GS, Rimm EB. Dietary and lifestyle factors in relation to plasma leptin concentrations among normal-weight and overweight men. *Int J Obes Relat Metab Disord* 2001 Jan;25(1):106–14.

9. Step 4: Break Craving Cycles

1. Berteus Forslund H, Lindroos AK, Sjostrom L, Lissner L. Meal patterns and obesity in Swedish women—a simple instrument describing usual meal types, frequency, and temporal distribution. *Eur J Clin Nutr* 2002;56:740–7.
2. Barnard ND, Scialli AR, Hurlock D, Bertron P. Diet and sex-hormone binding globulin, dysmenorrhea, and premenstrual symptoms. *Obstet Gynecol* 2000;95: 245–50.
3. Vanovski JA, Vanovski SZ, Sovik KN, Nguyen TT, O'Neil PM, Sebring NG. A prospective study of holiday weight gain. *N Engl J Med* 2000;342:861–7.

10. Step 5: Exercise and Rest

1. Poehlman ET, Tremblay A, Nadeau A, Dussault J, Thériault G, Bouchard C. Heredity and changes in hormones and metabolic rates with short-term training. *Am J Physiol* 1986;250:E711–17.
2. Jakicic JM, Winters C, Lang W, Wing RR. Effects of intermittent exercise and use of home exercise equipment on adherence, weight loss, and fitness in over-weight women. *JAMA* 1999;282:1554–60.
3. World Cancer Research Fund, American Institute for Cancer Research. *Food, Nutrition, and The Prevention Of Cancer: A Global Perspective* (Washington, D.C.: World Cancer Research Fund/American Institute for Cancer Research, 1997), 398–403.

12. Step 7: Use Extra Motivators

1. Thorogood M, Mann J, Appleby P, McPherson K. Risk of death from cancer and ischaemic heart disease in meat and non-meat eaters. *Brit Med J* 1994;308:1667–70.
2. Ornish D, Brown SE, Scherwitz LW, et al. Can lifestyle changes reverse coronary heart disease? *Lancet* 1990;336:129–133.
3. Kauppila LI. Can low-back pain be due to lumbar artery disease? *Lancet* 1995; 346:888–9.
4. Michal V. Arterial disease as a cause of impotence. *Clin Endocrinol Metab* 1982; 11:725–48.
5. Wabrek AJ, Burchell RC. Male sexual dysfunction associated with coronary heart disease. *Arch Sex Behav* 1980;9:69–75.
6. Nicholson AS, Sklar M, Barnard ND, Gore S, Sullivan R, Browning S. Toward improved management of NIDDM: a randomized, controlled, pilot intervention using a low-fat, vegetarian diet. *Prev Med* 1999;29:87–91.
7. Lindahl O, Lindwall L, Spangberg A, Stenram A, Ockerman PA. A vegan regimen with reduced medication in the treatment of hypertension. *Br J Nutr* 1984;52: 11–20.

8. Burkitt DP. Hemorrhoids, varicose veins, and deep vein thrombosis: epidemiologic features and suggested causative factors. *Canad J Surg* 1975;18:483–8.
9. Reddy ST, Wang CY, Sakhaee K, Brinkley L, Pak CY. Effect of low-carbohydrate high-protein diets on acid-base balance, stone-forming propensity, and calcium metabolism. *Am J Kidney Dis* 2002;40:265–74.
10. Barnard ND, Scialli AR, Bertron P, Hurlock D, Edmonds K, Talev L. Effectiveness of a low-fat, vegetarian diet in altering serum lipids in healthy premenopausal women. *Am J Cardiol* 2000;85:969–72.
11. Fraser GE, Shavlik DJ. Ten years of life: is it a matter of choice? *Arch Intern Med* 2001;161:1645–52.
12. Barnard ND, Nicholson A, Howard JL. The medical costs attributable to meat consumption. *Prev Med* 1995;24:646–55.

13. Foods That Love You Back

1. Barnard ND, Scialli AR, Bertron P, Hurlock D, Edmonds K, Talev L. Effectiveness of a low-fat vegetarian diet in altering serum lipids in healthy premenopausal women. *Am J Cardiol* 2000;85:969–72.
2. American Dietetic Association. Position of the American Dietetic Association: vegetarian diets. *J Am Dietetic Asso* 1997;97:1317–21.
3. Abelow, BJ, Holford, TR, Insogna KL. Cross-cultural association between dietary animal protein and hip fracture: a hypothesis. *Calcif Tissue Int* 1992;50:14–18.

ABBREVIATIONS

Am J Clin Nutr	*American Journal of Clinical Nutrition*
Am J Cardiol	*American Journal of Cardiology*
Am J Epidemiol	*American Journal of Epidemiology*
Am J Kidney Dis	*American Journal of Kidney Diseases*
Am J Med	*American Journal of Medicine*
Am J Physiol	*American Journal of Physiology*
Am J Psychiatry	*American Journal of Psychiatry*
Am J Publ Health	*American Journal of Public Health*
Annu Rev Nutr	*Annual Review of Nutrition*
Arch Intern Med	*Archives of Internal Medicine*
Arch Neurol	*Archives of Neurology*
Arch Sex Behav	*Archives of Sexual Behavior*
Biol Psychiatry	*Biological Psychiatry*
Br J Clin Psychol	*British Journal of Clinical Psychology*
Br J Nutr	*British Journal of Nutrition*
Brit Med J	*British Medical Journal*
Calcif Tissue Int	*Calcified Tissue International*
Canad J Surg	*Canadian Journal of Surgery*

Cancer Res	*Cancer Research*
Clin Endocrinol Metab	*Clinical Endocrinology and Metabolism*
Devl Psychol	*Developmental Psychology*
Eur J Cancer	*European Journal of Cancer Prevention*
Eur J Clin Nutr	*European Journal of Clinical Nutrition*
Eur Psychiatry	*European Psychiatry*
FEBS Lett	*FEBS Letters*
Intl J Eating Disord	*International Journal of Eating Disorders*
Intl J Food Sci Nutr	*International Journal of Food Sciences and Nutrition*
Intl J Obes	*International Journal of Obesity*
Intl J Obes Relat Metab Disord	*International Journal of Obesity and Related Metabolic Disorders*
J Am Dietetic Asso	*Journal of the American Dietetic Association*
J Clin Endocrinol	*Journal of Clinical Endocrinology*
J Clin Endocrinol Metab	*Journal of Clinical Endocrinology and Metabolism*
J Clin Psychiatry	*Journal of Clinical Psychiatry*
J Dairy Res	*Journal of Dairy Research*
J Lipid Res	*Journal of Lipid Research*
J Natl Cancer Inst	*Journal of the National Cancer Institute*
J Nurs Res	*Journal of Nursing Research*
J of Food	*Journal of Food Science*
J Pediatr Psychol	*Journal of Pediatric Psychology*
J Royal Soc Med	*Journal of the Royal Society of Medicine*
J Sci Fd Agric	*Journal of the Science of Food and Agriculture*
Life Sci	*Life Sciences*
Med Hypotheses	*Medical Hypotheses*
Metab	*Metabolism*
Monogr Soc Res Child Dev	*Monographs of the Society for Research in Child Development*
N Engl J Med	*New England Journal of Medicine*
Nutr Neurosci	*Nutritional Neurosciences*
Nutr Rep Intl	*Nutrition Reports International*
Nutr Rev	*Nutrition Reviews*
Obstet Gynecol	*Obstetrics and Gynecology*
Physiol Behav	*Physiology and Behavior*
Prev Med	*Preventive Medicine*
Schizophr Bull	*Schizophrenia Bulletin*
West J Nurs Res	*Western Journal of Nursing Research*

Recommended Reading

Nutrition Information

Barnard, Neal. *Food for Life*. New York: Harmony Books, 1993.

———. *Eat Right, Live Longer*. New York: Harmony Books, 1995.

———. *Foods That Fight Pain*. New York: Harmony Books, 1998.

———. *Turn off the Fat Genes*. New York: Harmony Books, 2001.

Davis, Brenda, and Vesanto Melina. *Becoming Vegan*. Summertown, Tenn.: Book Publishing Co., 2000.

McDougall, John. *The McDougall Program*. New York: Plume Books, 1991.

Moran, Victoria. *The Love-Powered Diet*. San Rafael, Calif.: New World Library, 1992.

Ornish, Dean. *Dr. Dean Ornish's Program for Reversing Heart Disease*. New York: Random House, 1990.

———. *Eat More Weigh Less*. New York: HarperCollins, 1993.

Physicians Committee for Responsible Medicine. *Healthy Eating for Life Series*. New York: John Wiley & Sons, 2000–2002. Includes the following titles: *Healthy Eating for Life for Children, Healthy Eating for Life for Women, Healthy Eating for Life to Prevent and Treat Diabetes,* and *Healthy Eating for Life to Prevent and Treat Cancer.*

Stepaniak, Joanne. *The Vegan Sourcebook*. New York: McGraw-Hill, 2000.

Weil, Andrew. *Natural Health, Natural Medicine*. New York: Houghton Mifflin, 1993.

Cookbooks

Barnard, Neal. *The Best in the World*. Washington, D.C.: Physicians Committee for Responsible Medicine, 1998.

Barnard, Tanya, and Sarah Kramer. *How it all Vegan*. Vancouver: Arsenal Pulp Press Ltd., 1999.

Bennett, Jannequin. *Very Vegetarian*. Nashville: Rutledge Hill Press, 2001.

Bronfman, David, and Rachelle Bronfman. *CalciYum!* Toronto: Bromedia, 1998.

Costigan, Fran. *Great Good Desserts Naturally*. Summertown, Tenn.: Book Publishing Co., 2000.

Davis, Brenda, Bryanna Clark Grogan, and Joanne Stepaniak. *Dairy-Free and Delicious*. Summertown, Tenn.: Book Publishing Co., 2001.

Keller, Jennifer. *The Best in the World II*. Washington, D.C.: Physicians Committee for Responsible Medicine, 2002.

Klein, Donna. *The Mediterranean Vegan Kitchen: Meat-Free, Egg-Free, Dairy-Free Dishes from the Healthiest Place Under the Sun*. New York: HP Books, 2001.

Kornfeld, Myra. *The Voluptuous Vegan*. New York: Clarkson N. Potter, 2000.

Krauss, Pam. *Moosewood Restaurant Low-Fat Favorites*. New York: Clarkson N. Potter, 1996.

McDougall, Mary, and John McDougall. *The McDougall Quick & Easy Cookbook*. New York: Plume Books, 1999.

Oser, Marie. *The Soy of Cooking*. New York: John Wiley & Sons, 1996.

———. *The Enlightened Kitchen*. New York: John Wiley & Sons, 2002.

Raymond, Jennifer. *The Peaceful Palate*. Summertown, Tenn.: Book Publishing Co., 1996.

———. *Fat-Free & Easy*. Calistoga, Calif.: Heart & Soul Publications, 1997.

Sass, Lorna. *Lorna Sass' Complete Vegetarian Kitchen*. New York: HarperCollins, 1995.

Stepaniak, Joanne. *The Uncheese Cookbook*. Summertown, Tenn.: Book Publishing Co., 1994.

———. *Table for Two*. Summertown, Tenn.: Book Publishing Co., 1996.

———. *Delicious Food for a Healthy Heart*. Summertown, Tenn.: Book Publishing Co., 1999.

———. *Vegan Deli*. Summertown, Tenn.: Book Publishing Co., 2001.

Stepaniak, Joanne, and Suzanne Havala. *Vegan Vittles*. Summertown, Tenn.: Book Publishing Co., 1996.

Index

I had it all, and then I nearly lost it because I couldn't stop drinking."

I studied him. He seemed so put together, so calm, even serene, as he told me his terrible story. He seemed free of all the guilt and shame I felt crowding around me.

"I am a drunk, Elizabeth, and so are you." I recoiled. His words felt like a slap in the face. "You may think you're special, or different, but you're not. You are just like me, and every other person here, trying to stay sober." I started to cry. He continued. "You need to take this chance and make the best of it. Many, many people relapse. You are not the first, and you will not be the last. The question is what are you going to do about it."

He was right, on so many levels. I was not the first person in the world to leave rehab and drink—not by a long shot. But I felt like I was. And now, I was right back in the same house, living under the same strict rules, feeling just as despondent and isolated as ever. I knew that this time I had to fight to save my life.

One of the first things I did was to try to alleviate the yawning abandonment I felt by being at the Center. I could not make it go completely away, but I began reaching out to people who would support me and talk to me: my parents, my brother, my sister, and my friends Dana and Michelle. I figured out that I could call my own work voice mail and access messages from that living room phone at the Center. I asked everyone to leave word for me on it. I could call it every night, if I made it to the phone sign-up sheet in time, and in five minutes I could hear what felt like a week's worth of love and encouragement.

My mom in particular left a message almost every single night. Echoes of those lunch box notes she would give me in third grade when I was tormented at school by the class bully. My priority still was calling Zachary and Sam, trying as best I could to connect with them, and that took most of my allotted phone time. But those other messages now left me better equipped to handle the heartbreak of the calls home.

One night, as I sat listening to my messages, I heard an unfamiliar voice. It was a friend of my sister's. She was in recovery. Aimie had given her my number.

"Elizabeeeeeeeethh! How are you? Hang in there! But hey, don't you know? *Getting* sober is so much harder than *staying* sober. Why do you keep doing the hardest part over and over?"

I had never looked at it that way. I have thought about that message almost every day since I heard it. Why had I stayed in that terrible spin cycle, over and over, emerging battered and disoriented, and then climbing back in for another go? Quitting is so very hard. "I'll stop tomorrow" is the worn-out refrain. But it feels herculean to resist drinking on day one. It's only once you have days, weeks, or months of sobriety under your belt that the siren call to drink is much less potent. It is easier to reject the temptation to drink if your mind is clear and you're not hungover or feeling hopeless because you drank the night before.

I worked hard with my therapist at the Center, trying to solve the mystery of why I kept going back to what was killing me. Once again, we dug deep into why my anxiety was so terrifying to me, and how I could calm it without wine. I listened to lecturers explain that alcoholism is a disease of the mind *and* body...that alcoholics cannot stop drinking or obsessing about it once they start. I went to the Center's trauma expert, who did something called brain spotting. I had to sit and stare at the tip of a stick that the therapist would slowly wave back and forth. When she explained it to me, I burst into a laugh.

"You're kidding me, right?"

The trauma therapist looked annoyed and mildly offended. "No, I am not kidding you. Are you ready to work or not?"

Yes, I was ready to work. She made me tell her about those mornings in Okinawa—when my dad was in Vietnam and my mom left for work. She made me describe in detail how I clung to her, begged her, was dragged to the car trying to stop her, my bare feet skidding across the rocks. I could barely tell anyone that story. Every time I started I would become overwhelmed, and have to stop. At that point, the therapist made me stare at that silly stick again, and she moved it slowly from side to side. I had to keep my head still, following it only with my eyes moving.

I honestly have no idea what she was doing or how it was supposed to work, but unbelievably, after several sessions, it did work. For the first time in my whole life, I can now tell the story of those panic attacks in Okinawa without crying.

There were other exercises, meant to build our trust in the world and in ourselves, and to make us believe that we could be okay. We were all led out to a small cliff one afternoon, high above a gully full of dead trees and rocks. One by one, we were strapped into a harness and told to stand on the very edge of the cliff and jump.

We all knew we wouldn't fall—that's what the harness and the safety ropes above were for—but trust me, it was scary. Because I am afraid of heights, I volunteered to go first. Why sit and wait and worry—just get it over with. I forced myself to look down. I wanted to feel fully afraid, and then I held my breath and jumped. For one second, the world, the trees, even I, all felt suspended in time, like a scene from the movie *The Matrix*. For a nanosecond it felt like I floated, and then I plummeted, my stomach lurching up into my throat. And then with a jerk, I stopped, swinging gently in my safety harness, laughing up at the sky.

My therapist also taught me how to meditate. She took Lin, Elaine, and me to Nashville one Saturday for a day-long silent retreat. No talking, just meditating.

"I don't think I can do it," Elaine said from the back-seat of the van. "What happens if we blurt out something? Are they going to kick us out?"

"I have never not talked for a whole day in my life!" Lin exclaimed. "This is epic!" We were giddy, mostly just to be allowed out of the Center for a day.

We were on our way to the gorgeous Vanderbilt campus, where one of our first exercises was a walking meditation. We all had to walk, very, very slowly, repeating one line of the mantra with each step:

May I be calm.
May I be peaceful.
May I be happy.
May I be healthy.

I put one foot out carefully in front of the other, so slowly I was barely moving. Lin and Elaine and I tried not to look at each other. We might start giggling. We felt like zombies, moving slowly and muttering chants to ourselves. But to my surprise, I liked it. We spent the day learning all kinds of meditation—standing, seated, with a mantra, and without.

I learned that day that I loved to meditate. It was the first time ever that I had been able to calm my anxiety without a drink or even a pill. Meditating would go on to become a key part of my recovery.

But the best part of the Center's recovery program, in my opinion, is when they have family weekends. Once or twice a month, everyone's husband or wife, children, parents, and siblings are invited to come to the Center and spend three days, learning about addiction and that it is a family disease. While the family has most certainly been profoundly hurt by the addict's actions, the Center therapists said, blaming and shaming the addict is the worst possible thing a family can do. Many alcoholics also drink because of deep dysfunction in families, and for the family to heal, every member of the family must recognize his or her part. On the last day of the family weekend, the addicts and their family members were to read to each other a list of regrets and requests. This was done in front of a group, with everyone else watching. It was an important and emotional part of the weekend.

"Now, family members," warned Teddy, the program leader. "This is not your chance to blame the alcoholic for every bad thing that has ever happened! You don't get to write 'I regret that you drank.' It has to be something you did. You can request they don't drink. But you have to own your own failures. Like, 'I regret I didn't listen to you when you tried to tell me you were unhappy,' or 'I regret I got defensive and lashed out at you when you tried to tell me what was wrong.'"

Teddy was a character. He was a strapping man with a booming voice and a thick southern accent, and I think he lulled everyone into thinking he was a good ol' boy. He was actually whip smart and could charm just about anyone to drop their defenses and listen. He was also a recovering alcoholic.

Hoping he would come and hear what Teddy had to

say, I invited Marc to every family weekend. He never came. But my parents did—all the way from Reno. So did my brother, Chris. Aimie would have come, but she is a single mother with three young children and couldn't. Even my friend Dana offered to come from Los Angeles.

Chris came first. We sat opposite each other in chairs, our list of regrets and requests in our laps.

"I regret I was not there for you more when we were growing up," Chris said.

"I regret I didn't ask you more about what was happening in your life."

"I request that you stop drinking." Then, Chris put down the paper and looked up at me.

"You light up a room when you walk into it, Beth. Don't walk into it drunk."

I started to cry. I picked up my paper and read what I had written.

"I regret that I hurt you. I regret that I let you and Mom and Dad and Aimie slip away from me."

"I regret not asking you about your new business. I know it's important to you, and I regret hurting you with my disinterest."

"I regret that I didn't tell you what was happening to me, how I was losing myself. I regret not asking for help. I didn't when we were little and I was so scared (and you must have been, too), and I didn't when we were grown up and could do something about it."

"I request you call me more."

"I request we try harder to stay closer."

Exchanging those regrets and requests, first with my brother and, later, with my parents, helped clear out some of the emotional clutter that had for years kept me and my family from truly talking. When my mother sat across from me and told me she regretted that she did not comfort me in Okinawa, and that she did not stop the bullies from tormenting me for years, it was like an enormous weight was lifted from me. Her simple statement that she knew what I had gone through, and was sorry she didn't do more, somehow eased the pain of those 40-year-old memories that I had been dragging behind me all my life, like bedraggled baggage.

Everything was on the table that weekend for everyone to explore. We drew an enormous family tree, labeling any ancestors who were alcoholic or depressed and any relatives who experienced trauma of any kind. Addicts are rarely spawned in a vacuum.

Each family weekend ended with a maze made of ropes. I went through it with Chris. We put on blindfolds and were led to a large room, which contained a series of ropes. We would have to feel our way along the ropes to find the exit.

"The rules are very simple!" Teddy boomed. "Do not let go of the rope! Do not duck under the rope! Do not climb over the rope! Do not try to walk on top of the rope! [*Seriously?*] Feel along the rope with your hands until you find the way out!"

We all looked at each other uneasily, some smiling, others searching around for a way out of doing this.

"If you have a question, or you need something, raise your hand!! One of us will come to you. *Do you understand?*" Teddy was especially thunderous on maze days.

Cue the music, don the blindfolds, and off we went. Shuffling and bumping, we were led into a large space, and our hands first touched a rope. We groped along. The ropes were stretched in what seemed to be a giant cat's cradle. Chris and I were in the crowd, fumbling around, when suddenly Teddy shouted, "Ladies and gentlemen, we welcome our first person home!"

There was applause from the staffers and residents watching. *Wow*, I thought. *Someone did it!* On and on I went, bumping into people, walking into walls. I could hear people swearing around me as they did the same thing. Teddy kept yelling every few minutes, "We welcome another person home!!" and then there was more applause for whoever figured the way out. I was beginning to feel frustrated, like I was going around in circles. How could all these other people find the way out and I could not? It was annoying to hear all that clapping as yet another person succeeded while I was still looking. I forced myself to focus. Think. Use your head. Count how many steps before turning left, stop, the wall is on the right, it must be forward. Finally, after walking into my fifteenth wall, it occurred to me. I raised my hand. Moments later I felt Teddy's hand on my back. "Do you need anything?" he asked.

"Yes, I need help." That, ladies and gentlemen, was the way out of the maze. The way out of alcoholism, the way out of any crisis. Asking for help. "No one can do it alone," Teddy said, as my brother and my housemates gathered around me (they had all figured it out long before I did). "We all need help. We can't think our way out of addiction. We can't will our way out. The first step to recovery is raising your hand and asking for help."

—⁂—

Unhappy Holidays

Christmas Eve, 2013. I am sitting in the living room window of the crowded house at the Center, watching the taillights of the last staffer to leave dissolve into the night fog. I am struck by a memory—sitting in my living room window in Stuttgart, Germany, watching the taillights of my parents' car recede as they drove away for a week's vacation. I feel a little of that terrible panic from that day decades ago...how could they leave me? Would they ever come back?

I usually love Christmas, but this year it is unbearable. We are all stuck inside. A misting rain clings to the tree branches and the eaves, droplets quivering, before falling to the sodden wooden deck below. My parents and my sister have both sent me gifts—a few books, body lotion, and some homemade gingerbread cookies. The cookies and the lotion are both confiscated. "Against the rules," says the staffer as she tosses them onto a shelf. I wince. Those little things mean the world to me. They are all I have this year. My nieces and nephews have all sent drawings of Santa Claus and Christmas trees. I hang them in my bedroom, next to my pictures of Zach and Sam, and I lay on my bed and wonder what my children are doing at that exact moment. I could not get much information from them on the phone. And I couldn't yet tell them when I would be home. Marc was insisting I stay until the therapists at the Center cleared me to leave. That date had finally been settled—for the second week of January. Now he was insisting I stay even longer. I felt like he was trying to whitewash me out of our life back in New York.

New Year's Eve was slightly better than Christmas, mostly because I was now counting the days until I would go back to New York. Since it was a holiday, we were allowed to watch movies. *Pitch Perfect* was playing for the fourth time since I had been there, so I wandered into the kitchen and waited for my turn on the phone. The boys answered when I called.

"Happy New Year, you guys!! Happy New Year! What are you doing that's special tonight?"

"Hi, Mommy! We are staying up until midnight!!"

"Midnight!? Oh my gosh, that's so late!" I said. "Are you going to watch the New Year's Eve Times Square show?"

"Yeah, but maybe a movie first. We're having dinner now." At that point I heard Bev, our nanny, call Sam to the table to eat.

"What's Bev doing there tonight?"

"Daddy's going out. He's getting all dressed up right now."

"Huh." I was taken aback. "Can I talk to Dad?"

"Sure—bye, Mommy!" I could hear Sam yelling, "Dad, pick up the phone!"

"Hello?" It was Marc.

"Hi. Happy New Year."

"Happy New Year to you." He was curt, overly formal.

"The boys said you were getting all dressed up. Where are you going?"

"I'm going out to dinner," he answered.

"With who?" My question was honestly innocent. It had never occurred to me to be jealous.

"That's none of your business!" he snapped. "I don't know what *you* are doing on New Year's Eve; you don't have any right to ask me what I am doing!"

I was stunned, completely taken aback. "What do you mean?" I stammered. "You know exactly what I am doing tonight. I am locked up in rehab."

I can't even remember how the conversation ended. It certainly wasn't with any wishes that 2014 be better than the last few years, or pledges to work together to at least try to heal our fractured marriage. I just remember hanging up the phone feeling shaken and absolutely certain in my core that something was very wrong.

Center Stage, Whether
I Liked It or Not

The first days of the new year, my final days at the Center, were mired in negotiations with Marc about coming home. He had finally brought the boys to Tennessee, not for the long promised visit, but because a therapist he was consulting told him they should see me before I arrived home in a few days. The Center had cleared me to return January 13th, but that date happened to fall while Marc was out of town. He wanted me to stay in Tennessee until he got home. Given what happened the last time I got out of rehab, I understood his request. But I argued that I was ready to come home, and to sit around in rehab doing nothing was ridiculous. I was paying for all this myself, along with all the bills in our household, while I was away. The financial burden was becoming a strain. So I agreed to sleep at my friend Michelle's apartment for ten days until Marc came back to town.

It was absolutely wonderful to come home. I hugged my sons long and hard, thrilled to see them, to feel them in my arms. I unpacked my suitcases and tossed all those loose-fitting clothes in the wash. I wandered around my apartment. I never felt luckier to live there. I spent all the afternoons and evenings with the boys after school, helping with homework, cooking their dinner, and putting them to bed, before heading over to Michelle's to sleep. I didn't allow myself even a whiff of resentment at the arrangement.

Besides, I loved sleeping at Michelle's. Her spare bedroom was in the back—facing a courtyard. It was dark and quiet, and I slept longer and harder than I ever had. I luxuriated in her big bed with its plump pillows and crisp sheets.

I was exhausted and bone weary from all those months in a twin bed, in a crowded house, rising at seven a.m. I slept in until ten or eleven every day that first week, for the first time in twenty years...maybe more. By that time, Michelle had gone to work. I'd rub the sleep from my eyes and pour myself a bracingly strong cup of coffee, lingering over a second cup, treasuring the solitude and the quiet after three months of communal living.

I felt like someone who had been sealed away for a very long time and had just returned to life. I got my hair cut and my nails done for the first time in three months. It felt like the best manicure and blowout I had ever had. I drank green juice and ate sushi. It never tasted so good. In the hours before picking up the boys from school, I read newspapers and watched CNN, starved for information about the world and what had happened while I was gone. I was like Rip Van Winkle, emerging from a long sleep and discovering that my old life felt brand-new again.

Most important, every day I met with other alcoholics, to keep my recovery going strong. I also joined an outpatient group at a recovery center, and I met there three days a week. I stayed in close touch with my therapist back at the Center, and with my friends Lin and Janie from Tennessee who were also now home. I was determined that this time, I would succeed.

I returned to work at ABC while Marc was still away. I was nervous. The whole world now knew my dirty little secret, and as I rode up the elevator on my first day back, I was afraid to meet people's gazes. It was strange, walking the hallway to my office, like it was any other day, like my wine-soaked meltdowns and three months in rehab never happened. My heart was thumping in my chest. I was afraid people would shun me, that everyone was thinking, "Oh look who's back—*20/20*'s resident lush."

But the people who tapped on the door to say welcome back or give me a quick hug were wonderful and empathic. Maybe they already knew what was true: that behind our carefully contrived exteriors, we all have something we're dealing with. No one walks through the world immune to insecurity, worry, failure, heartbreak. It was just that all of mine had been laid out for everyone to see.

It was only a few hours into that first day when there came a tap on the door. It was Jeff Schneider. He gave me a warm smile and a big hug, and then shook his head ruefully.

"Darlin', I hate to do this, but Page Six just called. They heard you were back to work today and are going to run a story." My heart sank. No one outside ABC knew when I was returning. Someone at the network must have called in the tip.

I sighed.

"What do you want me to say?" Jeffrey asked. We came up with a brief statement saying I was indeed home, back at work, and grateful to be there. We both knew we could not let the drip-drip-drip of stories continue. Piecemeal statements in response to tips—"Yes I am an alcoholic. Yes I am home from rehab. Yes I am back to work."—were only fanning the buzz and the interest. I was inundated with requests for interviews from talk show hosts and magazines.

"The best thing you can do now is pick someone, sit down, and tell them everything," Jeffrey advised.

It's the first lesson of damage control: tell the truth, tell it all, and put it past you. Hedging, delaying, hiding, and denying will just drag a story out. Better to get it out early and completely. I already knew that and had planned on eventually doing an interview, but not now. I had just come home. I wasn't ready.

"The stories will just continue," Jeffrey warned. "Put it to bed." So that day, my first day back at work, we began making arrangements to do a tell-all sit-down interview.

Initially, the plan was just to air it on *GMA*, the show I had been hosting as I filled in for Robin, just one year before. I picked George Stephanopoulos, with whom I had shared the anchor desk over the years for hundreds of hours of live television. I knew he was tough but fair, and he had integrity. He would ask hard questions, but I trusted him.

The arrangements were made to tape the interview that Thursday. It would air Friday morning.

At nine thirty a.m. on January 23, I arrived at the *GMA* studios in Times Square and sat down opposite George. As we had countless times before, we both pinned tiny microphones to our clothes while the crews adjusted the focus on their cameras and checked the enormous lights around us. This time, only he had some papers in his lap, a list of questions and notes he had jotted down. I arrived to the studio empty-handed. It felt very, very different to be the subject of the story instead of the journalist reporting it.

For the first time I really understood why nearly everyone I interviewed confessed they were nervous to be on camera. I was terrified. My heart was pounding; my hands were cold and clammy. I felt distracted by my own anxiety, by the sensation of being completely out of control of the next twenty minutes. I was unable to make any small talk with the people around me, people with whom I had worked a thousand times. As the makeup artist powdered my shiny forehead I wondered yet again, *Is this the right thing to do?*

"Are you ready?" George asked. I nodded and took a deep breath. I had no idea what he was going to ask. I had no idea what I was going to say. All I knew was that I had to be honest.

G: So, you're an alcoholic.

I nearly died. *You're going to start with that question? The hardest question, right out of the box?* For a moment, I thought about stopping the interview, asking for some time to warm up, some space to compose myself. Then I swallowed and said,

> E: I am. I am an alcoholic. It took me a long time to admit that to myself. It took me a long time to admit it to my family, but I am.

Okay—it was out there.

> G: And it must have taken so much effort to keep that secret.
> E: The amount of energy I expended keeping that secret and keeping this problem hidden from view, hidden from my family, hidden from friends, from colleagues, was exhausting.

George's face was compassionate, and yet his expression was baffled.

G: I mean, you and I have spent literally hundreds of hours this far apart anchoring live television. I would have never guessed this in a million years.

E: I mean, George, it's a staggering burden to walk around with. And you become so isolated with the secret and so lonely because you can't tell anyone what's happening. And yet it was a fact of my life. I spent most of my childhood having almost daily panic attacks and most of my adulthood, um, having a lot of panic and dealing with a lot of severe anxiety. I dealt with that anxiety and with the stress that that anxiety brought by starting to drink.

G: Did anyone close to you realize?

E: My husband. My husband knew I had a problem.

G: What did he say?

E: You have a problem. You're, you're an alcoholic. And, and it made me really angry. Really angry. But he was right.

G: So when Marc first said something to you, did you immediately go and seek professional help, go to rehab?

E: No. It took a long time. I mean, denial is huge for any alcoholic, especially for any functioning alcoholic, um, because I, you know, I'm not living under a bridge. I haven't been arrested.

No arrests. Just a bunch of other really horrible things, like waking up in an emergency room after a thirteen-hour blackout.

E: I had a panic attack on live television when I was anchoring the local news in Chicago. I had to take beta blockers because I was so nervous and so anxious and, and you know, that's exhausting to, to live like that. And it becomes very easy to think, I deserve this glass of wine. I'm so stressed out, and I'm keeping it hidden. I can't tell anybody, not even you, sitting next to me...I felt like I had to be, you know, perfect, which is ridiculous. Um, nobody's perfect.

Except I thought I had to be. All the while I was failing miserably.

G: So what happened?

E: I went to a rehab that specializes in treating trauma.

G: How long did you stay?

E: I—I stayed for twenty-eight days and left against their advice and came home because I really wanted to come home. And they said, we think you need to do more work, and I came home for five days and realized they were right, and I went back and finished and stayed until the doctors there said I was ready to come back. Um, and I, you know, this isn't what I want to be known for, um, but I'm really proud of what I did.

G: How did you know you were ready to come back, to come home?

E: You know, it's, it's a psychic change, I think. I mean, it's learning to accept that I'm human, that there's nothing wrong with failing, that there's nothing wrong with feeling anxiety.

Anxiety can't kill you, even when it feels like it can.

G: Marc must be relieved too.

To be honest, I don't really know. I haven't seen him yet.

E: Yes. And my kids. You know, my kids, too.
G: Is it hard not to drink?
E: Yes.

George looks surprised. People who don't have this disease really don't fully understand the need to blot out the feeling that I don't quite fit into this skin...the need for immediate relief.

E: Right now, I feel really strong, and I've got a great support system in place. I have great, great friends who, um, who I love and who love me.
G: What are your triggers? What are the stress points?
E: Daily stress. Listen, there are lots of people who feel a lot of stress. Not everybody turns to a glass of wine or three like I did, or four, like I did on some occasions. What I learned to do when I was away was to feel the feelings. You know what? They're

not gonna kill you. You have to experience them, and I never learned that skill and it makes it tough some days. Alcohol, for me, is no longer an option.

G: Well, what are the tricks now? So when you feel that, what do you do instead?

E: Call a friend. Um, meditate. Pray. There's been a real spiritual component for me in all of this. Reach out to somebody who can talk you through that rotten day and support you in that.

I hate talking about myself like this. I feel naked in front of the world.

G: Telling your story, sharing it now, do you think it makes a difference in how you live your life?

E: It's always embarrassing to have the entire world know your deepest, darkest secret and yet, I think in the long term it will be, ultimately, a blessing because I can be free about it.

Ultimately. Not quite yet.

G: Well, you look great and you sound great. Are you ready to get back to work?

E: I feel great. I am! [*laughs*] I'm really ready to get back to work.

G: Welcome back.

George could not have been nicer. I thanked the crew and left the interview suite in a bit of a daze. My legs felt wobbly. I felt like I had just run ten miles. Later that day, I learned the segment would run for seven minutes on *GMA*...twice as long as the time originally allotted for it. I could not remember ever doing a segment on the show that ran as long.

Friday morning, I woke up early at Michelle's, poured myself some coffee, and curled up on the couch to watch. I was gripping my mug with both hands, afraid I would spill it. *What if I sound ridiculous? What if I sound defensive? What if the interview is edited in a weird way and I don't make sense? What if I look as sweaty and nervous as I felt?*

But before I could spin out any further, Robin and George were introducing the story, and moments later, my face loomed in the screen stating, for all the world to hear, "I am an alcoholic."

I wondered, in that moment, about all the people in my life who I had not yet had the chance to tell...people who might be shocked, or who might say, "I always knew." I wondered if my husband was watching it somewhere, in a hotel room, on the road, and what he thought of my long-overdue, televised admission.

It was excruciating to watch, but I did it, and when it was over, the response was enormous. I was flooded with calls and emails from friends and colleagues; I received letters from people all over the country—wishing me luck, praising my courage, sharing their own battles with addiction.

My *20/20* co-host, David Muir—who had been one of the most supportive people at the network the whole time I was in rehab—decided to do a story about me for our show, using parts of my interview, along with new interviews with my mother and my friends. As I stood on the set with David my first night back, he warmly welcomed me. I was able to fully take in how lucky and happy I was to have this job. But I knew harder days were ahead. Marc was coming home. I had a lot of work to atone for everything I had put him through with my drinking, and to try to save our marriage.

In my final days in Tennessee they had told me, over and over, do not make any big life changes in your first year of recovery. Your sobriety is too new, too fragile. All the ordinary feelings you have been numbing with alcohol can seem overwhelming. It's advice every addict hears. I, however, never had the chance to take it.

—⚋⚋—

The wheel of life takes one up and down by turn.

—KALIDASA

I am perched on the edge of my bed and my husband is sitting on the floor in front of me, his legs crossed, his voice low and calm. I cannot feel my body, and my face feels numb. "I have feelings for someone else," he tells me. "We want to explore being together." I am shocked, reeling, as I struggle to process what he is saying. My mind feels—well, it feels drunk. Drunk and clumsy. Like I am underwater, moving in slow motion, trying to fit pieces into a puzzle, but the pieces keep floating away and I am too slow to grasp them and put them where they belong.

Too soon, the warning not to make big life decisions feels quaint. Life has outpaced me. Just days after moving back into my apartment, my husband told me he wanted a divorce. Weeks after unpacking my cheerful cards from my housemates and my books of daily reflections, I learned Marc had been sharing holidays and intimate dinners with another woman...a woman I had introduced him to, a woman I had thought was my friend. While I was away in Tennessee, Marc had hired a divorce lawyer and started legal proceedings.

I sit there in my nightgown, unable to say a word, even as the pieces finally thud into place—his refusal to come to any family weekend, his fury when I asked where he was going New Year's Eve—and still, I cannot believe it. I look down at my hands and I realize they are shaking. Our children are asleep in the next room, and it is all coming to an end. This. Our life together. Our marriage. I had thought when he first mentioned a divorce that he was just angry. He had every right to be. I had hurt him so very much. But hearing him talk about this other woman and their feelings for each other left no doubt in my mind: Marc had moved on.

In the days, weeks, and months that followed, I seesawed between disbelief and fury. Without alcohol, the pain was brittle, sharp-edged. While I didn't yearn for the hazy soft-edged fog of wine, I needed something to escape the pain, or at least dull it. I spent hours cleaning closets, organizing cabinets, cooking, baking—anything to try to divert and distract me from the cyclone of questions: *How could this really be happening? How can I fix this?* I kept banging into the same wall, the one that has "you're not in control anymore" spray-painted on it.

I clung to my new sobriety like a life raft. I went to meetings with other alcoholics and raged about my crumbling life, sharing how seared I felt by the rejection, but nothing could blunt it or alter the course of events. By May, Marc had found a new apartment and bought himself new furniture, and at the end of the month he moved out and on to his new life. Left behind were closets crammed with his clothes and guitar cases, shelves filled with photos of birthdays and beach vacations...all no longer wanted or needed, shed like an old skin. He had a clean slate, with no reminders of the past. I was confronted with the memories and the wreckage every time I opened a drawer.

We all learned to navigate our new reality and the painful new routines: the walks with Zachary and Sam to Daddy's new house, the awkward pickups after school with other parents' pitying smiles, the dropoffs on the nights the boys were sleeping with him—their empty beds and the screaming silence in my home. I didn't know what to do with myself those nights. I would wander around the apartment, straightening photographs, picking up toys and socks they had left lying on the floor. It was physical, this ache I had for them. I still could not believe this was how life was going to be.

It was summer when it all began to fall apart for me. I don't know exactly what it was that pushed me over the edge, sent me tumbling back into the swamp of addiction. Was it another long weekend without the boys? News from my divorce lawyer that as the "moneyed spouse" I would have to pay for Marc's lawyer, too? Someone thoughtlessly tattling that they had seen Marc strolling up Broadway holding hands with another brunette?

Maybe it was just everything—the fighting, the worry, the financial strain of supporting two households—it was all pressing down, too hard. At some point the misery of those months in Tennessee and the memory of what drinking had done to me was eclipsed by my daily distress. I forgot to meditate and pray—they seemed like flimsy weapons in this battle. I forgot what I had told George in that *GMA* interview—that my feelings couldn't kill me. I felt like I was dying of grief. I would do anything not to feel that. And I did. A few times that summer, I did what I swore I would never again do: I drank. It was just a handful of times, but it was enough to set me on a terrible course as August, and my first vacation as a single parent with my boys, loomed.

—⁓—

Half measures availed us nothing. We stood at the turning point.

—ALCOHOLICS ANONYMOUS

I hit bottom on August 16, 2014. It was Sam's birthday. I had rented a beautiful house in the week leading up to it, on the beach in Malibu. It had wraparound decks and stunning views of the waves roaring and crashing just below. I had planned this trip for two months, my first ever vacation trip with just my two sons.

I had wanted these ten days at the beach to be a balm, a salve to all our pain. I had wanted us to be happy even though we were now three instead of four. Looking back, I shudder at how high I pinned my hopes for this trip: how much I wanted to erase all the pain and heartbreak and loss and betrayal I had felt, and had inflicted on my children. What I should have done was steel myself for the hard times that would also come far away from home, even in paradise.

For Sam's birthday, I had carefully selected an iPad

Mini and wrapped it in shiny gold paper. I had planned to bake him a vanilla coconut cake, his favorite, and had bought eight blue candles—and a red one for luck—to put on top. But on that bright sunny Saturday, with the salt from the ocean thick in the air, eight years after I brought my freckle-faced redhead into this world, I was drunk. I was upstairs, throwing all my clothes into my suitcases. The dresses I had planned to wear to dinner with friends, the bathing suits I packed to surf with the boys, the flip-flops, the sandals, the sun hats, the cashmere wraps—all the things I meticulously laid out six days ago, I now shoved back in with abandon. Downstairs, my friend Dana loaded the boys into her car to take them to her house to play with her daughters while they waited for Marc to fly from New York to pick them up. My brother, Chris, who had flown down from San Francisco with my sister, to save me yet again, waited to drive me to a detox facility in Pasadena.

In two short hours I traded those thousand-dollar views of the Pacific Ocean for a tiny room in a Las Encinas lockup. I had a single bed and a small window that was bolted shut. There was no door to the tiny bathroom, no hooks on which to hang towels out of fear that someone would try to hang themselves. There was a single fluorescent overhead light buzzing faintly, and the sharp, cloying smell of industrial detergent.

Every hour, day and night, an orderly would open the door and shine a light to see if you were in your bed (at night) or still breathing (day or night). Once I sobered up, I spent every waking hour outside in a small common courtyard. I was told by one of the staff that this place was once called the Marilyn Monroe Center, because it was here that she would come to privately detox. If true, the place was definitely showing its age.

Outside, where I spent the next four days, there was a collection of picnic benches. Styrofoam cups and used paper plates sat on tables, and in the desiccated grass were cigarette butts...mounds of them. All matches and lighters had been confiscated upon check-in, so hour after hour I sat and watched person after person stand in front of a rusty metal box mounted at eye level on the wall and lean their face in close. Embedded inside it was one of those old-fashioned cigarette lighters, the kind you would see in an old Buick in the 1970s. I was sure one of those smokers was going to ignite his eyelashes instead of his Marlboro Gold. And that is how I spent the week of my son's eighth birthday. Instead of watching Sam blow out his birthday candles, I was watching nameless addicts light up their smokes.

I had plenty of time in those four days in Las Encinas to think about what I did when we arrived in Malibu. I had worked the first day of our vacation, on Monday, shooting an interview for a story that would air that week on *20/20*. I was scheduled to record the audio for my script on Friday, from the house, so it could be fed via satellite to New York and edited into the story. But when the crew arrived to our Malibu rental that day, I was under the influence, unable to properly read the script. A few days before, while shopping for groceries, my cart loaded with fruit and cereal and chips and salsa, I had found myself wheeling it past an enormous display of wine. I stopped in front of it, gazing at all those bottles. *That would make me feel better*, I had thought. *Just one bottle, just one glass tonight.* Then, forgetting every hard lesson I had learned, I reached out and picked a nice California chardonnay.

That night, I drank more than half of that bottle. The following night, after draining it, I looked around the rental house for more. I could not drive to the store again—I had sipped a glass and a half already. I would never dare drive after drinking—a singular moment of lucidity in an otherwise insane episode. I opened every cabinet, searched every shelf. Finally, way in the back of the pantry, next to a container of margarita mix, I found a bottle of tequila. Hard liquor was not my thing, but it was all there was, so I poured myself a glass. The tequila was strong—too strong. Very quickly my head was spinning, and I had to go to my room to lie down. The boys and our nanny were already asleep, thank God, but by Friday, I was hopelessly ensnared...it was clear to everyone that I had relapsed.

This time, my bosses at ABC had had it. The network had stood by me through two lengthy stints in rehab and through two relapses already. This time, I nearly lost my job. But most crucially, I had hurt my children—deeply. As I sat on that picnic bench and watched the smokers light up I wondered bleakly if they would ever forgive me, ever trust me again.

I had two visitors during those four days in Las Encinas—my sister, Aimie, was the first. She flew down a second time from the Bay Area to offer her support and her love.

"Beth, you have got to stop doing this."

"I know, I know," I said miserably. "I have really messed up this time. I may lose everything and everyone."

Aimie looked around the yard, taking in the depressing scene in which I was now a player.

"You have to fight for yourself. This has to be the most important thing you do."

I was deeply grateful she came, and when she left, it was really hard to see her go...her small back, her head held high. She had not had an easy time of life, either—she had had her own painful divorce to go through. She had gone through it without drinking herself into oblivion and, I realized in that moment, had done it without sufficient support from me.

I called out to her as she reached the locked door to the outside world. "Bye, Aimie! I love you!"

She turned and waved. "I love you, too."

My second visitor was someone I had just met on my trip to Malibu. He was an actor and director who had gone through his own highly public battle with alcohol. He had taken me to a meeting in Malibu with other alcoholics, at the beginning of my vacation, before I fell into the bottle. He had come that Friday morning, too, when it all fell apart, and with my brother and Dana had helped get me to this facility. When they talk in recovery about alcoholics helping other alcoholics, this man's name should be at the top of the list. He arrived in Las Encinas on my third day, and he brought someone with him. Her name was Polly.

"Elizabeth, meet Polly. This woman got me sober, and kept me sober. She saved my life."

Polly had big brown eyes, long hair, and a warm smile. She was lovely. "It's nice to meet you!" she said.

The three of us sat down in a pretty, secluded area apart from the common yard—a concession by the staff to my visitor's fame.

"How are you doing?" he asked.

"I am okay," I sighed. They both knew I was lying. They knew exactly how I felt. Hopeless.

The three of us sat and talked for half an hour, Polly telling how she helped our friend get sober, telling me her own story of addiction. She had been sober now for more than twenty years. Her wisdom and her strength awed me.

"You can stay sober, Elizabeth. I have helped many alcoholics who are worse than you." She was offering me a ray of hope I had by then denied myself. "All you have to do is follow some simple steps. If you are willing, I can help you."

She seemed so serene, so sure. As I looked at her that day, I saw my only lifeline. I grabbed it with both hands. By the end of the visit, we came up with a plan. Polly would come home with me to New York and live with me.

I knew going to another rehab was not the answer for me. Instead, this time I resolved to work with Polly every day.

Polly flew home with me two days later and moved into my guest bedroom. I returned to a very different life than the one I left, on my way to Malibu, where I turned that dream vacation into yet another nightmare. I was no longer working. ABC had agreed to give me one last chance to get it together, but this time without pay. I returned to my outpatient group. I slept every night for a month at a sober house, where I was tested daily to prove I had not been drinking. But most important, I worked each and every day with Polly.

She laid out a meticulous timeline of my entire adult life and showed me how I had used alcohol for years in an unhealthy way, almost always to escape something, or someone, usually myself. She wrote out, in wrenching detail, every episode in the last eight years when I had gone to a hospital, or blacked out, or missed work, or missed moments of my own children's lives. It was the first time someone had laid it out for me to see, every awful episode in its entirety, and it left me shaken. We took turns reading aloud from the book of Alcoholics Anonymous, full of stories of other people who had fallen hopelessly at the feet of this disease, only to find redemption.

Over and over, she hammered it home: "You cannot safely drink. Every attempt at controlled drinking ends disastrously. Your very life is at stake." Time and time again, she would pull out that timeline and point to it. "Do you see how powerless you are over alcohol? Where did your best thinking get you?" There was no denying my life had become unmanageable. It was right in front of me, in black and white.

But most important, Polly talked a lot about God. I am Catholic, and my parents are devout in their faith. I have always considered religion to be a personal matter, and I was frankly embarrassed when Polly started talking about prayer, and God, and how we have to turn it all over and ask for His guidance. She was unshakeable in her devotion to God. If she was aware of my discomfort, it didn't matter to her: her faith was that strong. Maybe she just knew I had to find my way to embracing it. I had spent my life praying in times of crisis. I wasn't an atheist convert in the foxhole, but I didn't pray regularly, and I sure didn't pray when times were good. Polly set out to show me a different way—and it has become a cornerstone in my recovery. When I was tearful about meeting with Marc to negotiate our divorce, she would say serenely, "Hand it over to God. He will guide you." When I had to go to ABC to meet with the president of the news division and persuade him to give me one last chance, she nodded and closed her eyes. "Pray. God will show you what to do."

Today, when I feel anxiety start to overtake me, I pray. When I feel angry, or resentful, or just cranky, I list every thing in my life that is a gift. And now I pray when times are good. I end each day by making a gratitude list—all the things I am grateful for that night. They can be big things like a long trip that went smoothly, or an interview I conducted at work that went really well. They can be small things, like a moment of laughter with my son, or just the way the sun sparkled on the river that evening, like a million shards of glass. And every single day, I thank God for my family, my health, my home, and a job that I still love.

I went back to work in November, fully aware there would not be another chance. I could not get back all the opportunities I had squandered, and I needed to stop looking with regret and shame over my own shoulder. I could only look forward and do my very best, every single day.

My recovery this time was different because I was not in a bubble at rehab; I was not in an alternate universe. I was home, confronted every hour of every day with what I had done. I could look into my sons' faces and see how I had hurt them. There was no escaping it; there was no denying it. The full extent of my disease and what I had done while in the throes of it was front and center in my life. I could not run away from it, as I had run away from every uncomfortable, anxious moment in my life. I had to navigate all the consequences of my drinking—the painful divorce, the two months off work, the incredulous glances I seemed to see everywhere from people who had read the news or heard the gossip. "She relapsed yet again? Can't she get it together?"

I took a class in Transcendental Meditation and learned

how to stop twice a day, center myself, and meditate. That and prayer have helped slow down the escalation of anxiety into panic, helped me not to take every single thing in life so personally. But these tools only work if you use them every single day, several times each day. They are not flimsy tools, as I had thought during that last summer and that terrible relapse. They are powerful weapons. They gave me the power to at last say no to drinking. The power to say yes to life.

Finally, I began once again going to meetings with other alcoholics, this time without my mantle of shame. I no longer hid in the back under a baseball cap. I sat up front. I listened to the stories I heard there, of other people's journeys and tragedies—the blackouts, the rehabs, the DUIs, the divorces, the children lost in custody battles, the livelihoods and the lives all lost to this disease. I listened to those stories with empathy and compassion, hoping someday I could learn to show myself those same qualities and gain some form of absolution. I heard their stories of redemption and victory, of how they now lived lives they never imagined possible—were happier than they ever dreamed—because they stopped drinking. And when it came time to share at the end of the meeting, I raised my hand and said out loud, "Hi, I'm Beth. I am an alcoholic."

—⚍—

Fall seven times. Stand up eight.

—Japanese proverb

No little girl lays awake in bed at night, dreaming of what she will become, and says fervently to herself, "I hope I grow up to be an alcoholic!" No wife and mother wakes up in the morning, stretches and yawns and says casually to herself, "This would be a good day to get so drunk I have to go to the emergency room." She doesn't pour breakfast cereal into a bowl and think, *Maybe I will even flirt with death and drink so much my blood alcohol level will be lethal.*

There are a lot of people who think alcoholism is a character defect, a weakness or a lack of self-discipline. I know, because I was one of them, even when I was deep into the disease. I kept thinking, *I will just cut back.* Later, I would berate myself: *For God's sake, get it together.* I was so disciplined in so many areas of my life—my work, my exercise, my diet, my budget. But all that focus and effort and willpower were useless for me when it came to alcohol. Because it truly is a disease, as the American

Medical Association said way back in 1966. Perhaps it is because we hurt so many others, as well as ourselves, when we drink. We do so much damage. Our loved ones and those near us recoil, or worse, bail altogether. Sometimes, we deserve that. But I can tell you that nearly every addict I know drank or took drugs because there was something else bigger that felt wrong, that hurt so much, it was unbearable. Numbing that "something else" became the only way to survive. We were, many of us, tormented souls who needed to find our way, however possible, to a place of grace.

Alcoholism and addiction have touched millions of people in this country. If you don't suffer from it, you know someone who does. We are your wives, your mothers, your daughters, your sisters. We are your children, your colleagues, your employees, your friends. We are Emmy award–winning journalists, Grammy award–winning singers, and Oscar-winning actors. We are diplomats and doormen, presidents and accountants, housewives and handymen. In the face of this disease we are all equal, the playing field leveled. If we are truly fortunate, we have employers who did not abandon us, family who stood by us, and perhaps someone who helped us find our way back, who never forgot that beneath all the appalling behavior there was a human being.

I am so very lucky for my family and my friends who stood by me. For years, my parents and my brother and sister were sick with worry...terrified that one day a call would come that I was dead. My family spent countless hours on the phone together, trying to figure out how to help me. My friend and producer Terri Lichstein was on many of those calls—and at my side during some of the worst times. I am deeply grateful to Ben Sherwood, James Goldston, Barbara Fedida, and David Sloan for giving me another chance at ABC News, for allowing me to return to the work I love. I am so fortunate that the producers and staff at *20/20* forgave me, and worked with me this past year. I am grateful Marc took such good care of our children during the times I could not, and that he tried his best to take care of me. I am thankful that he and I have found a way to be good parents to our boys together, even if we are now apart.

I wrote this book because when I first worried I had a drinking problem, I read other peoples' books about their battles with the disease—mostly women. I spent my whole life looking at other people and thinking their lives were perfect and easy and wonderful, while mine was not. Maybe someone watching me on television, or seeing me in an airport, or walking down the street, thought the same thing about me. Perhaps my story will show them everyone has something they struggle with, something difficult and painful. There is a saying in recovery that you are only as sick as your secrets. Now my secrets are out. Part of me is absolutely terrified. I know some people have already heard a different narrative about the blackout, the visits to the emergency rooms, the drunken vacations, the trips to rehab. I have lived in fear that those stories would leak out to the press, as tiny bits of it already have. Now the narrative is mine. I must own my story, and I must take responsibility for my role in the end of my marriage. I still feel enormous guilt and anguish over what I did, and the people I hurt. I will never get back all the precious moments I lost with my sons, and that is perhaps the most bitter pill of all. I remind myself every day that I cannot undo what I have done, that I need to focus on what I can do now and be the best mother possible to these two incredible boys I am so lucky to have. They tell me they have forgiven me for what I did while drinking. I pray someday I will find the power to forgive myself.

Today, am I cured of alcoholism? No, one is never cured. It is a daily battle, a daily choice. I have heard alcoholics with twenty-four years of sobriety say, "Thank God I am sober today," and mean it. They have learned and embraced a valuable lesson. Today is all we have. That's all anyone has, really. When I walk down the street, past restaurants and wine bars, I still sometimes glance at the tables of people enjoying what I cannot. I take in their glasses, half filled, and their easy camaraderie, and I feel envious. I still sometimes pass a liquor store and shudder with memories of my secret trips there to stock up. But that happens less and less now. Even more surprising to me is that my anxiety—my lifelong nemesis—has waned. Somewhere in my journey, the alcohol that I used to calm myself turned into kerosene—igniting small blazes of worry into bonfires of panic. It is still amazing to me how manageable my anxiety is, now that I am not drinking.

Every day I make the choice not to drink, the choice to be present in every moment, even the difficult ones. And every night I thank God for another day of sobriety. I do not take it for granted. Not now, when I have seen how quickly everything good about my life can dissolve in a glass of wine, never to be recovered. I am responsible for my own sobriety, and my own happiness. I cannot expect other people to fix my problems, or blame them when things go wrong. Learning that lesson has helped me take ownership of my own life again. It's not perfect, it's sometimes really hard. But it's mine, and it's up to me to make the most of it, and there is so much to be so thankful for.

I think back often to that hike I took up that mountain in Utah on my last day at Cirque. How I thought so many times that it was too hard, that the journey to the top was too far. I remember how I looked around at the beauty all around me and decided then to soldier on, timing my breath to my steps. Slow and steady, breathing in, breathing out. And between breaths, never forgetting the lesson I learned that day about recovery, about life, a lesson I now remember every single day. One step at a time, one day at a time. Be strong. Be grateful. Just do the next right thing, and you will arrive.

—m—

Acknowledgments

I would like to thank Peter Kaminsky for his help and expert guidance in this last year—I could not have written this book without him. My deepest thanks to my editor, Gretchen Young, and my agent, Cait Hoyt, for their endless patience and encouragement to be brave and honest in these pages. They never let me forget that I am not the only one in the world who has struggled with anxiety and addiction, and that there are others out there who might feel less alone by reading my story.

About the Author

ELIZABETH VARGAS is the co-anchor of *20/20* on ABC News. She resides in Manhattan with her two children.